The Child Survivor

MW00356443

The Child Survivor is a clinically rich, comprehensive overview of the treatment of children and adolescents who have developed dissociative symptoms in response to ongoing developmental trauma. Joyanna Silberg, a widely respected authority in the field, uses case examples to illustrate hard-to-treat clinical dilemmas such as children presenting with rage reactions, amnesia, and dissociative shutdown. These behaviors are often survival strategies, and in *The Child Survivor* practitioners will find practical management tools that are backed up by recent scientific advances in neurobiology. Clinicians on the front lines of treatment will come away from the book with an arsenal of therapeutic techniques that they can put into practice right away, limiting the need for restrictive hospitalizations or out-of-home placement for their young clients.

Joyanna L. Silberg, PhD, psychologist at Sheppard Pratt Health System, is an international expert on dissociation in children and adolescents, and past president of the International Society on the Study of Trauma and Dissociation.

The Child Survivor

Healing Developmental Trauma
and Dissociation

Joyanna L. Silberg

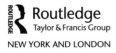

Routledge
Taylor & Francis Group

NEW YORK AND LONDON

First published 2013
by Routledge
711 Third Avenue, New York, NY 10017

Simultaneously published in the UK
by Routledge
27 Church Road, Hove, East Sussex BN3 2FA

Routledge is an imprint of the Taylor & Francis Group, an informa business

© 2013 Taylor & Francis

The right of Joyanna L. Silberg to be identified as author of this work
has been asserted by her in accordance with sections 77 and 78 of
the Copyright, Designs and Patents Act 1988.

All rights reserved. No part of this book may be reprinted or reproduced or
utilised in any form or by any electronic, mechanical, or other means,
now known or hereafter invented, including photocopying and recording,
or in any information storage or retrieval system, without permission
in writing from the publishers.

Trademark notice: Product or corporate names may be trademarks
or registered trademarks, and are used only for identification
and explanation without intent to infringe.

Library of Congress Cataloging in Publication Data

Silberg, Joyanna L.
The child survivor : healing developmental trauma and dissociation /
Joyanna L. Silberg.
  p. cm.
  Includes bibliographical references and index.
  ISBN 978-0-415-88994-0 (hardcover : alk. paper) —
ISBN 978-0-415-88995-7 (pbk. : alk. paper)   1. Dissociative disorders
in children.   2. Dissociative disorders—Treatment.   3. Psychic
trauma—Treatment.   I. Title.
RJ506.D55S55   2012
618.92'8523—dc23   2012017123

ISBN: 978-0-415-88994-0 (hbk)
ISBN: 978-0-415-88995-7 (pbk)
ISBN: 978-0-203-83027-7 (ebk)

Typeset in Times New Roman
by Apex CoVantage, LLC

SUSTAINABLE
FORESTRY
INITIATIVE

Certified Sourcing
www.sfiprogram.org
SFI-00555
The SFI label applies to the text stock.

Printed and bound in the United States of America by
Walsworth Publishing Company, Marceline, MO.

For Ayla Rose, Judah Samson, and the promise
of healthy children.

Contents

Appendices D, E, F, and I are instruments and checklists provided to clinicians for use in their practice. They are available for downloading at www.routledge.com/9780415889940.

List of Tables and Figures

TABLES

FIGURES

x   *List of Tables and Figures*

Acknowledgments

First, I would like to thank my family—Richard, Naomi, Shira, Dahlia, Adam, and Avi—for their love, support, and patience that spurred me forward during the long process of writing this book. I would also like to thank my mother, the late Edythe Samson, and my father, Norman Samson, who cultivated in me compassion for the vulnerable and pursuit of justice, which motivates my work with traumatized children.

I am indebted to the creative ideas and therapeutic skill of my colleagues in the Child Committee at the International Society for the Study of Trauma and Dissociation—Els Grimminck, Sandra Wieland, Sandra Baita, Renée Marks, and Na'ama Yehuda. I am particularly grateful to Frances Waters for her leadership in the field, collegial support, and case consultations over the years. Our collaborations have enriched my thinking and my work.

I am lucky to be part of a rich and diverse community of mental health providers at the Sheppard Pratt Health System who have provided a setting for these ideas to be nourished. Dr. Richard Loewenstein originally opened my eyes to the field of dissociation and Dr. Steven Sharfstein has always made the treatment of trauma-related disorders a high priority. I am grateful to the service chiefs of the child inpatient units at Sheppard Pratt who welcome my treatment input—Dr. Laura Seidel, Dr. Michael Bogrov, Dr. Meena Vimalananda, and Dr. Desmond Kaplan.

My colleagues locally and around the world have always been supportive of my work and helped me refine ideas with stimulating discussions, probing questions, and invitations to teach. I want to thank the late Elaine Davidson Nemzer, Phyllis Stien, Joshua Kendall, Lisa Ferentz, Susan Straus, Bethany Brand, Bradley Stolbach, and Arne Blindheim.

I also want to thank my colleagues at the Leadership Council, especially Dr. Philip Kaplan, Toby Kleinman, Dr. Ruth Blizard, Nancy Erickson, Dr. Noémi Mattis, and Dr. Paul Fink, who have served as a cushion of support and a safe community in a world that is not always friendly to victims of child abuse and their supporters.

I was supported in the technical details of writing this book by my assistants Elan Telem and Betsy Samson, and I am grateful for their patience and attention to detail. I am deeply grateful for the friendship, knowledge, editorial skill, and scholarship of my cherished colleague Stephanie Dallam, without whom this project would have been impossible.

Finally, I would like to thank the many clients and their families who taught me so much and gave me permission to share their stories with you.

* * *

Many of the children and teens described in the book, such as Angela, Balina, Timothy, Jennifer, Lisa, and many others, gave permission for their stories to be shared, but names and identifying information were changed to protect their identities. However, some of the cases are fictionalized composites of clinical experiences from 30 years of practice that illustrate important concepts but are not intended to directly relate to any individual client or their family. In these cases, any similarities in names or individual circumstances to real clients is coincidental and unintentional.

Preface

Traumatized children and the mental health systems designed to help them often seem to be in a standoff, a virtual battle of wills. The children develop symptoms that resist medication and restraint and seem impervious to all of the treatments we try to offer them. Logical consequences don't seem to matter, and these survivors of trauma are often caught in what seem to be repeated cycles of self-harm, provocation, and self-destruction.

Our classification systems are often hard-pressed to come up with the right labels, and many times these labels cast judgment on what appear to be inevitable consequences of the hard lives they have lived. Those who work regularly with children in our mental health systems will be familiar with what I mean. Children from serial foster homes are often diagnosed with attachment disorders. Yet, these children in their wisdom have not risked attachment, knowing that foster homes change as quickly as each new approaching birthday. Is this an appropriate adaptation or a symptom of a psychological disorder? Children exposed to extreme abuse and trauma are often labeled "bipolar," as their moods seem contradictory and shifting. Yet, shifting moods may be adaptive when a child's environment can quickly shift between being safe and appropriate, and being unpredictably frightening and abusive. Some traumatized children hear voices commanding them to fight back or voices consoling them with comforting words. They are often labeled psychotic. Yet, lacking consistent parental guidance and support, children adapt by providing themselves with the soothing or protection that they so desperately need. The labels we give traumatized children often restrict our thinking and prevent us from acknowledging the internal wisdom and logic of the symptoms our clients have "chosen" as their only hope of survival in the war zone of their haphazard and violent lives.

For many chronically traumatized children, the symptoms learned in a lifetime of thwarted goals remain their only comfort. These symptoms represent the tools they developed to navigate the unpredictable worlds of their childhood—tools that they do not want to give up, despite our interventions. In this book, you will learn how to understand the symptoms of the severely traumatized child or teen as adaptive mechanisms to help them cope with the chaotic world that is their habitat. This book will focus on the young survivors of early trauma—sexual abuse, physical abuse, neglect, abandonment, multiple placements—who often rely on dissociative strategies to cope with the dilemmas in their world. They use automatic programs such as rage, retreat, or regression that help them avoid authentic emotional engagement. Often, these children adapt to the conflicting pulls of their hidden emotional world by attributing blame for their behavior on internal characters who represent their contradictory feelings or attitudes. They sometimes have amnesia for recent events, because they have learned that remembering the reality of their own behavior and that of others may result in overwhelming anxiety that they are unable to soothe.

Understanding the child as an adaptive survivor provides the necessary key for unlocking tools that promote healing. A simple solution emerges: Provide for them a world where remembering what happened, trusting your caregivers, distinguishing the past from the present, and regulating emotions is adaptive. As a therapist, your own office becomes that new resource-rich habitat, and with your guidance, leaving their survival symptoms behind becomes both possible and worthwhile. In this book, guided by the knowledge of the child survivor's resourcefulness and adaptive potential, we will look at each of the many symptoms that severely traumatized and dissociative children and teens may display. The techniques discussed promote healing and encourage new ways to cope with the stresses of their lives.

Balina, like many of the children you will meet in this book, displayed significant dissociative symptoms at the age of 9 when I met her. She went into shutdown states during which she had trouble being aroused, and her behavior fluctuated from calm to rage-filled, without apparent precipitants. Her history of sexual abuse, multiple placements, and inconsistent caregiving was typical of the many children you will encounter in these pages. When faced with difficult interpersonal and academic challenges, she would curl into a fetal position under a desk in her classroom. When faced with rules or directives that she felt limited her unfairly, she would attack in rage. Balina accumulated diagnoses with each new placement—bipolar disorder, oppositional defiant disorder, major depression with psychotic features. As she moved through nine different foster homes, Balina learned to understand her behaviors, not in terms of diagnoses, but as adaptations to life's circumstances. Her changing moods were understood as reactions to rapidly changing circumstances. Oppositional behavior was Balina's way of mastering the helplessness induced by her traumatic circumstances. Balina learned that dissociative retreat was her method of escape from untenable demands. With therapy, she learned that her reactions did not make her "sick" but, rather, a "survivor." The problems she encountered were solvable, and her own strengths, learned in an environment of struggle, could help her navigate the ups and downs of her life.

At 18 and a college-bound high school graduate, Balina was asked by her foster care worker to speak at a conference for social workers as a "success" of the foster care system. Balina's oppositionality, now an expression of her renewed self-confidence, kicked in. She refused. "I won't be your poster child," she said.

"I did well, despite what you did to me." She never accepted the implicit message of her foster care placements: that she should be grateful she had a home at all. Her therapy helped her to internalize the message that she deserved safety, love, and a promising future, as did the other children she had encountered going through similar struggles. Her therapy helped her to understand her dissociation as a helpful survival tool, not as a symptom of severe dysfunction.

Dissociation, a well-described clinical phenomenon among adults, has only in the last two decades started to gain increasing attention in the clinical and research literature. Dissociation presents in traumatized children with dazed states, confusion in identity, voices or imaginary friends that influence behavior, and a variety of dysregulations in behavior, mood, cognitions, somatic experiences, and relationships. Initially described in contemporary literature by Kluft (1984) and Fagan and McMahan (1984), dissociation in children and adolescents has been increasingly documented by a variety of researchers and clinicians who have found that dissociative symptoms are often associated with histories of significant trauma (e.g., Bonnano, Noll, Putnam, O'Neill, & Trickett, 2003; Collin-Vézina & Hébert, 2005; Hulette, Fisher, Kim, Ganger, & Landsverk, 2008; Hulette, Freyd, & Fisher, 2011; Macfie, Cichetti, & Toth, 2001; Putnam, Hornstein, & Peterson, 1996; Teicher, Samson, Polcari, & McGreenery, 2006; Trickett, Noll, & Putnam, 2011).

The experience of clinicians around the world who are treating young people with dissociative symptoms and disorders suggests that many dissociative children are not responsive to the standard techniques for trauma treatment currently available (Wieland, 2011a). Memory problems may make it difficult for conventional forms of therapy to be effective, and some of the most severe dissociative symptoms, such as profound dissociative shutdown, may be misdiagnosed as neurological symptoms. Dissociative children present unique treatment challenges, as the intensity of their acting out and destructive behaviors are difficult to handle in outpatient and even inpatient settings (Hornstein & Tyson, 1991; Ruths, Silberg, Dell, & Jenkins, 2002).

There is emerging research evidence that dissociation is indeed a predictor of clinical severity in child and adolescent populations. In a study of 2,450 children entering the child welfare system, the presence of significant dissociation was a key predictor of psychiatric hospitalization, and significant dissociation was the symptom that predicted the most rapid need for hospitalization for children in care (Kisiel and McLelland, unpublished findings, personal communication, March 28, 2012).

This book introduces a set of therapy interventions called Dissociation-Focused Interventions (DFI) (see Appendix A). Dissociation-Focused Interventions uniquely address the needs of children and adolescents who have dissociative symptoms that are resistant to more conventional approaches to treatment. The approach described in this book can be used alone, or combined with many of the new and developing practices that have shown promise in remediation of the symptoms of traumatized children (Arvidson et al., 2011; Blaustein & Kinniburgh, 2010; Busch & Lieberman, 2007; Cohen, Mannario, & Deblinger, 2006; Ford & Cloitre, 2009; Perry, 2009).

Although more research is needed focusing specifically on children, there is reason to believe that, when properly utilized, treatment of dissociation in children can be efficacious. In 1998, my colleague Frances Waters and I presented preliminary results of our treatment of 34 dissociative clients (Silberg & Waters, 1998) and found moderate or significant improvement for clients who stayed in treatment. The positive outcomes possible with techniques focused specifically on dissociation have been confirmed by the work of a group of international clinicians who participate in the child committee of the International Society for the Study of Trauma and Dissociation (Baita, 2011; Grimmink, 2011; Marks, 2011; Silberg, 2011; Waters, 2011; Wieland, 2011b; Yehuda, 2011), and a set of guidelines for treatment of dissociative symptoms and disorders in children and adolescents has been developed by the International Society for the Study of Trauma and Dissociation (ISSTD, 2003).

A consensus practice model for the treatment of adults with dissociation has demonstrated that when patients with dissociative disorders are treated by trained clinicians, they show a significant reduction in dissociation, posttraumatic stress disorder symptoms, reduction in hospitalizations and disabling symptoms, and overall increase in adaptive behaviors and feelings of well-being at follow-up assessment (Brand et al., 2012). The 29 younger patients in the sample (ages 18–30) made even more progress in decreasing self-destructive behavior and suicide attempts relative to those who were over age 30 (Myrick et al., in press). Consistent with this research finding, my clinical observations confirm that the younger the client, the easier it becomes to achieve significant remediation for dissociation. Developmentally informed interventions geared to the unique symptomatology of this population may have the potential to reverse the severe and disabling effects of early trauma across the life span.

The approach in this book is not focused specifically on Dissociative Identity Disorder (DID), as the DSM-IV (*Diagnostic and Statistical Manual*) criteria requires observation of personality states and amnesia, which are not always present in the child forms of the disorder (American Psychiatric Association [APA], 2000). Instead, the manifestations of dissociation in children are found across a continuum of severity, and in some ways resemble normal developmental processes, such as the phenomenon of vivid imaginary friends in young children. All-or-nothing labels that view the client as having a rigid disorder are less helpful than is a view of dissociative phenomena as spanning a range of severity across a continuum. As such, adult models that present a normalizing view of dissociation have been particularly influential in the development of this approach (see, e.g., Chu, 1998; Gold, 2000; Rivera, 1996). Also influential to the theoretical basis of this approach are treatment models based on affect theory (Kluft, 2007; Monsen & Monsen, 1999; Nathanson, 1992; Tomkins, 1962, 1963), models that stress attachment disruption (Hughes, 2006; James, 1994; Kagan, 2004), and models focusing on a relational approach to clients exposed to early trauma (Pearlman & Courtois, 2005). The work of clinicians who are part of the Child Committee of the International Society for the Study of Trauma and Dissociation has also played an important role in the development of the ideas and concepts presented here (see, e.g., Wieland, 2011a).

The acronym EDUCATE organizes a sequence of steps of Dissociation-Focused Intervention. These steps begin with psychoeducation about trauma and dissociation (E: Education), and assessing the child's motivations to hold on to their dissociation (D: Dissociation motivation). The next group of interventions assists the child in (U) understanding what is hidden and (C) claiming the hidden parts of the self. The "A" in EDUCATE stands for regulation of Arousal, Affect, and Attachment. The techniques covered under the "A" include managing hyperarousal, hypoarousal, and regulating affect in the context of attachment relationships. Traumatic processing and understanding triggers are the "T" in the EDUCATE model. Processing traumatic events involves attending to the content of early trauma, its sensory and affective associations, and its meaning to the child. The final E of the EDUCATE model (E: Ending Stage of Therapy) organizes techniques that help the child survivor face new developmental challenges, while fully accepting the self and the meaning of their traumatic history. As an integrated self, the true survivors learn to leave the past in the past and come to appreciate who they are, despite where they have come from.

People in other fields often ask me if it doesn't sometimes become depressing, working with children who have been so badly hurt and abused. "No," I answer. "It is exhilarating, discovering anew the amazing resiliency and potential of each new client." I hope you will find the same exhilaration as you apply some of these techniques to the children on your caseload, and admire the strength and adaptive potential of the children you will meet in these pages and the children you will treat. Through your treatment of each individual child, you have the potential to reverse cycles of abuse and help create for the next generation the safe, tolerant, loving world that all of our young clients deserve.

1   Trauma and Its Effects

"It's like you're on autopilot and someone else is controlling the switches," stated Shawn Hornbeck, kidnap victim and sexual abuse survivor. With these words to a reporter, he explained the dissociation, helplessness, and terror that kept him tied to his kidnapper for four years and three months until his rescue by the FBI in 2007 outside of St. Louis, 50 miles from his home (Dodd, 2009). When interviewed later about his trauma, Shawn stated, "Most people would say their greatest fear is probably dying, but that's not mine. I would have to say my greatest fear is probably not being understood" (Keen, 2008).

At the age of 11, Shawn was abducted from his neighborhood and forced to live with a sex offender, who enrolled him in school, gave him a pseudonym, and enforced his enslavement with threats and rewards for compliance. Shawn felt his healing from the trauma of his abuse and captivity was directly tied to people understanding the helplessness and terror that kept him trapped with his abuser, enduring repeated trauma and humiliation.

Like Shawn Hornbeck, the children in this book have felt the helplessness and terror of their plight, felt like they have been on "autopilot" and their behaviors misunderstood even by well-meaning people; but unlike Shawn's trauma, their stories captured no headlines. They have endured their trauma in isolation, but yearn to be understood, and hope that healing can follow from that understanding.

Trauma has been defined as events that are outside of the individual's normal, expected life experiences and are perceived as a threat to "life, bodily integrity" or "sanity" (Pearlman & Saakvitne, 1995, p. 60). The individual faced with trauma feels at that moment or multiple moments in time that they will not be able to survive, and that experience of intense powerlessness is a hallmark characteristic of trauma. Martha Stout (2001) explains, "These events open up a corridor of essential helplessness and the possibility of death" (p. 53).

These feelings of being overwhelmed beyond the limits of one's capacity can be mitigated when the experience is shared with others. Traumatic experiences endured in isolation and secrecy, which is often the case for the traumatic experiences of the children and teens you will meet in this book, are some of the hardest experiences to overcome. Protecting the secret, as well as enduring the multiple effects of these experiences, causes children's internal resources to become overtaxed, leaving fewer resources for the difficult work of healing.

As research about the early effects of trauma has proliferated, the field has made an important distinction between the traumatic results of single-incident events (Type I) and long-term chronic trauma (Type II) whose onset is during early development (Terr, 1994). Herman (1992) uses the term "complex trauma" to refer to early onset, relational trauma that leaves enduring effects on the traumatized person's basic capacities. Herman identifies six key areas of functioning that are impacted by early trauma, including alterations in affect regulation, consciousness, self-perception, view of the perpetrator, relationships, and systems of meaning. Later researchers and clinicians describing both adults and children have continued to refer to long-term early chronic relational trauma as complex trauma.

One source of information we have about the prevalence of trauma comes from the Adverse Childhood Events study. Felitti et al. (1998) studied thousands of patients through the Kaiser Permanente Health system and determined that 60% of the adult population had experienced at least one "Adverse Childhood Experience," including neglect, physical abuse, emotional abuse, sexual abuse, observing violence, or having parents with histories of mental illness or drug abuse. Most importantly, the number of the traumatic events experienced correlated with a variety of negative health outcomes, showing that exposure to trauma has long-term and serious implications for individual health.

The prevalence of multiple forms of trauma in the lives of children has been confirmed by the ongoing data collected from the National Child Traumatic Stress Network database. The more than 14,000 children referred for services through this national network endured an average of 4.7 different types of trauma—including physical abuse, sexual abuse, emotional abuse, neglect, exposure to domestic violence, illnesses, losses or exposure to natural disaster, violent assaults, or community violence (Kisiel et al., 2011).

DENIAL

Despite the emerging knowledge of how widespread trauma is to the individual, children we meet in our practices often come to us having internally absorbed society's message of denial. Their demoralization and disbelief in the possibility of change often is rooted in the fact that their disclosures were not believed, or as with Shawn Hornbeck, they may feel blamed for their apparent complicity. Often, the crimes committed against them were never prosecuted, and important adults in their life failed to appreciate the harm they suffered. Discomfort with trauma can lead adults to quickly change the topic, ask doubting or minimizing questions, or challenge children about why they did not tell sooner.

Traumatized children are hyperalert to any messages that appear to minimize or discount their experiences, and they will often reject with anger and then tune out any adults whom they suspect don't understand their suffering. Twelve-year-old Deborah, adopted from a Romanian orphanage at age 3, told me with disdain that her previous therapist had called her "a liar" when she discussed her memories of the Romanian orphanage. Upon inquiry, the therapist stated that she had responded to Deborah's horrific memories by saying, "You were so young, are you sure you are remembering it right?" This seemingly mild, but questioning, response made it impossible for Deborah to trust her therapist. Children who encounter skeptical police officers, defense attorneys, or department of social service workers often emerge from these interviews feeling retraumatized by the doubting response they often encounter. While most avoidance or denial of children's traumatic experiences is inadvertent, sometimes adults have a vested professional, legal, or monetary interest in refuting or disputing known traumatic events.

Unfortunately, there is a fervent backlash to deny or minimize the effects of trauma and sexual abuse. This denial appears to serve powerful vested interests, including defense attorneys and their defendants, as well as the organized pedophile movement, which tries to justify the abuse of children by "minor-attracted" individuals (the "neutral" term they prefer). In 1998, Rind, Tromovitch, and Bauserman published an article in which they claim to find that the sexual abuse of boys, which they retermed "adult-child sex" was not harmful. My colleagues and I discovered that the article was riddled with scientific reasoning errors and blatant misreporting (Dallam et al., 2001). The article was quickly touted by pedophiles as vindication for their lifestyle and cited in their writings to justify their sexual exploitation of children under the guise of an alternate lifestyle (Dallam, 2002).

Often slickly packaged as if scientific, these denials of the harm of abuse and trauma ring hollow, as increasingly persuasive research data document long-term health outcomes, psychological comorbidity, and even brain impairment as a measurable effect of a variety of traumatic events.

PSYCHOLOGICAL EFFECTS OF MALTREATMENT

Sexual Abuse

Sexual abuse may affect from 12% to 35% of girls and 4% to 9% of boys (Putnam, 2003) and is found in all socioeconomic levels and cultures. Research suggests that sexual abuse, particularly when it is more invasive, is associated with a variety of psychiatric sequelae, such as sexualized behavior and sexual risk-taking, depression, eating disorders, self-harm, drug and alcohol abuse, and significant risks of subsequent revictimization (Putnam, 2003; Trickett et al., 2011).

Finkelhor and Browne (1985) identify that the harm of sexual abuse may relate to the stigmatizing effects of the experience, the experience of powerlessness, and the boundary violations associated with sexual abuse. It is difficult to develop a sense of self-worth and autonomy when one's experience of one's body is as an object of another's pleasure. Compounding these effects are the psychological experiences of the child survivor as they internalize and react to the messages of the perpetrator. Self-justifying rationalizations are typical of the sexual offender (Courtois, 2010), such as, "This is an expression of love," "You made me do this to you," or "This is what you deserve."

When a parent or close family member expresses these ideas, it becomes hard for child survivors to extricate themselves from these beliefs, because their attachment to the family member would be jeopardized. If even Shawn Hornbeck, abused by a stranger who became his caregiver over four years of captivity, felt this loyalty and fear of escape, imagine the bind felt by children abused by their own parents. The sexual abuse perpetrated by family members often occurs at night, thus disrupting the child's privacy, and interrupting the soothing and restorative rest that bedtime can provide (Courtois, 2010).

Trickett et al. (2011) followed 84 sexually abused girls for 23 years and found significant physiological sequelae of sexual abuse, including obesity, gynecological abnormalities including early onset of puberty, major illnesses, increased health care utilization, cognitive deficits, abnormal levels of the stress hormone cortisol, and disruption of the hypothalamic-pituitary-adrenal axis, the part of the neuroendicrine system that is reactive to stress. Of significant concern, the next generation born to abused girls was also at risk, showing more referrals to child protective services, primarily for neglect.

A new form of sexual exploitation that therapists are just beginning to see in their practices is children forced to pose in the creation of pornographic materials, often at the instigation of family members. Once released into cyberspace, these materials can never be recovered. These children suffer with the awareness that their crimes continue into perpetuity in the virtual world of the internet. These survivors are dealing with unique issues as they are often plagued by guilt that their images may be used to induce others into sexual exploitation, and the forced smiles captured in still or moving images make them feel a sense of ongoing complicity with the crimes (Leonard, 2010). The fact that their abusers are for the most part anonymous and nameless makes it hard in therapy to deal with specific episodes of exploitation, and these survivors may become increasingly inhibited because they feel continually exposed, with computers themselves becoming triggers of overwhelming anxiety (Leonard, 2010).

This new area of child exploitation has created provocative legal questions, such as whether each new viewer of a child's images owes restitution to that individual victim. Federal appeals courts are still debating this issue with the test case of "Amy," one of the first identified child victims of internet photographic exploitation, who has applied for restitution in federal court against multiple perpetrators who have viewed her image since the early 1990s, when a family member first posted pornographic pictures of her online (Kunzelman, 2012). The Supreme Court is likely to eventually hear and resolve the central controversy created by this test case—can a "perpetrator" who viewed her image long after Amy's sexual abuse as a child, and who never met the real Amy, still be a cause of her harm?

For Amy the answer is obvious. In her victim impact statement, she wrote:

> I am there forever in pictures that people are using to do sick things. I want it all erased . . . But I am powerless to stop it just like I was powerless to stop my uncle . . . How can I get over this when the shameful abuse I suffered is out there forever and being enjoyed by sick people? (Amy, 2009)

Research on sexually abused children and teens documents high levels of dissociation in this population (Bonnano et al., 2003; Collin-Vézina & Hébert, 2005; Macfie et al., 2001), and dissociative symptoms in sexually abused children are related to early onset of sexual abuse, multiple perpetrators (Trickett et al., 2011), and risk-taking behavior (Kisiel & Lyons, 2001). As Amy wrote, "Sometimes I just go into staring spells when I am caught thinking about what happened and not paying any attention to my surroundings . . . Forgetting is the thing I do best since I was forced as a little girl to live a double life and 'forget' what was happening to me."

Like Amy, survivors often vividly describe their experiences of dissociation— "I floated to the ceiling and watched myself from above," or "I split into two people, and let the other me feel the pain." Many of the children you will meet in these pages developed dissociative coping tools to handle the trauma of sexual abuse. Sexual abuse experiences, because of their invasiveness, the associated arousal that induces an unfamiliar physiological state, and their association with the betrayal from attachment figures (Freyd, 1996), may readily trigger dissociative coping strategies.

Physical Abuse

Physical abuse may affect as many as 23% of children and, like sexual abuse, has broad-ranging implications for later adjustment (Kolko, 2002). In addition to the physical effects of early physical injury, such as scarring, or feeding problems, the physically abused child is likely to suffer a variety of cognitive and emotional consequences, as well. Physically abused children have been found to have academic and attentional problems, with lower scores in both reading and math, and higher risk of repeating an academic grade (Kolko, 2002). Physically abused children have significant problems with anger, and are two times more likely than their peers to be arrested for violent crimes when they reach adolescence (Widom, 1989). In addition to problems with aggression and antisocial behavior, physically abused children have higher levels of depression, anxiety, suicidal ideation, and suicide attempts (Silverman, Reinherz, & Giaconia, 1996).

There appears to be a particularly robust relationship between a history of physical abuse and dissociation (Hulette et al., 2011; Macfie et al., 2001). The children I have worked with who have been victims of physical abuse describe learning how to disconnect their experience of the physical sensation of pain, and this dullness in their sensory experiences generalizes to other physical sensations as well. Boys who have been physically abused struggle greatly to control their aggressive reactions to even minor provocations, and may seem to turn these aggressive responses "on" and "off" dramatically, to the consternation and confusion of those around them. The realization that someone chose to hurt them consciously often becomes a prominent theme that must be addressed in their treatment. Relationships tend to be fraught with suspicion and hypervigilance about potential harm, and this may affect the development of intimate relationships as these children grow older. Recent research suggests that when sexual abuse is associated with physical abuse, the long-term effects on later adjustment are more severe (Fergussen, Boden, & Horwood, 2008).

Neglect

Of the 3.3 million reports of child abuse that came into child services in the United States in 2010, 78% were for suspected neglect (U.S. Department of Health and Human Services, Administration for Children and Families, Administration on Children, Youth and Families, Children's Bureau, 2011). These numbers likely underestimate the incidence of neglect, which is often unreported and affects a high percentage of infants and young children.

Neglect has profound long-term implications for development, with neglected children having difficulties with cognitive development and early language skills, insecure attachment, peer difficulties, problems with modulation of emotional arousal, negative self-perceptions, early signs of depression, lack of enthusiasm, and low frustration tolerance (Erickson & Egeland, 2002; Hildyard & Wolfe, 2002). Emotionally neglected children tend to have difficulties with peer relationships with low levels of popularity, a variety of school problems, and high incidence of later psychiatric problems including suicide risk and delinquency (Hildyard & Wolfe, 2002). Neglectful caregiving is also associated with high levels of dissociation in children. Longitudinal follow-up studies have measured significant dissociation in children of parents who are psychologically insensitive and avoidant (Dutra, Bureau, Holmes, Lyubchik, & Lyons-Ruth, 2009), neglectful (Ogawa, Sroufe, Weinfield, Carlson, & Egeland, 1997), or punitive (Kim, Tickett, & Putnam, 2010).

The clinician may find a child who has been a victim of early neglect to relate to the therapist in odd ways, sometimes overly friendly and solicitous, and other times distant and avoidant. The relational components of therapy become particularly significant when working with children who have been victimized by early neglect.

Witnessing Domestic Violence

In the United States, approximately 15.5 million children live in households experiencing intimate partner violence (McDonald, Jouriles, Ramisetty-Mikler,

Caetano, & Green, 2006). Children's exposure to violence in the home, whether or not they were the direct victims of this violence, has been shown to predict a variety of subsequent mental health problems, including posttraumatic stress, aggression, and negative affect (Kitzman, Gaylord, Holt, & Kenny, 2003). The higher the level of violence between the parents that is observed by the child, the worse the outcome.

Many of the children described in this book were exposed to domestic violence in their homes. The unpredictable nature of sudden eruptions of violence in their homes have led many of these children to be hypervigilant and reactive to raised voices and angry faces, fearing that these might signal a sudden escalation in danger to themselves or to their loved ones.

While each of the forms of early trauma has known consequences, it is the repeated exposure to multiple forms of trauma for children that produces the most severe and long-lasting consequences. Some recent evidence suggests that multiple kinds of trauma are associated with the highest levels of dissociation (Hulette et al., 2008, 2011; Teicher et al., 2006). Other types of trauma, such as early abandonment, death of parents, painful medical procedures, and exposure to community violence and natural disaster, may lead to long-term consequences, which are magnified when compounded with the other forms of early trauma.

DEVELOPMENTAL TRAUMA

The phrase "developmental trauma" has been used to describe early relational trauma, particularly when the study population is children and adolescents (van der Kolk et al., 2009). Researchers often count the number or duration of caregiver-related traumas when assessing complex or developmental trauma and have consistently found that the higher the exposure to multiple forms of trauma, the more the severity of symptoms across a variety of developmental domains increases. Increased exposure to multiple forms of trauma affects multiple affective and interpersonal domains (Cloitre et al., 2009), creates significant disturbances in children's affect regulation, aggression, impulse control, and negative self-images (Spinalzola et al., 2005), and affects the overall severity of mental health symptoms (Kisiel et al., 2011).

The documentation of deficits in multiple domains of functioning among those who have suffered from more severe forms of chronic trauma led Bessel van der Kolk to propose a new diagnostic category called Developmental Trauma Disorder for the DSM-5, the new *Diagnostic and Statistical Manual* put out by the American Psychiatric Association (van der Kolk, 2005; van der Kolk et al., 2009). This diagnostic category aptly describes children who have had exposure to chronic early trauma by focusing on the multiple dysregulations in behavior, affect, perception, relationships, and somatic experiences that are typical of chronically traumatized children. This diagnosis is undergoing field trials and structured interviews have been developed to assess symptoms (see e.g., *The Developmental Trauma Disorder Structured Interview for Children (10.3)*, and

The Developmental Trauma Disorder Structured Interview for Caregivers (10.3) [Ford and The Developmental Trauma Working Group, 2011a, 2011b]). Developmental trauma, as defined on these measures, requires that the traumatic events last at least a year and assesses affective and physiological dysregulation, attentional or behavioral dysregulation, and self and relational dysregulations.

Table 1.1 lists the symptoms measured on these tools for evaluating developmental trauma. While it is unclear if Developmental Trauma Disorder will appear in the new DSM-V, this conceptualization has advanced our clinical understanding of the multiple deficits commonly found in chronically traumatized children. As you read case histories throughout this book, many of the symptoms listed in Table 1.1 will come to life in vivid ways.

Table 1.1 Symptoms of Developmental Trauma

Affective or Body Dysregulations

Can't tolerate or recover from negative affect states

Can't recover from or modulate negative body states

Perceptual sensitivity to noise or touch

Physical complaints that are not easily explained

Diminished awareness of body or emotions

Diminished ability to describe emotions

Attention or Behavioral Dysregulation

Avoidance of threat-related signals

Hypervigilance about future danger

Risk-taking

Impaired or inappropriate self-soothing (i.e., compulsive masturbation)

Self-harming behaviors

Inability to follow through with plans

Self and Relational Dysregulations

Seeing self as damaged, helpless, impaired

Worries about caregiver

Extreme distrust of caregiver

Oppositionality

Aggression

Inappropriate attempts to get physical intimacy or extreme dependency in relationships

Lack of empathy

Inability to tune out distress of others

Adapted from Ford and The Developmental Trauma Working Group (2011) and van der Kolk (2009).

For the purpose of this book, I will use the term *developmental trauma* to refer to the children and adolescents who have suffered multiple forms of early onset trauma. Some of the children have been removed from their homes of origin after physical abuse, sexual abuse, or neglect. Some have chronic medical conditions, which, combined with other forms of trauma, have reduced their ability to cope. The term *child survivor* will refer to children and adolescents who have experienced multiple forms of trauma and experienced some disruption in caregiving, often because a caregiver was also the source of trauma.

NEUROLOGICAL EFFECTS OF TRAUMA

Martin Teicher (2010) of Harvard University explains that early maltreatment alters the trajectory of brain development in traumatized children in predetermined ways, dependent on the child's age and type of maltreatment. One of the most consistently documented effects of maltreatment on the brains of maltreated children and adolescents are changes in the corpus callosum, the brain "superhighway" that connects the right and left sides of the brain (De Bellis et al., 1999; Teicher et al., 1997, 2000, 2003). Teicher and colleagues (2003) found that boys who suffered neglect had the most profound damage to the corpus callosum, while for girls the experience of sexual abuse was associated with a more depleted corpus callosum. Remarkably, research by Teicher, Samson, Sheu, Polcari, and McGreenery (2010) also found abnormalities of the corpus callosum in young people exposed to verbal abuse from peers, particularly during their middle school years.

The finding of an underdeveloped corpus callosum in maltreated children may suggest a potential neurological underpinning of the disconnections, flashbacks, and dissociative phenomena observed in traumatized children. The undeveloped corpus callosum may inhibit the ability to integrate visual information (right side) with verbal encoding (left side), or may lead the individual to respond to events in contradictory ways, depending on whether the right or left side of the brain is being stimulated. Research supports the notion that traumatized individuals show a preference for processing traumatic content on the right side of the brain, compared to normal comparison subjects (Schiffer, Teicher, & Papanicolaou, 1995). If information cannot be integrated across the corpus callosum and processed verbally, the result may be the recurrent reexperiencing of traumatic sights and sounds, a problem frequently found during flashbacks.

Anomalies of memory associated with sexual abuse, both hypermnesia (vivid memory that feels like it is really happening) and amnesia for traumatic or autobiographical events, may be associated with abnormalities in the hippocampus. Deficits in the hippocampus have been traced to excessive cortisol, which affects the hippocampus's ability to turn off an excessively stimulated amygdala (Teicher et al., 2003).

Another region of the brain that appears to be disrupted by trauma is the amygdala, the center for conditioned fear responses. Research on the brains of Romanian orphans shows a comparatively larger right amygdala (Mehta et al., 2009). Similarly, reduction in the size of the left amygdala has been reported among sexually abused young adults (Teicher et al., 2003). The amygdala appears to be on a hyperalert mode among traumatized people. Joseph LeDoux (1996), a well-known neuroscientist, explains that there are two "roads" for response to fear. The "low road" involves processing fear instantaneously from the thalamus to the amygdala, with resulting immediate physiologic reactivity. In contrast, the "high road" involves the processing of fear responses through the prefrontal cortex, which allows careful matching of how close this stimulus resembles the original source of trauma, and allows ongoing analysis inhibiting immediate reactivity. Those who have been traumatized repeatedly may have limited access to the "high road," and as a result, trauma responses are immediate and uninhibited.

When this fear pathway is stimulated over and over again, the amygdala becomes sensitized, so that lower levels of stimuli can trigger conditioned fear responses. Throughout this book, you will meet young people who show unthinking reactivity—fighting, rages, shutting down, hypersexuality—to stimuli in their environments, demonstrating this difficulty in inhibiting the conditioned responses to their traumatic past.

Also impaired by the effects of trauma are the more primitive areas of the brain, such as the cerebellar vermis, which is involved in coordinating intentional body movements and associated with cognitive, linguistic, social, and emotional skills (Teicher et al., 2003). Teicher's work demonstrates that abused individuals show decreased blood flow in this area of the brain compared to normal subjects. Teicher et al. (2003) note that Harlow's famous baby monkeys, deprived of tactile stimulation with their mothers, showed deficits in this area of the brain. However, when provided with rocking stimulation, even with wire mother surrogates, these deficits appear to be minimized.

The higher centers of the brain located in the prefrontal cortex appear to be particularly vulnerable to the effects of traumatic stress. The prefrontal cortex contains regions that help evaluate current experiences and determine their relevance to past experience. Without input from the prefrontal cortex, the activated amygdala cannot easily calm down the fear response. Evidence of cortical abnormalities in children suffering from posttraumatic stress or histories of abuse has been demonstrated repeatedly (Carrion et al., 2001; De Bellis, Keshavan, Spencer, & Hall, 2000; Teicher et al., 2003). Teicher et al. (2010) found that sexual abuse disrupts the development of gray matter in both the right and left primary and secondary visual cortex. Corporal punishment appears to specifically affect the medial and dorsolateral prefrontal cortex (Tomoda et al., 2009).

Some evidence suggests that brain abnormalities on the right side of the cortex may be uniquely related to the development of dissociative phenomena (Lanius et al., 2002; Schore, 2009). According to Schore, this area of the brain is particularly sensitive to stimulation from an attuned caregiver, and may suffer impairment due to the lack of this stimulation. Schore explains that the right orbito-frontal cortex in traumatized dissociative patients may have impaired connectivity to limbic structures, leading to the "inability to flexibly shift internal states and overt behavior in response to stressful external demands" (p. 119).

Ford (2009) differentiates between the child's survival brain—the brain in emergency survival mode—and the learning brain, the brain poised for taking in new information and growing. Deficits in the cortical areas of the brain, particularly the ventral and medial prefrontal cortex, affect peoples' overall ability to observe themselves, talk about their experiences objectively, and put their experiences into context. These areas are underdeveloped in traumatized people, in part, because the "survivor brain" is too busy protecting itself from incoming threats. At the same time, these metacognitive skills are the exact skills that we want to encourage in our traumatized clients.

Besides the structural changes in the brain associated with early trauma, children exposed to chronic stress develop imbalances in the brain's chemical makeup, with excesses of stress hormones, or catecholamines, such as epinephrine and norepinephrine, which lead to increased startle responses, irritability, and high heart rate. As the child's brain becomes sensitized and is reactivated into stress reactions by signals that remind him of the original trauma, over time, this hyperarousal may become an enduring trait (Perry, Pollard, Blakely, Baker, & Vigilante, 1995). Hyperactivity, anxiety, impulsivity, sleep difficulties, and tachycardia may be some of the symptoms observed in children in these states of chronic hyperarousal. Alternatively, the child might experience hypoarousal, which involves a surrender or freezing response with circulating epinephrine but accompanied by increased vagal tone with decreasing blood pressure and heart rate. Perry and colleagues note that in this state there is a special increase in the dopamanergic system so that the body may release endogenous opioids and induce desensitization to pain (see Chapter 10).

In summary, the brains of traumatized children are affected both structurally and chemically by the effects of enduring stress. Multiple areas of function are compromised, and disconnection and dysregulation is the result. The healthy brain is a brain that is well integrated, where communication through brain chemicals flows freely in cascades of arousal and inhibition. The brain of a traumatized child lacks integration, as communication horizontally (between the right and left) and vertically (between the higher centers and lower centers) is less fluid. The hippocampus and prefrontal cortex do not communicate with the amygdala. Barriers to integration result from structural and chemical effects of repeated traumatic experiences and the resulting use-dependent pruning and selection of brain cells.

The child's traumatized brain has a dual handicap: Reactivity is enhanced while regulation is impaired. As a result, the sensitized brain over-responds to any suggestion of trauma, and the regulating effects of higher brain processes and chemical inhibiters are minimal.

This research on the neurobiological effects of trauma also hints at multiple directions for the remediation of symptoms. The brain grows by pruning and discarding underused pathways, while strengthening new ones. Thus, the dysregulated and stress-affected brains of traumatized children are uniquely adapted to the traumatic, chaotic, and unpredictable environment in which the child finds himself. Getting out of the way quickly is important for a child frequently exposed to danger. To survive, there is no time to reflect or perform careful matching functions to compare a new stimulus to an older source of fear. Disruptions in memory may be adaptive for an organism if trauma and caregiving emanate from the same source, as often happens in the environment of abused children.

Understanding that certain abnormalities may be necessary to survive trauma can help us appreciate what direction the child survivor must move in to try to adapt to a healthier, more regulated, and loving environment. The parts of the brain affected by early trauma thus become the indirect target of our efforts, while the symptoms, behaviors, chronic reactivity, and protective behaviors of the "survivor brain" become our direct targets. By being aware of the ways in which these children's developmental trajectory in many domains is moved off course by the exposure to chronic trauma, we can aim interventions to those domains. The children you will meet throughout this book are a testament to the potential of the brain to absorb and respond to the new healing experiences we offer them in our therapeutic interventions.

The overarching goals of therapy are summarized in Table 1.2, with speculation about how those interventions might affect the developing brains of traumatized

Table 1.2 Goals of Therapy

Treatment Goal	Intervention	Associated Brain Structure
1. Be safe (stop any current trauma)	Environmental management (Chapter 14 and throughout)	Prevent further brain compromise
2. Stay calm in the face of triggers	Regulate affect and arousal (Chapters 9, 10, and 11)	Connectivity of the medial prefrontal cortex with the limbic areas, cerebellar vermis
3. Increase self-awareness	Practice grounding; memory, body awareness (Chapters 8, 9, and 10)	Connectivity of left prefrontal cortex
4. Tell the trauma story	Understand what happened and what it means about the self (Chapter 13)	Activate brain function in the hippocampus and connect to prefrontal cortex
5. Develop reciprocal relationships	Family therapy Relationship to therapist (Chapters 5 and 12)	Interpersonal attunement may stimulate the right orbital-frontal cortex
6. Turn helplessness into mastery	Behavioral practice, or imagery work (throughout)	New brain pathways emerge through practice
7. Develop coherent and integrated consciousness	Dissociative focused interventions (throughout)	Both vertical and horizontal neural integration; corpus callosum connectivity and connectivity of prefrontal cortex to limbic and lower brain functions

children. This book will address many of the interventions summarized in Table 1.2, with a special emphasis on Dissociation-Focused Interventions, which address disruptions in the children's continuity of awareness. Most of the children and teens you will meet in these pages have significant symptoms of dissociation as well as the well-described features of developmental trauma. Like Shawn Hornbeck, they see themselves as living their life on autopilot, feeling little control over their choices or behavior. Exploring their dissociation can give us further insight into the disruptions in affect regulation, somatic experiences, cognitions, self-views, behaviors, and relationships that we see in these children. The nature of this dissociation that we see in chronically traumatized young people will be the focus of the next chapter.

2   An Integrative Developmental Model of Dissociation

Sonya moved like a puppet on strings when I first met her in a group home for traumatized girls. *"Why do you move in that slow, robotic way; does it feel like something or someone else is controlling you?"* I asked, fishing for something to help me establish rapport with this mostly mute 12-year-old who had a history of violent and assaultive behavior. She suddenly turned to me and answered, "Yes, we don't let her move on her own. It is too dangerous." I clarified slowly: *"Did you just use the first person plural, we?"* I asked. *"Who would that be?"* "The three men who turn my feelings on and off," Sonya answered. With this statement, Sonya finally began to reveal her hidden imaginary world, peopled by "helpers" who controlled her moods and actions and were now holding back her dangerously escalating behavior.

As has become commonplace in my practice, simple direct questions that reflected my observations of the child's behavior opened up a previously hidden dissociative process that gave me a powerful entrée into Sonya's treatment. The information Sonya provided allowed me to enter her private world, and help her take the first steps towards freeing herself from the hold of these imaginary characters. *"How wonderful that they help you,"* I said. *"Maybe they could also learn how to help the feelings calm down, so your behavior won't be dangerous at all."*

Dissociation has been a controversial concept from both a diagnostic and theoretical point of view. Yet controversies about its definition and its causes have not prevented multiple children and teens, such as Sonya, from coming to the attention of clinicians around the world. Case studies and case series since 1984 have documented children and adolescents with severe psychiatric symptoms, including self-harm and suicidality, who show problems of memory, identity confusion, rapid fluctuations of mood and behavior, and belief that imaginary friends or other selves are responsible for unremembered actions (see, e.g., Albini & Pease, 1989; Bowman, Blix, & Coons, 1985; Dell & Eisenhower, 1990; Fagan & McMahon, 1984; Hornstein & Tyson, 1991; Jacobsen, 1995; Klein, Mann, & Goodwin, 1994; Kluft, 1984; Laporta, 1992; Malenbaum & Russell, 1987; Putnam et al., 1996; Riley & Mead, 1988; Weiss, Sutton, & Utecht, 1985; Zoroglu, Yargic, Tutkun, Öztürk, & Sar, 1996). In-depth case descriptions of dissociative children and adolescents have been included in a variety of books

(Putnam, 1997; Shirar, 1996; Silberg, 1998a, 2001a; Silberg & Dallam, 2009; Wieland, 1998), and finally in 2011, an entire book was devoted to clinical case descriptions and therapeutic interventions for children and adolescents with dissociative symptoms and disorders from around the world (Wieland, 2011a).

These articles and books show that while traumatized children and adolescents have some of the features of adult dissociative disorders, they tend to display less amnesia and more awareness of the identity states—which often take the form of vivid imaginary friends. Because adult criteria for dissociative disorders have not provided an accurate overview of the presentation of dissociative children, some clinicians have suggested that dissociative children be given a diagnosis unique to their developmental presentation, such as Incipient Multiple Personality Disorder (Fagan & McMahon, 1984) or Dissociative Disorder of Childhood (Peterson, 1998).

Despite careful documentation in the literature, and sometimes observation in their own child clinical practices, there is often hesitancy in professional circles to accept dissociation—in part based on a fear of being associated with an unscientific or invalidated treatment "fad." Well-publicized critics of the dissociation field (e.g., McHugh, 2008; Nathan, 2011) have portrayed dissociation as a "misdirection of psychiatry" promulgated by misguided practitioners. Media portrayals of flamboyant cases of DID, formerly Multiple Personality Disorder (MPD), have led to a professional squeamishness about this topic and fear of criticism or rejection from the mainstream of psychiatry and psychology. Simplified portrayals of theories of dissociation, such as those that emphasize "shattering of the self" or "fragmentation of the personality," may appear too mechanistic and irrelevant to a child or adolescent population, and may have led to avoidance of dissociation and its treatment in child clinical work.

In this book, I will introduce you to a theoretical understanding of dissociation that views dissociative behaviors of your young clients as understandable adaptations to environments that have caused a level of affect arousal so painful that the clients learn to habitually avoid this arousal. Over time, these affect avoidance strategies may become increasingly well organized, impervious to interpersonal influences, and may begin to take on their own behavioral, emotional, and identity features.

The DSM-IV-TR definition is a good starting point for developing an understanding of the concept of dissociation and the limits of our current understanding. *The Diagnostic and Statistical Manual* (APA, 2000) tells us that dissociation is "a disruption in the usually integrated functions of consciousness, memory, identity or perception" (p. 519). Unfortunately, this definition appears to originate from an adult perspective. By stating that these functions are "usually integrated," this definition appears to be describing an adult mind that became "disrupted," rather than a child's mind that is in the process of development and integration of its functions. A comprehensive theory of dissociation will have to account both for any apparent "disintegration" as well as the developmental roots of these processes.

Unfortunately, the terms "dissociation" and "dissociate" are used in multiple ways by clinicians and researchers, and clarity about the meanings of these words is sorely lacking (Dell, 2009; Spiegel et al., 2011). Dell suggests there may be several distinct mental processes that we have come to lump together as "dissociation" that may stem from different etiological pathways and serve different functions. For example, dissociative shutdown responses are reminiscent of animals' responses to predators in the wild and, thus, may be evolutionary based. This type of physiological and mental shutdown may be very different than the blocking of unwanted mental content and the later intrusive reemergence of these thoughts or images. Yet, currently, we tend to term all of these as examples of dissociation. Optimally, dissociation should be defined in such a way as to accommodate the variety of clinical manifestations and lead to an organized treatment approach that remediates dissociative symptoms.

Another problem with our understanding of dissociation in children is that much of the empirical data upon which our theorizing is based comes from different measures that may not all be tapping the same dimensions. Studies of large groups of children or adolescents diagnosed with dissociative pathology based on a standardized assessment procedure have yet to be conducted (Boysen, 2011).

One of the leading theories explaining dissociation is the Structural Dissociation Model. Developed by van der Hart, Nijenhuis, and Steele (2006), the model considers the key feature of dissociation to be the splitting of the personality at the time of trauma into functional systems, so that the brain's adaptive system involved in daily activities and the defensive system involved in fear reactions and self-defense become disconnected from each other. According to the Structural Dissociation Model, further trauma can further divide the split parts of the personality, resulting in what is called secondary and then tertiary dissociation. The therapeutic approach suggested by the model involves reconnection of these separated elements through encouraging attachment and security of the adaptive part of the personality and reducing the fear and avoidance of the emotional part of the personality. While this theoretical model has yielded a promising therapy approach for adults suffering from the most severe dissociative disorders, the language used and the theory underlying it may not be as relevant for a child and adolescent population.

In children and adolescents, the earliest manifestations of dissociative phenomena do not involve "splitting of the personality" as the personality is still in an early developmental phase. What we see in children manifesting dissociative symptoms are early precursors to this kind of "splitting of the personality," and their clinical appearance only begins to resemble that of their adult counterparts over time (Putnam et al., 1996). Thus, theories of dissociation relevant to children must be sensitive to the development and early manifestations of dissociative-like phenomena. Ultimately, we need to understand dissociation from the "bottom up" rather than the "top down." In other words, we should not base our theories of dissociation in children on the clinical presentations of adults, but instead on the clinical manifestation of children and adolescents.

AFFECT AVOIDANCE THEORY

The theoretical approach that I will describe here is the Affect Avoidance Theory, which is a refinement of the Integrative Developmental Perspective (Silberg, 2001a, 2004). This theory relies on developmental literature, specifically Putnam's (1997) Discrete Behavioral States Model, attachment theory, affect theory, and interpersonal neurobiology to explain how and why traumatized children develop dissociative coping strategies. The Affect Avoidance Theory provides an organizing theoretical framework for a variety of dissociative phenomenon. This framework views dissociative phenomenon from a normalizing and adaptive perspective. That is, this model is attentive to the ways in which the child's deviations in consciousness, identity development, affect, or behavior have served to protect the child, and this model provides a framework for redirecting the child incrementally back to behaviors seen in a more normative developmental trajectory.

Putnam's Discrete Behavior States Theory

Putnam (1997) made significant advances in our developmental understanding of dissociation through his "Discrete Behavioral States" model of dissociation. Putnam based his theories on observations from the infant observation studies of Peter Wolff (1987), who identified the basic states of infants observed throughout the day. He noticed that infants tend to move predictably from deep sleep, to REM (Rapid Eye Movement) sleep, to crying, to fussy, to alert. As the babies developed, Wolff observed increasing flexibility between states and more likelihood that steps could be skipped. Putnam theorized that the traumatized child develops states that are fear-based and that may be associated with unique state-dependent memories. Putnam explains that in chronically traumatized children, these states can become impervious to regulation, and increasingly segregated over time, rather than more flexible, as is characteristic of the general process of state changes in children. Putnam noticed that dissociative children seem to lack the meta-cognitive integrative skills that could counter this lack of integration of traumatic states. Putnam's theory provides valuable insight as it recognizes that normal development involves a process of alternating and shifting states, and that flexibility and freedom to move within states is a hallmark of health and normal development.

Attachment Theory

Attachment theory provides the next central insight that informs the Affect Avoidance Theory of dissociation presented here. Bowlby (1988) proposed that infants developed "Internal working models" or organized expectations of caregiver behaviors that determine how infants and young children relate to their caregivers. If a parent is consistent and attentive, and promotes secure attachment, the infant develops an internal working model of predictable, loving behavior and interacts with the world based on this expectation. If the parent is inconsistent, rejecting, or unavailable, the infant may develop an insecure attachment, with an associated internal working model. This internal working model helps the infant to predict the kind of response they will likely get from their caregiver and to modify their behaviors accordingly.

Original attachment researchers identified three kinds of attachment styles—secure, insecure-avoidant, and insecure-ambivalent (Ainsworth, 1964). Later research identified a fourth kind of attachment, "disorganized attachment," characterized by contradictory behavior patterns, incomplete and interrupted movements, freezing and stilling, asymmetrical movements, and indications of apprehension (Main & Solomon, 1990). The behavioral characteristics of disorganized attachment show similarities to clinical descriptions of dissociation. Research, in fact, provides some evidence that disorganized attachment in toddlers, particularly in combination with parenting deficits or traumatic experiences, may predict dissociation in teenagers (Dutra et al., 2009; Ogawa et al., 1997). Most importantly, both of these studies show the important role of impaired caregiving in the development of dissociation.

Liotti is an attachment theorist who has focused on disorganized attachment in maltreated youngsters. Liotti (1999, 2009) hypothesized that caregivers who are fearful and frightened may elicit multiple, competing internal working models in the developing infant. Sometimes the infant may react with a high expectancy of avoidance, retreat, and fear, and at other times may seek attention and expectation of nurturing. These competing schemas may be experienced simultaneously or in rapid succession, leading to confusion, impaired integration, and the "freezing" or dissociation observed in young children with disorganized attachment. Liotti further hypothesized that this impaired attachment style makes it increasingly more difficult for a child to be able to seek comfort after a traumatic event. A feedback loop of increasing fear is created by the child's attempt to seek comfort while simultaneously being stymied by the unavailability of consistent comfort. Liotti emphasized that the dissociative reaction may be seen as a failure in the child's ability to develop an organized response to the dilemma of the need for attachment and soothing, particularly when such soothing is inconsistently available.

Like the shifting states described by Putnam (1997), research on disorganized attachment provides one of the building blocks for understanding dissociative behaviors in children. The competing internal working models described by Liotti (1999, 2009) may be the genesis of the alternating and shifting behavioral states seen in children with dissociative symptoms. Putnam's work explains how these states become rigid over time, rather than showing the flexibility and malleability seen in the development of normal children without a traumatic history.

Affect Theory

Affect theory contributes to the Affect Avoidance Model by providing insight into the affective underpinnings of the internal working models described by Liotti (1999, 2009). Tomkins (1962, 1963) proposes that there are nine discrete, biologically based, native affect states. Six affects are negative (anger-rage, fear-terror, distress-anguish, disgust, dissmell ["turning up one's nose"], and shame-humiliation). Surprise-startle is a neutral affect and the two positive affects are interest-excitement and enjoyment-joy. Tomkins considers affects to be the "psychic glue" that holds the experience of self together (Monsen & Monsen, 1999). According to Tomkins, affects serve to provide internal signals to a developing child about what is beneficial or harmful to their survival. Tomkins considers affects to be amplifications of the child's lived experiences—making positive experiences more positive and negative experiences more negative—so that the child has a method for rapidly learning what is beneficial or harmful to his welfare.

Over time, these various affects become associated with stimuli and responses, and eventually get organized into affect "scripts." Affect scripts are collections of learned associations between affect, what stimulated them, and behaviors that provide useful responses to these affects. Nathanson (1992) and Kluft (2007) have applied Affect Theory clinically and found that practiced scripts begin to take on a life of their own and people increasingly rely on them for dealing with affect in rote and automatic ways. For example, the affect of shame, which can represent the experience of the loss of positive connection with a caregiver, becomes particularly painful when aroused repeatedly by an inadequate caregiver. Avoidance of this affect through practiced behavioral scripts of attack, or avoidance, provides a successful method for learning to deal with the pain associated with shame.

Living in a world of trauma-based affect scripts is where our child survivor finds herself. Multiple triggers evoke affects, which are amplified and may become more aversive than the original event. New scripts evolve to develop avoidance to the arousal of affects associated with trauma—terror, humiliation, disgust—as these painful affects are soon mistaken for the sources of trauma themselves, and thus in turn provoke avoidance scripts of their own. The child survivor then displays a phobia to the arousal of affect, which was originally associated with the traumas or disruptive attachments endured at an earlier time, and engages in practiced, automatic behavioral scripts evoked by multiple triggers in the environment.

Neuroscientist Antonio Damasio (1999) confirms the fundamental role of affective experience for building consciousness, as his research suggests that it is the basic awareness of our affects, which we experience as "feelings," that allows the conscious self to emerge. The development of affect becomes the central building block for conscious awareness, as each affect colors our interactions, and helps us tie them together to build continuity of the self. This process is disrupted in traumatized children, as affects of terror, humiliation, or grief become something to be avoided. As a result, affect becomes a signal of avoidance, memory loss, initiation of nonconscious action plans, and disorganization. Emotions become stimuli for avoidance, rather than for processing and integration of self.

Research on the mind and brain tells us that much of our behavior occurs prior to the experience of conscious awareness (Damasio, 1999; Norretranders, 1998), and that there is much that we process automatically without conscious awareness or full engagement. This is often called "nonconscious" responding to distinguish it from the "unconscious" used as a psychoanalytic term. I will use this term *nonconsicous* in this book to describe behaviors or responses about which the child survivor is unaware. Research evidence suggests that nonconscious responding to emotional triggers may be common among traumatized children. For example, research on dissociation in abused preschoolers suggests that children who heavily rely on dissociation may find ways to keep perceived threats out of their awareness by using divided attention (Becker-Blease, Freyd, & Pears, 2004). Pine et al. (2005) found that abused children with posttraumatic stress disorder were more likely to shift their attention away from threatening faces, suggesting that immediate perception may be accurate, but it is followed by avoidance.

Interpersonal Neurobiology

The final theoretical building block that informs the Affect Avoidance Theory of dissociation is the new science of interpersonal neurobiology. Interpersonal neurobiology has described how the interactive relationships between children and their caregivers promote the growth of neural pathways that regulate affect and create a stable sense of self. The development of self from the interpersonal neurobiology framework is a dyadic process where another person's responses to a child's actions shape the child's mind. Schore (2009) and Siegel (1999, 2010) theorize that the healthy brain builds adaptive connections through interpersonal experiences with an attuned caregiver, who responds empathically to the needs of the young infant. The self grows through the process of interpersonal interactions that validate, reflect, mirror, and regulate our affect states, to the point where we learn to become aware of our shifting affect states and to regulate them ourselves.

It is the interpersonal environment in which our child survivor finds herself that shapes and solidifies the shifting affect scripts and internal working models into rigid patterns of behavior. What is tragic for the child engaging in rigid and repetitive patterns of destructive, oppositional, or avoidant behaviors is that caregivers and others respond to these behaviors in ways that reinforce these very behaviors, and serve to make them even more likely.

When is the last time a parent came to your office, telling you how her 10-year-old son trashed the house and she responded with, "Come here honey, you must be hurting, tell Mommy what is wrong"? The extreme behaviors of their children provoked into automatic dissociative programs evoke reciprocal states in parents, who may become even more belligerent and angry—the very thing that provoked the child in the first place. As the minds of the child and parent react to each other, the rigidity of responses in each is shaped. In this case, the child's behaviors, and the reaction his behaviors provoke in others, can shape the child's mind to increasingly disconnect from the important relationships he needs.

Putting It All Together

Combining the insights of Putnam, Bowlby, Liotti, Tomkins, Nathanson, Shore, and Siegel, let us review what we see in the traumatized child. Experiencing early trauma combined with lack of consistent or attentive caregiving can cause the child to develop multiple competing internal working models, sometimes seeing the parent as nurturing and sometimes as rejecting and harmful. In traumatized children, the cessation of positive attention is not always predictable, and shame (an affect associated with the cessation of positively experienced nurturance) is triggered very frequently. If the child experiences terror or distress in connection with the caregiver, this too becomes an alternate internal working model, setting off other avoidance programs. The affects aroused by interaction with caregivers are often so intense and distressing that a pattern of avoidance of affect emerges, and planned scripts with associated behaviors of fighting, hiding, or acting out are practiced. As Putnam described, it is the rigidity and impermeability of shifting states that make them maladaptive. The rigidity and impermeability of these affect scripts, stimulated by multiple triggers in the environment, make them highly resistant to intervention. These rigid patterns are further reinforced by reciprocal reactions in the parents who often withdraw from children displaying these behaviors. As these children, deprived of appropriate caregiving and overwhelmed by trauma, enact learned patterns of behavior with origins in their early trauma history, these patterns of responding may become organized as shifting identities, "ego states" (Watkins & Watkins, 1993), or as imaginary friends that influence behavior.

The mind becomes organized around the principle of dissociation from affect, which generalizes to not remembering experiences related to the affect, or to not feeling pain related to the affect. In the normal mind, affect is a signal for memory retrieval, approach or avoidance, action plans, assessment, and reorganization. Affects are like the road signs of the self's navigational system—go closer, go farther, fight, retreat, yield. For the dissociative child, the navigational system is turned off and autopilot programs, responding to only partial information, control behavior.

We wonder why our chronically traumatized clients don't respond to our reassurances, their new caregiver's affection, or to our standard interventions. Dissociative processes in children and adolescents organize the brain in such a way as to inhibit the healing effects of corrective experiences, as even attempts to soothe can trigger avoidance programs.

Treating dissociation involves unraveling those hidden islands of segregated affect and experience and integrating them into a cohesive experience of self.

The reversal of dissociative states from this perspective requires an interpersonal process—the presence of an attuned therapist and an engaged family. According to Siegel (1999), "Interpersonal processes can facilitate integration by altering the restrictive ways in which the mind has come to organize itself" (p. 336).

The specific neurological underpinnings for dissociative processes are not yet well described, but an emerging body of research is making these processes more understandable. Most likely, dissociative processes in the brain involve multiple barriers, structural and chemical, to neural integration across hemispheres, and integration vertically of the more primitive structures of the brain with the planning and organizing centers of the brain. One of these barriers to integrative functioning may be the intensity of shifting states of hyperarousal or hypoarousal, which may become increasingly rigid, and impermeable. Recent research using contemporary neuroimaging has documented evidence for alternating cortical or limbic inhibition depending on the type of symptom (Brand, Lanius, Vermetten, Loewenstein, & Spiegel, 2012). During intrusive flashbacks, for example, there is evidence of limbic activity without cortical inhibition. In contrast, during symptoms of analgesia, depersonalization, or derealization, there is limbic inhibition and increased cortical activity, termed "emotional overmodulation." This "emotional overmodulation" is one way to describe the nonconsicous and automatic disconnection from affect observed in the dissociative clients I will be describing in this book.

As we know, brain connections are strengthened through use and repetition, and brain connections that are not reinforced are soon pruned. PET scans show that at one year, the prefrontal lobes of the brain reflect millions of potential capacities and connections that will dwindle by the age of two. This pruning and selection is based on the individual experiences of what may be needed in a given environment. An environment of trauma and impaired caregiving elicits overwhelming negative affect; consequently, the brain selects and reinforces pathways that encourage avoidance of affect and associated traumatic content. A traumatic environment can make memory itself maladaptive, as the growing child does not want to remember experiences that result in behaviors that threaten their ability to get their needs met. Moreover, bodily sensations, such as pain or pleasure, may also become maladaptive, especially when one has little control over being able to increase good sensations and decrease unpleasant ones.

Definition of Dissociation

Affect Avoidance Theory defines dissociation as: *The automatic activation of patterns of actions, thought, perception, identity, or relating (or "affect scripts"), which are overlearned and serve as conditioned avoidance responses to affective arousal associated with traumatic cues.* As these patterns of behavior are practiced and rehearsed, they become more rigid and inflexible, reinforcing themselves as they shape the interpersonal environment around them. The dissociative child may display memory problems, fluctuating behaviors, perplexing shifts in consciousness, a sense of shifting identities, and somatic abnormalities as a result of these practiced patterns of avoidance.

Eight-year-old Adina came to my session clearly frightened about something that had happened on a weekend visit with her father. Every time she opened her mouth to explain to me what happened, she became tense, frozen, and mute. Finally, she described to me what she thought was happening in her mind while trying to recall the painful experience: "It's like a brain seizure," she said. "Your brain does this so you don't have to remember and don't have to have thoughts." Adina's insightful description reflects an awareness of the nonconscious nature of the avoidance program her mind initiated to escape from painful reminders of the visit.

Which Children Become Dissociative?

You might notice that Adina seems particularly articulate and able to describe her psychological processes. Some have speculated that people who develop dissociative coping tend to be more intelligent than the average, but this has not been borne out in research (see, e.g., Putnam, 1997). Nonetheless, I have noticed that many of the children with significant dissociative symptoms I have assessed and treated tend to have certain special abilities, and I have speculated that these individual differences may predispose them to a dissociative coping style (Silberg 1998a, 2001a). In addition, I have treated siblings from the same traumatic environments, where only one shows dissociative pathology. Clearly, there must be some unique predispositions that encourage this method of adapting to trauma.

Kluft (1985) has suggested that a biological predisposition to dissociate when coupled with early exposure to trauma, unavailable caregivers for soothing, and an environment that perpetuates dividedness, may contribute to the development of dissociation. This underlying biological predisposition may include a variety of capacities that seem to separate the dissociative youth from others in my practice. One quality I have noted is that they seem particularly facile with symbolic expression, using dolls, creating pictures, or using imagery in symbolic ways. This ability makes them particularly sensitive to therapeutic approaches involving symbolic imagery. While the literature is conflicted regarding whether dissociative individuals may be more hypnotizable (Dell, 2009; Putnam, 1997), it is my impression that dissociative children are suggestible and are receptive to hypnotic suggestion even when formal hypnosis is not used. I have hypothesized that this capacity with hypnosis allows dissociative children to transform evolutionary-based shutdown states into dissociative states over which they have more control (see Chapter 10).

I have observed that dissociative children are more tuned in to others and have a well-developed appreciation of other's minds. Sometimes referred to as "theory of mind," this ability may predispose dissociative children to adopting multiple conflicting self-attributions as they readily internalize the conflicting information about themselves that they hear from others in their environment. This quality may also make it difficult for them when they first recognize that someone is hurting them on purpose, and may predispose them to self-harm as they internalize the understanding that someone "intends" harm to them.

There is some research evidence that the ability to appreciate others' minds is associated with the development of imaginary friends (Taylor, Carlson, Maring, Gerow, & Charley, 2004), which can be a precursor to the development of dissociative symptoms in traumatized children (see Chapter 3). Traumatized children may have higher levels of "fantasy-proneness" (Rhue, Lynn, & Sandburg, 1995). That is, they are particularly interested in fantasy and able to become absorbed in it. It is my impression that children who are particularly skilled with fantasy are also more prone to develop dissociative coping mechanisms.

The capacities that appear to typify the children who develop dissociative symptoms are important, as they may be the substrates on which dissociative symptoms may be built. For example, the capacity for hypnotizability may lead children who experience biologically based hypoarousal from stress to harness that hypnotic capacity to develop more executive control over these states and find ways to utilize hypoarousal more frequently to avoid affect-arousing situations in the future. Those with a high capacity for fantasy and absorption may develop imaginary worlds and imaginary friends, and then utilize these capacities to develop affect-avoidance coping tools. There is some evidence that the inner dispositions associated with dissociation may be based on genetic differences (Jang, Paris, Zweig-Frank, & Livelsey, 1998), but this remains controversial (Grabe, Spitzer, & Freyberger, 1999).

THE HEALTHY MIND

The brain is our hardware, the structural landscape that sets the boundaries for our potential; however, our interventions are aimed at the "software"—the mind. Tor Norretranders (1998) in the *User Illusion* uses this computer metaphor to help us appreciate how different our experience of the mind is from what is actually happening internally outside of our awareness. For example, when we experience the illusion of willing something, often the motivated action happened in the microseconds preceding our cognitive narration of what we did and why we chose to do it. Our belief in the reasons for our behavior is thus really just a "user illusion," a contrivance that helps us attach meaning to our actions. This is an important insight with regard to trauma survivors, as often they feel lacking in free will, deeply convinced that their future is predetermined to be as traumatic as their past. Their "user illusion" has broken down. They see themselves as victim, as an object of forces beyond their control. Sometimes, when faced with a patient so listless and hopelessly buried in this philosophy of determinism, I will suddenly jump on my chair and start to squawk like a chicken, or engage in some other ludicrous and equally improbable event. Then I ask them: Was my behavior predictable? Could they have predicted it? Could I have predicted it? They agree they did not predict it. I use it to help illustrate for them the infinity of choices that one has at one's disposal when one appreciates one's own power to choose. This little exercise dissembles most armchair determinists, or at least amuses them and shakes them from their sense of powerlessness as they ponder how to predict themselves and others.

To further explore the connection between human will and planned action, imagine two cars on a train, connected by a long tether. When one goes around a bend, it takes some time before the other can catch up. Imagine that the first of these cars is your brain and the second is your mind being pulled along with the ongoing illusion that it is driving itself. In a nontraumatized person with normal mind-brain connectivity the connections between the mind and brain are "seamless," and the experience of willed action feels authentic and purposeful. The will of the individual is clearly aligned with the choices of the brain, based on flexible response to the world and learned by experiences that facilitate increasing adaptation. Conversely, the traumatized brain has a sloppy, long tether and automatic responses happen before there is an opportunity to process choice. As a result, the traumatized individual feels helpless, pulled against her will, or driven without purpose. The deep helplessness of the traumatized person is reflected in a sense of loss of will. Traumatized persons often feel they have no choices, because their perception of choice is so minimal. We must help strengthen the mind to overcome this deep-seated feeling of powerlessness, which is a kind of mindlessness.

What is a healthy mind and how can we promote movement in our clients to this healthy mind? My definition of the healthy mind portrays the opposite of dissociation, emphasizing flexibility and adaptability:

> *The healthy mind effectively selects the information that will allow it to seamlessly manage transitions between states, between affects, between contexts, and between developmental challenges in a way that is adaptive to each shifting environmental demand.*

While this definition may seem complex, it contains all of the elements that dissociative children need to develop in order to become adaptive and flexible when facing the ongoing challenges of their world. This definition emphasizes a mind in charge of what it attends to and how it responds to the environment. The internal and external environment is constantly shifting, and adaptation involves managing these shifts in context-dependent ways. Understanding the development of a healthy mind allows new doors to intervention to open. Treatment must emphasize how to avoid trauma-based cues and select information from the environment that facilitates increasing self-determination, and freedom from automatic responses learned in the traumatic past.

TRANSITION MOMENTS

What overrides the autopilot program of dissociative actions, shifts, or memory lapses, and what initiates these programs? Focusing in on those transition moments is the opportunity to build up the "psychic glue" that will build the healthy mind we are aspiring to create in our young clients. As Daniel Siegel (1999) writes, "It is at the moments of transition that new self-organization forms can be constructed. Indeed, integrating coherence of the mind is about state shifts" (p. 316). Those are the unique moments in time when the mind is moving from one state or experience to another, signaled by some stimulus. The stimulus that provokes these shifts in the normal mind is the healthy experience of affective states that signal approach or avoidance, such as fight or flight, or reunion with loved ones through the affective signal of love. In the dissociative mind, it is as if there is a program that sets off dissociative disconnection whenever affect is aroused, with a rehearsed procedure to handle that affect without central awareness. Affect itself becomes so painful that avoidance programs take over, triggering automatic behaviors, which may have been learned at a time and place where it was adaptive to engage in those behaviors. Let's revisit Sonya, introduced at the beginning of the chapter, to illustrate how these automatic programs can hijack a young person's functioning.

Sonya was adopted at 9 years of age from one of the worst orphanages in Siberia. Her behaviors were difficult from the start, with parental reprimands or even mild-mannered guidance provoking aggressive or combative responses. It was often unclear what exactly was triggering a particular behavior, but Sonya got increasingly better at identifying precipitants to her acting out behavior and befriending the internal voices that she had perceived as controlling her. One day in therapy, Sonya's adoptive mother came in, frantic about Sonya's behavior the night before. Sonya's mother reported that Sonya—a strong, athletic, now-14-year-old teen—had broken her bed, apparently triggered into rage by something unclear to either one of them. I asked for them both to focus on what happened right before this event. Both agreed that nothing particularly remarkable had occurred. They had been sorting through clothing, looking to see which items could be donated to Goodwill, as it was time to shift clothes for the next season. They both remembered a conflict over a particular shirt. Sonya said the t-shirt still fit, while her mother stated that it was too small, and it was time to discard it. They argued for a while, grabbing the shirt between them for a few moments until Sonya let go of the shirt, and then went upstairs and broke her bed.

I worked with Sonya individually, focusing intently on this transition moment, the moment that went from participation with her mother, to retreat and destruction. I believed that affect would be the key to understanding the trigger, as her destructive behavior appeared to be a way of avoiding the troubling affect and associated memories elicited during the argument with her mother. I asked Sonya to think about what it felt like to have her mother take away from her something that she desired, and asked her to focus on the origins of any similar feelings from earlier in her life. To assist her, I amplified the feeling, *"You really want this; it is being taken away. How dare someone deprive you, how horrible to be deprived."* A sudden brightness appeared in Sonya's eyes. "You will not believe what I just remembered," she exclaimed. "When I was at the orphanage, there were only a few night shirts to go around and they would be put in the dryers to warm before bed. I was so fast I always was able to get one of these. But one day when, as usual, I ran to get the night shirt, a staff person said to me, 'No, Sonya, you are strong and quick and the other children smaller than you often don't get one, so today we are going to give your shirt to another child.'" Sonya remembered that she had gone to her bedroom at the orphanage and broken her bed in a fit of rage and deprivation. Immediately, Sonya exclaimed, "Bring my mother in here and tell her I am not crazy!" Sonya was excited to have discovered the connections between her past memory and current behavior.

Therapy involves highlighting these transition moments and learning substitutions of new behaviors at these critical transition moments. The origin of Sonya's seemingly mindless behavior was rooted in a traumatic moment from her past that aroused similarly intense affect. In the present, Sonya was still too triggered by affects of deprivation and rage to handle these with trust and discussion with her mother. Instead, she was thrown back into time with an automatic program that reacted to her emotional triggering with a built-in behavioral program, "Break the bed!" Yet, in her new more adaptive environment, discussion, making her case, even getting a new shirt, might all be options that could provide logical resolutions.

After her mother heard her story, I asked Sonya to work with her mother to process a new solution. Sonya's mother responded by tenderly explaining that she had no idea how much that shirt had meant to Sonya, and that she would have been happy to buy her a new one like it, or let her keep the old one if she had understood. Sonya's mother promised in the future to give Sonya more opportunities to explain what things mean to her. At the same time, Sonya promised to try to use words to counter the automatic effects of triggering.

This automatic affect bypass illustrated with Sonya's story is an example of the dissociative moments we will be talking about throughout the book. These moments may be short-lived, as dissociative fragments, or longer procedural programs involving identities or self-states. They may even involve dissociative shutdown states, where an overlearned conditioned response to affect stimulates the most profound avoidance possible, a state of complete unresponsiveness to the surroundings, which I will discuss in Chapter 10. Now let us turn our attention to the early assessment phase with traumatized children, during which we must establish an alliance with deep respect for the adaptiveness of the child's symptoms.

3   Diagnostic Considerations

Where do you start when a new child client comes to your office? Insurance companies may require you to find a label for the child in the current *Diagnostic and Statistical Manual*, but does that assist you with knowing what is really troubling your client and, most importantly, how to move your client toward health? I have previously argued (Silberg, 2001b, p. 4) that at their most useful, our "classification schemes are a mutually agreed on narrative, an abbreviated story that distills the essence of the problem, about which the client and therapist share mutual assumptions." The most useful naming and classification schemes would be "healing stories" that potentiate grown and recovery. So this chapter will not discuss questions of differential diagnoses or debate whether traumatized children are best characterized as having Posttraumatic Stress Disorder, Dissociative Disorder Not Otherwise Specified, or even Developmental Trauma Disorder.

For filing insurance or filling out necessary forms, I will often utilize a combination of Posttraumatic Stress Disorder (PTSD) and Dissociative Disorder Not Otherwise Specified (DDNOS) for many of the traumatized children I work with—sometimes adding additional diagnoses for presenting problems, such as eating disorders, depression, or somatization disorder. While the proposed diagnosis, Developmental Trauma Disorder, is very descriptive of traumatized children's behaviors, the dissociative dimension is not well developed in this diagnosis. The newer features of Posttraumatic Stress Disorder proposed for the DSM-5 may capture developmental trauma more accurately, as the new definition describes flashbacks as dissociative reactions and includes more affect dysregulation features—such as presence of shame, horror, grief, or terror. It also specifies that hyperarousal can include aggressive behaviors that are often found with children exposed to developmental trauma (Sar, 2011). Some preliminary data support the addition of these PTSD criteria, showing that they better capture the symptoms found in children and adolescents exposed to chronic early trauma (Ford, van der Kolk, Spinazzola, & Stolbach, 2011). However, the important point for this discussion is not the label we choose, but whether the therapist and client can devise mutually shared constructs that both describe the problems and potentiate healing and growth. A model that understands symptoms as survival tactics developed in response to traumatic environments provides clinicians a way to view their client's problems that is both affirming and empowering to traumatized children and their caregivers.

In order to develop a therapeutic relationship, it is important for young clients to agree with the basic assumptions upon which you base your diagnostic formulation. I base my diagnostic formulation of trauma on three assumptions. First, whatever symptoms the traumatized children display have been developed out of necessity. Everything the child is doing, whether it is cutting, lying, hitting, stealing, or fighting, is based on good and important reasons. Secondly, children have the ability to change their behaviors and develop new coping strategies that are suited to a less traumatizing environment. My third assumption is that finding new coping tools will help each child reach his or her own goals, whatever they may be.

When a teen initially comes into my practice, I often begin therapy with an explanation of these basic assumptions. With younger children, the explanation of the necessity for symptoms will happen at the time we discover together the reasons for a certain behavior pattern. The task for therapist and client in the diagnostic phase thus becomes an analysis of why the particular symptoms have evolved, and what functions they have served for the child or adolescent. The process of exploration into the motivations or reasons for symptoms and behaviors is a delicate process that must proceed with an attitude of sensitivity and honest curiosity. The clinician needs to be guided by a scientific approach of curiosity, respect, an awareness of the symbolic meanings that people can attribute to behaviors, and knowledge of the physiological roots of many traumatic symptoms and responses. This is a freeing and empowering exercise, as the child and adolescent realize that they are not going to be blamed, diagnosed, or labeled in this process, but rather profoundly understood. This process escapes the judgmental tone that may often come across in diagnostic interviews that focus on pathologizing children's behaviors.

Is it always possible to find reasons behind even the most provocative and entrenched symptoms? What about lying, stealing, self-harm, flashbacks? Can all of these have some meaning or purpose related to trauma? I have found that all of them do, as the symptoms provide a comfort zone, a familiar and safe approach to deal with painful information from the past. In fact, behaviors that may seem on the surface the most self-destructive often turn out to be profoundly self-preservative.

Barbara was brought to see me after having told members of her after-school competitive swim team that she had a brain tumor and she would require expensive surgery to cure her possibly fatal condition. Her swim team and coach took up a collection and when they went to give the money to her parents, found out that the whole story was a lie. Barbara was deeply ashamed of her lie and fearful of the condemnation that she thought she deserved from having told it. Condemnation and shame are antithetical to the kind of joining process necessary to find survival reasons for that kind of elaborate lie. But how can you join with a client who is already condemning herself more strongly than she deserves? I figured that any teenager who would develop this kind of elaborate hoax in order to get sympathy from her teammates must feel invalidated. I asked Barbara to simply write an essay starting with the phrase, "My life feels to me like I have a brain tumor because . . . "

Through the completion of that sentence, Barbara was able to write about a sexual assault from an older brother, something she had felt forced to keep secret. The weight of this secret and the knowledge that at some point the information would "kill" her family led her to express her fears in an oblique and dramatic, yet highly symbolic way. The weight of her secret felt like a brain tumor, and her lie allowed her to symbolically join with this lie and express her suffering to the outside world. My joining with the meaning behind her symptom allowed her to experience the feelings underlying this elaborate lie, and allowed us to develop a plan to handle the difficult situation in which she found herself. Had I approached her behavior from the diagnostic standpoint of pathological lying or the diagnostic criteria for sociopathy or antisocial personality disorder, I would have missed entirely the opportunity to find out the symbolic meaning of her behavior, and the associated trauma in her life that her dramatic lie served to camouflage.

During our first diagnostic session, besides seeking to join with the child or teen around the reasons for behaviors, I seek to assess a variety of dimensions that will help guide my treatment. These dimensions include motivations, beliefs about the self, trauma and its meaning, family messages, the severity of symptoms, receptivity to intervention, transition moments (the chain of feelings, thoughts and behaviors that precede the onset of symptoms) and the extent to which a child harbors a secret dissociative world. The following list of questions covers what I seek to answer in that initial session (see Table 3.1). This list can be used as a shorthand

Table 3.1 Questions to Guide the Initial Assessment of a Traumatized Child

What is motivating the child and what keeps him or her stuck in traumatic adaptations?

What are the central beliefs that guide what seems at first to be self-destructive behavior?

What messages from the family interfere with health?

How disruptive are the symptoms to the trajectory of normal development?

How receptive to intervention are the child and family?

What precedes and precipitates acting out, episodes of dissociative shutdown, self-harm, or other entrenched habits (transition moments)? Can the child name or describe his or her emotional reactions?

What traumatic events happened to the child and how are they understood by the child and the family?

In what ways does the child still perceive him- or herself as unsafe?

Who, if anyone, does the child trust and how can that circle be secured and expanded?

Does the child have a secret dissociative world that can help explain his or her puzzling behavior?

guide to structuring the initial assessment of children who come into your office. The questions are complex and multilayered and may not all be answered right away, but focusing on these kinds of questions will move the therapy toward the target of a healthy mind and aid in overcoming traumatic adaptations.

Throughout the book, case examples are provided that illustrate in detail how to find and build on the answers to these important questions. For now, we will focus on building that early alliance, assessing motivations, and uncovering the roots of the traumatic adaptations.

BUILDING ALLIANCE AND ASSESSING MOTIVATIONS

The initial assessment involves joining first with what the child likes or dislikes, including how they are feeling about the interview with the evaluator. Many children and, especially, teens are resentful of even having to meet with an evaluator and will make their displeasure known by refusing to talk, avoiding eye contact, or giving rote unelaborated answers. Immediately encouraging them to talk about how they feel about being forced to see you tends to cut through some of this initial resistance. In addition, while finding out what they are upset about in the evaluation process, you can collect important information about how to fine-tune your approach in order to secure your young client's trust.

If you can get the client to talk about things that make her happy or excited, you can find ways to connect progress in therapy with motivating goals or experiences. It will also serve as a big relief to the client to talk about things they like and enjoy before having to delve into more painful information. Once you understand what the client authentically enjoys, you are in a position to evaluate how the behaviors or symptoms are interfering with the client's attainment of more opportunities to derive life satisfaction. Furthermore, finding out what motivates the client in an authentic way can help you figure out what secondary motivations may be derived from holding on to traumatic patterns.

Remembering the child's goals and reminding him of these goals even as he changes through the years helps to provide the child with a motivation to continue in treatment that makes sense to him. Even the most demoralized child can tell you something that she wants to attain in her future. Although trauma can create a sense of a foreshortened future, early talk about the distant future makes your sense of hope for the child clear and ignites a spark of hope, even if it is small.

ASSESSING TRANSITION MOMENTS

As described in the previous chapter, transition moments provide an immediate window into the onset of affective experiences, along with subsequent behaviors that can derail a client's functioning. Because of the importance of understanding these moments, I want details, lots and lots of details, of the events that precede transitions into symptoms, bad moods, or acting out behaviors. Of course, most children will simply say "I don't know" in order to get the evaluator off track. While the children have learned that this is generally effective in most psychiatric interviews, I never allow "I don't know" to be the last word. I use many comebacks to refocus the child toward answering my probing questions in order to illuminate the triggers for a transition moment. I might say, *"That's fine to start with not knowing, but even when we think we do not know something, something in our mind knows more than we think."* Or I might say, *"Well, let's talk about what we do know. Do you remember what you had for lunch before you threw something in the cafeteria?"* If the child tells me what was for lunch, I might ask, *"How did it taste?"* Asking many questions that surround the experience right before the transition into the new behavior helps engage the child's affective memory, and ultimately we will be able to uncover the emotions underlying the onset of a destructive action or symptomatic behavior. Questions about what precipitated certain behaviors will help you assess how fluent the young person is with an affective vocabulary to name, describe, and understand his or her emotional reactions.

While this inquiry into the microscopic level of detail of their lives may initially seem annoying and invasive, if this inquiry is done with sincere curiosity and a nonjudgmental tone, children are often more than willing to comply. The client must be made to feel that nothing is more interesting or more important than fleshing out that particular event, so that together the two of you can derive insight into the behaviors in question. The assumptions are that the information is there, that it is valuable and instructive, that all of the client's behavior has purpose and meaning as a necessary adaptation to her life's circumstances, and together client and therapist can work to understand it and ultimately to change it.

Ten-year-old Sam, a newly adopted boy who had experienced multiple foster placements, was caught stealing money from his mother's wallet, along with trinkets from the lockers of boys at school. Sam was uninterested in discussing his behaviors, let alone what happened in the moments before those behaviors. I helped Sam by suggesting for him what children with histories like his often feel like before stealing property—"I can take care of myself. I can get what I need, and no one can stop me." We discussed what a *wonderful* feeling it is to be in charge of yourself, and I wondered if he might like that feeling and seek to obtain that feeling by taking what he thinks he needs. Because I made it clear that I understood what his positive feelings before stealing might be, he was able to share that he was unsure he could trust his new mom. I told him that it made sense to me that he would steal things for himself, if his new mom could not be trusted to take care of him. At the same time, I was able to help Sam recognize how these behaviors might interfere with the trust he wanted to build with his new mother and with developing good relationships with peers at his new school. By avoiding judgment and recognizing his stealing as a traumatic adaptation, I was able to motivate Sam to work with me on decreasing his stealing behaviors so that he could enjoy better relationships with those around him.

ASSESSING TRAUMATIC EVENTS

In the early assessment phase, sometimes the traumatic event or events that a child has suffered appear to be the "elephant in the room": an enormous reality that no one wants to refer to or talk about. There is fear that the child will decompensate if the trauma is mentioned, and, often, evaluators must deal with their own discomfort about hearing the details of horrific trauma. It is important in the very first session to acknowledge this "elephant" and to invite discussion at the child's level of comfort. If the traumas occurred before the current placement, I usually acknowledge the information like this: "*I know before you lived with your mom and dad (or before you came to this placement, or several years ago), some pretty scary things happened to you, and I have worked with children who have been through things like this and won't mind us talking about some of that when it feels like the right time.*" If the event was more recent, I might say, "*I heard from your social worker that the distress you are feeling is because of an attack that happened to you a few months ago. I want you to know that it is ok with me for us to talk about that, and it may even feel better for you when you are able to share more about that.*"

Sometimes, the traumatic information is not fully known. In that case, the evaluator needs an attitude of open inquiry and to give the child the sense that any information that is shared is acceptable, and there will be no judgment or overreaction if traumatic information is revealed. If a child is currently in a situation of abuse, it may take months of testing the waters before the information is finally revealed. Adina, an 8-year-old with severe dissociative symptoms (see Chapter 2), alluded to a secret she wasn't able to reveal for the first six months of therapy. One day she told me that a fairy in her brain told her "today is the day," and she revealed a longstanding history of sexual abuse during weekend visits with her father. Through calling social services, I was able to prevent any further visitation. Adina needed to be confident of my capacity to protect her before revealing the trauma.

When a child discloses a trauma in the assessment phase of therapy, the important information to glean is how the experience made the child feel about herself and the meaning derived from the traumatic event. How the child made sense of the event has the greatest impact on the child's subsequent symptomatology. Does the child believe that he deserves bad things and the trauma was his fault? Does the child believe that she is powerless against traumatic events and always will be? Does the child believe there is something essentially flawed about him that allowed this to happen? (The sensory details are less significant, but may be more important as therapy progresses, see Chapter 13.)

The other important piece of information to derive from the revelation of a traumatic experience is how the child's own symptoms and behaviors serve to help that child adapt post traumatically. Does the child let her mind go blank so she doesn't have to think about the experience? Does stealing from her stepfather help her handle some of the rage she feels about things not being fair? Does fighting with kids at school make him regain a sense of power when he had no power during the abuse? These connections are important to process in the early assessment phase so that the child knows that, rather than judging them, you believe that there is a logical meaning to that behavior. This understanding will set the stage for a logical path to remediation.

For the survivor of early trauma, a new stressor, such as a recent placement, change in school, or a loss of a friend, can precipitate symptoms because it is reminiscent of the helplessness that comes from a life filled with uncontrollable events. Thus, the therapist should explore recent events that may be a source for the exacerbation of symptoms. In inquiring about current stressors, it is important to be aware of new sources of trauma for children and adolescents that come from electronic media. Increasingly, the children and teens I encounter are experiencing some form of electronic bullying. Sometimes, the onset of severe symptoms, suicidal behaviors, cutting, or eating disorders is accompanied by an electronic communication of some kind that shames a child or teen in front of his friends. For example, a Facebook message sending false information, a picture of your client in a compromising position broadcast to friends, or a rumor that she is gay broadcast via text or on the Internet can cause the onset of disabling symptoms. Because these events feel uncontrollable, they can reinforce the child's sense of helplessness. Young people often feel that this world of the Internet and text communication is private and unknowable by adults and therefore it isn't something that they are likely to spontaneously bring up in therapy. Because electronic bullying can evoke extreme distress, it is important to always ask about whether the child has experienced trauma from any source of electronic media.

Having established an alliance with the client, understood the client's interests and goals, and found ways to emphasize the client's strengths and adaptiveness of coping choices, the therapist is ready to explore the possibility of a more hidden dissociative world. This exploration will be the focus of the next chapter.

4   Assessing Dissociative Processes

Eight months after having seen me for an initial assessment, Cameron asked his foster mother, "Can you take me back to the lady who knows about voices?" Children who have developed private worlds with elaborate imaginary friends, voices that talk to them, and secret identities that take over and influence their behavior are deeply relieved when this information is uncovered, and feel a strong and intense bond with the therapist who has finally understood them.

In order to create this profound level of understanding, the therapist must become familiar with the common classes of symptoms found among dissociative children and teenagers. These symptoms can be found in a variety of checklists, such as the Child Dissociative Checklist (Putnam, 1997), the Adolescent Dissociative Experiences Scale (Armstrong, Putnam, Carlson, Libero, & Smith, 1997) or the Child Dissociative Experiences Scale/Posttraumatic Stress Index (Stolbach, 1997), all of which are reproduced in the online appendices.

Symptoms of dissociation have commonly been organized into five categories. The SCID-D (Structured Clinical Interview for DSM-IV Dissociative Disorders) (Steinberg, 1994), a structured interview that assesses dissociation in adults, organizes five symptom classes to evaluate adult dissociation, which include depersonalization, derealization, identity confusion, identity alteration, and amnesia. This measure has been successfully used with adolescents, as well (Carrion & Steiner, 2000), but in my experience, depersonalization and derealization are less pronounced and significant in a child and adolescent population, and my organization of symptomatology reflects the more common behavioral manifestations of dissociation in children and adolescents. These symptomatic areas all relate to the central insight about dissociation described in Chapter 2: that the dissociative child or teen has developed elaborate systems of affect avoidance. The secondary by-products of this avoidance are aberrations in consciousness, perceptions, and body experiences, along with fluctuations of behavior, associated affects, and memory. The experience of overwhelming trauma rewires the trajectory of the child's development, resulting in the dysregulation in these multiple systems of daily functioning.

Shifts in consciousness may be rooted in biologically based states of hypoarousal augmented by autohypnotic capacities. Rapid fluctuations in behavior may reflect shifting "affect scripts," so that wide arrays of stimuli evoke these automatic responses. Unusual perceptual experiences such as visual and auditory hallucinations may reflect the child's absorption in an internal world of fantasy. This absorption provides another means of avoiding the overwhelming stimuli in the real world. Memory difficulties may reflect the nonconscious avoidance of trauma-related autobiographical information associated with intense affect arousal. Asking questions about the child's experiences in five primary domains will allow you to get a comprehensive understanding of the phenomenological world of the chronically traumatized child with dissociative symptomatology. These primary categories and associated areas for further inquiry are detailed in Table 4.1. An interview guide in Appendix B includes the questions that are helpful in assessing these symptoms.

Table 4.1 Five Classes of Symptoms Related to Dissociation

---

1. Perplexing Shifts in Consciousness
   Momentary lapses in consciousness or shutdown states that could last for hours
   Entry into flashback states where present and past are confused
   Sleep anomalies including sleepwalking, difficulty being aroused, sleeplessness, or
      having personality changes upon awakening from deep sleeps
   Feeling in a fog, or not in one's own body, depersonalization
   Feeling that one's sense of self shifts markedly

2. Vivid Hallucinatory Experiences
   Hearing voices
   Seeing ghosts, or other imaginary entities that interact with them
   Vivid imaginary friends, and belief that these can "take over" or influence behavior
   Feeling younger or markedly older than one's chronological age

3. Marked fluctuations in knowledge, moods, or patterns of behavior and relating
   Feeling one's moods have a "mind of their own"
   Extreme changes in relationships with family members
   Skills and abilities are inconsistent
   Sense of one's self as divided
   Extreme behaviors that seem uncharacteristic—sexual promiscuity, extreme aggression

4. Perplexing memory lapses for one's own behavior or recently experienced events
   Cannot remember what happened during an angry episode
   Cannot remember whole months or years of life (after age 4 or 5)
   Cannot remember assignments that one has completed
   Cannot remember experiences with friends or family that others report

5. Abnormal Somatic Experiences
   Shifting somatic complaints
   Self-harming behaviors
   Conversion symptoms
   Pseudoseizures
   Pain insensitivity
   Bowel or bladder incontinence

While gathering information from informants to assess these categories of symptoms is important, gathering this information from the children or teens themselves is the key to a comprehensive assessment. Dissociation is, at its core, an idiosyncratic experience of the self, a view of the self as disjointed and disconnected in a fundamental way. No one can provide the details of this idiosyncratic experience better than the child experiencing it.

ASSESSING PERPLEXING SHIFTS IN CONSCIOUSNESS

These momentary or lengthy episodes of disconnection from the world may span a range of severity. Children experiencing these symptoms may have momentary lapses in awareness where they may not respond to their name, or may appear to be involved in their own fantasy world even while others are talking to them. At the more severe end of the continuum, children may lose apparent consciousness, sometimes for hours at a time. These dissociative shutdown states at the most severe end of the continuum are described in depth in Chapter 10.

Some parents describe that when they look into their children's eyes, it looks as if "no one is home." There is a far-off gaze or a look of nonrecognition in response to people or places with which they are usually familiar. These sudden moments of disconnection often seem out of context to what is happening around the child. For example, children may freeze in the middle of playing with a toy or while engaging in conversation; or suddenly, they seem to lose the thread of what they were doing or saying. While for young children, this may look like the inattention seen with Attention Deficit Hyperactivity Disorder (AD/HD), there are differences that allow an astute clinician to distinguish between AD/HD and dissociative phenomena. The dissociative child is more likely to be distraught by the momentary lapse, and the lapse in attention may be accompanied by a rapid shift in mood. When dissociative children appear to not hear a question or comment asked, they often seem to be in another world. It may be harder to get their attention back than is typical with a child with AD/HD.

I have found it helpful to be very specific in my questions about what is going on during "blank" moments. I try to use direct questions to get around the "I don't know" response. For example, I ask questions such as: *"Are you spending time thinking about videogames you like to play, wondering when this interview will be over, or remembering something someone told you?"* Sometimes, the evaluator may observe lapses that are accompanied by odd repetitive movements such as a foot shaking, tapping, or even movements in the jaw or face. The following list of questions may assist with finding out more about these apparent lapses in consciousness.

Questions to Assess Lapses in Consciousness

When observing a momentary lapse:

> *What are you doing when you are spaced out like that? What were you think-ing just before you blanked out? Have you noticed what your thoughts or feelings are right before you space out?*
>
> *Do you ever finding yourself blanking out, not paying attention at all? What are you doing at those times? What are you thinking, hearing, seeing, and feeling?*
>
> *Do you have an imaginary place you like to go to in your mind? Do you have imaginary friends you like to talk to?*
>
> *Where are you when you are not paying attention?*
>
> *Do you ever have times when you feel like you are reliving something from the past? What does that feel like?*
>
> *Have you been told you do strange things in your sleep?*
>
> *Do you have trouble waking in the morning? Tell me about that.*
>
> *Do you sometimes feel like you change after going into a deep sleep?*
>
> *Do you ever feel like you are not really there, like you are watching yourself from a distance?*
>
> *Do you ever feel like you are looking through a fog?*
>
> *Do you have long periods of time where people tell you that you seem to have been in a trance or even a coma?*

ASSESSING VIVID HALLUCINATORY EXPERIENCES

Mental health providers have been taught to ask about hearing voices and this has traditionally been understood as the hallmark of a psychotic process. How-ever, in recent years contemporary researchers and clinicians have come to un-derstand the experience of hearing voices as more commonplace than originally thought (Altman, Collins, & Mundy, 1997). Arsenault and colleagues (2011) re-cently documented the presence of "psychotic symptoms," such as hearing voices, in children who experienced the common phenomenon of peer bullying. Others have questioned whether the features generally used to diagnose psychosis even in adults, especially hallucinations, are better understood as dissociative experi-ences resulting from traumatic events (Moscowitz, Read, Farrely, Rudegeair, & Williams, 2009). Dell (2006) argues that these intrusive symptoms of dissocia-tive disorders have not been stressed enough in the adult model of dissociation and are far more typical than are "switching" phenomenon, the sudden transition between identity states, which is more commonly perceived as the hallmark fea-ture of dissociation. This observation is consistent with my own clinical observa-tions in work with children. If the voices are associated with a psychotic process rather than a dissociative process, I find that the client shares rather disorganized information about the voices. Psychotic voices seem to be constantly shifting, do not seem to have organized personality traits or identities, and discussing these voices with a psychotic client may, over time, seem to be disorganizing. The finding of psychotic processes in my practice is unusual but most commonly seen with teenagers, evidencing a sudden deterioration in functioning, often with a family history of schizophrenia.

In my clinical practice, it is very common for children to report to me that they hear voices, and rarely does it seem to be associated with the extreme levels of psychopathology seen in schizophrenia. Often, when separated from loved ones by death or other traumatic circumstances, children report hearing the sound of the loved one talking to them in their mind. Abused children often report hearing perpetrators who harmed them continuing to harass or criticize them internally. Working with inner voices to minimize their negative power is one of the most important interventions when working with these children. When asking about inner voices, it is best not to ask directly, "Do you hear voices," as children are often prepared for this question and give the reflexive "no" to avoid a hospitalization or being labeled as crazy. Instead, I try to normalize the experience for them, stating, "*Many times children who have lost someone special to them, still hear them talking to them in their mind. Does this happen to you? What does he/ she say?*" Other helpful questions are listed here.

Questions About Voices and Imaginary Friends

Some children feel like their brain is fighting with itself. Does yours? Do you ever hear the fight?

Sometimes mean words that children heard over and over again seem to be stuck in the children's minds. Does this happen to you?

Sometimes children do things they wish they had not done. Has that happened to you?

Sometimes children feel like they didn't want to do something but someone or something made them feel like they had to. Have you felt anything like that?

Some children have toys that they have had for a long time that are particularly special to them. Do you have one? Can you talk to it? Can you hear it talk to you?

Some children have invisible friends that others can't see. Do you have this now? Did you have this when you were younger? Do you feel sometimes like the friends are still there? Can you see your friends?

Do you see things sometimes that others can't see? What do you see?

If the child reports hearing the voices of personalized objects, such as toys or stuffed animals, it is often helpful to invite the child to bring a stuffed animal or toy that is particularly meaningful to him or her to an initial interview. Some children see their imaginary friends vividly, and other forms of visual hallucinations, such as seeing ghosts or odd shapes, may accompany the experience of dissociation in children. Children tell me of imaginary presences that play a huge role in their behavior, sometimes directing from the background the child's every move. Yet, this internal process has stayed hidden from view, as no one has bothered to ask about it. This type of vivid and personalized imaginary friend or transitional object is common among normal preschool children. Four-year-olds may carry around their favorite dolls, hear them answer their questions, and set places for their imaginary friends at tea parties or even at the family dinner table.

Clinicians and theorists have noted the similarities between the imaginary friends of normal preschoolers and the hallucinated voices and dissociated identities of traumatized dissociative children. In fact, the DSM-IV-TR specifically mentions the presence of normal imaginary friends as an exclusion criterion for the diagnosis of a dissociative disorder in children: "In children the symptoms are not attributable to imaginary playmates or other fantasy play" (APA, 2000, p. 529).

Donald Winnicott coined the term *transitional object* in 1951 as a designation for any material object (typically something soft—a piece of cloth or a toy) to which an infant attributes a special value. Developmental psychologists view transitional objects as the basis upon which the child first learns to make distinctions between body boundaries of the self and others (Winnicott, 1953). Developmental psychologists also view imaginary friends as transitional objects that are projective manifestations of the child's experimentation with aspects of the self (Singer & Singer, 1990). Taylor (1999) found imaginary friends to be surprisingly common, in 28% of her sample of normal children, and notes that some children will impersonate their imaginary companions, acting them out and adopting their characteristics. Employing a broader definition of imaginary friends, Singer and Singer found imaginary friends in 65% of the children they studied. Imaginary friends are found to be most common between the ages of 4 and 7, but in some children last through age 10. Children tend to feel protective of their imaginary friends and do not like interference from adults (Klein, 1985). Imaginary friends assist children with a variety of developmental challenges—the practice of social skills, or an outlet for projecting difficult feelings or unacceptable impulses. Other imaginary friends help with feelings of loneliness or help embody traits the child wishes to have.

Trujillo, Lewis, Yeager, and Gidlow (1996) did a preliminary investigation comparing the imaginary friends of school children with those of dissociative children being treated in an inpatient setting. Trujillo and colleagues found that the dissociative children's imaginary friends were more likely to have malevolent characteristics attributed to them than those of normal children. Based on a review of the literature, McLewin and Muller (2006) concluded that dissociative children were more likely to have imaginary friends, had more imaginary friends than normal children, and the dissociative children were more likely to impersonate them. They also reported that dissociative children's imaginary friends were more likely to have more complex roles in the children's lives.

Adult and adolescent patients have frequently reported that imaginary friends were the first developmental manifestations that later became dissociated identities (Dell & Eisenhower, 1990; Putnam, 1991). Pica (1999) argued that all dissociated identities have their roots in the normative imaginary friends of childhood. While it is unclear if imaginary friends are the only pathway for the development of dissociative identities, retrospective studies of individuals diagnosed with dissociative disorders tend to report a much higher incidence (ranging from 52% to 100%) of imaginary friends in childhood than found in the normal population (McLewin & Muller, 2006). My experience with interviewing dissociative children suggests that concrete transitional objects such as dolls, stuffed animals, or even blankets, as well as more typical imaginary friends, can harbor the first self-projections, which over time become dissociated.

To better understand the role of imaginary friends in traumatized children, I conducted research examining the differences between the imaginary friends of normal children and those of inpatients with dissociative symptoms. A review of the literature, along with my own clinical experience, led me to hypothesize the following differences between normally developing children with imaginary friends, and dissociative children I was seeing in my practice.

1. Dissociative children are more confused about whether the friend is only pretend.
2. Dissociative children feel bossed or bothered by the friend.
3. Dissociative children feel the friend can take over their body.
4. Dissociative children believe there are conflicting imaginary friends who make them feel conflicted about how to behave.

To test these hypotheses, I developed the Imaginary Friends Questionnaire (see Online Appendix C), a version of which has been piloted on a sample of 149 normal preschool children in England (Frost, Silberg, & McIntee, 1996). The normal children's performance on this questionnaire was then compared with the performance of 19 inpatients on the Children's Unit at Sheppard Pratt Health System who were identified as dissociative. All of the hypotheses were confirmed, and some other interesting findings emerged.

Among the normal preschool children, 78% acknowledged that their imaginary friends were "just pretend friends," while only 37% of the hospitalized dissociative children agreed that these voices, dissociated identities, or characters in their mind were really pretend. This is particularly surprising when you realize that the evaluator began each interview explaining that the purpose of the interview was to explore the child's imagination, and that some children have friends, voices, or other imaginary companions that others can't see. Nonetheless, for these hospitalized dissociative children, the belief in the reality of these phenomena trumped the instructions given at the onset of the interview. One surprising finding was that normal children (84%) acknowledged that their imaginary friends kept secrets even more often than did the dissociative children (41%).

Dissociative children perceived themselves as having less control over their imagination than did their nondissociative counterparts. Dissociative children were significantly more likely to report that their "friends" took over and made them do things (74% versus 37%, respectively) and more likely to feel "bossed" by the imaginary friend or voice than their normal counterparts (72% versus 27%, respectively). They were also more likely to wish that their imaginary friends/voices/dissociated identities would go away (58% versus 17%, respectively). When asked if their imaginary friends argued about them, 94% of the dissociative children reported this, while only 25% of the normal children reported hearing arguments from imaginary friends.

Another difference between the experiences of the dissociative and normal children was the emotion that was predominant when their imaginary friends "visited." For normal children, the predominant emotion was happiness; among dissociative children, the dominant emotion reported was anger. The results of the study are provided in Table 4.2.

These results portray a picture of children with imaginary companions that have gotten out of their own control. Dissociative children report imaginary presences that argue with them, boss them around, take over, and in general cause

Table 4.2 Imaginary Friends in Normal Preschoolers Compared to Dissociative Inpatients

Questions about Imaginary Friends (IF)	Normal Children (N=51) % responding yes	Dissociative Inpatients (N=19) % responding yes	Confidence Level
IF comes whenever you want	76%	47%	$p < .02$
IF comes when you are happy	94%	58%	$p < .00$
IF knows a lot of things you don't	82%	58%	$p < .05$
IF is only a pretend friend	78%	37%	$p < .00$
IF takes over and makes you do things	37%	74%	$p < .01$
IF tries to boss you	27%	72%	$p < .00$
IF does bad things and blames you	41%	74%	$p < .05$
IF tells to keep secrets	84%	41%	$p < .00$
IFs argue about you	25%	93%	$p < .00$
IFs come when you are angry	41%	79%	$p < .00$
Wish IF would go away	17%	58%	$p < .00$

them difficulties. My research suggests children's experiences with imaginary friends fall on a continuum. Children who report a loss of control over their relationships with their internal companions suggest that this experience may have taken an ominous turn, and a dissociative process may be occurring. The presence of imaginary friends past age 8 should raise suspicion, and past 11 or 12 should be considered a red flag that suggests the need for more in-depth investigation. Many of the traumatized children I work with describe imaginary friends that are still present during adolescence.

One child described to me in vivid detail an elaborate four-part progression in the transformation of imaginary friends into dissociative phenomena (Silberg, 1998b). This child described that at first she had normal imaginary friends, and then noticed they could talk to her and do things without her conscious input. In the third stage, she perceived that the imaginary friends could control her actions for long periods of time. Finally, in the fourth stage, she experienced amnesia for her actions, and her dissociative experiences resembled DID as seen in adults. She reported that once the imaginary friends progressed in this way, she lost a sense of control over their influence, which became frightening to her. Online Appendix C provides a tool for clinical assessment of imaginary friends based on these research and clinical findings.

ASSESSING PERPLEXING FLUCTUATIONS IN BEHAVIOR

Assessing perplexing shifts in behavior is a subtle process. Sometimes, fluctuations that a parent or teacher find surprising are not surprising to a child or teen. By focusing in on what children themselves find surprising, you may get more clues to understanding their divided sense of self.

Asking about shifts in relationships is often a very fruitful area for inquiry, as these shifting relationships often feel surprising and uncomfortable for dissociative children. Changes in level of attachment to their mothers are very common in children with significant dissociation. They may have a dissociated identity who feels attached and loving toward a caregiver, along with one that holds their traumatic memories and is angry and resentful. Asking about these shifts, when you suspect that you are hearing only one aspect of their complex and conflicted feelings, can be very illuminating.

Thirteen-year-old Sandy described having an unusually close relationship with her mother. They would go shopping together and Sandy would ask her mother to help with homework and often climbed into her mother's bed to sleep when she had nightmares. At the same time, the mother reported that Sandy would intermittently go into argumentative states where she cursed at her mother and refused to do chores. I asked Sandy if sometimes she just felt that she could not stand another moment spent with her mother. Through asking this question, I was able to discover Sandy's perception of "the other Sandy," who was angry with her mother for years of not protecting her from her father's episodes of manic rage.

Awareness of "the other Sandy" remained dissociated from Sandy's consciousness much of the time.

When children talk about their fluctuating moods, they often describe these as "happening to them" with no apparent precursors or onsets. Dissociative children not only fluctuate in their moods, but also in their ability to function in day-to-day life. Some useful questions to tap fluctuations in behavior and mood are listed here.

Questions to Assess Fluctuations in Behavior and Mood

Do you feel sometimes like you can do something one day, and have great trouble doing it the next day?

Does it surprise you when your moods change? Give examples.

Do your tastes change from day to day?

Do your feelings about family members seem to go through changes? What are some examples of this?

ASSESSING AMNESIA

The assessment of amnesia often creates some logical paradoxes when assessing a young person with memory difficulties. The goal, after all, is to encourage as much memory as possible, rather than to substantiate that amnesia exists. Thus, assessing amnesia may be the very process that reverses the amnesia! A further difficulty in the assessment of amnesia is that children and teens frequently use "I forgot" as a distraction and avoidance technique, so it is hard to distinguish between actual memory gaps and willful avoidance. Certainly, no child wants to be held responsible for aggressive or destructive behavior, and if they can deflect responsibility by saying "I forgot," they may believe they can avoid consequences. It's important to recognize that memory and amnesia exist on a continuum. Memory, like the mind, is in a constant state of flux, with shifting accessibility to information that receives priority at any given moment. Dissociative amnesia may be seen as a practiced habit of mind that has led the child to repeatedly push unpleasant information out of central awareness. This habitual avoidance is often cued by unpleasant affect with avoidance becoming strengthened over time through repetition.

Laboratory research in cognitive science has recreated a model of the type of practiced forgetting associated with dissociative amnesia. Subjects asked to memorize associations between words can be trained to selectively forget certain words through a variety of incentives introduced by the experimenter (Anderson & Huddleston, 2012). This same process of selective memory, probably motivated by avoidance of shame and other painful affects, often occurs among children for recent behaviors associated with traumatic events. Selective amnesia is particularly common for their behavior when angry or for flashbacks in which they relive some traumatic event from the past. Over time, children whose minds are basically practicing forgetting may display sporadic memory for many recently experienced events, leading them to forget their homework or even plans made with friends.

Presuming that memory is always in flux, the goal of the assessment is to determine to what extent the evaluator can stimulate memory about things the young person has forgotten. When positive incentives are offered for remembering, children will sometimes surprise themselves with what can be remembered. It is the clinician's job in this initial interview to create an environment that feels so safe, secure, and embracing that even behavior that they have dissociated from awareness can be acknowledged without fear or shame. Whether the forgetting is due to nonconscious or willful avoidance is unimportant, and not really necessary to determine, as motivated forgetting falls on a continuum, and both can be reversed over time with positive incentives. More severe dissociated memory difficulties may take weeks or months to reverse, while the less-practiced memory deficits based on willful avoidance may be reversed sooner.

Arguing with clients about whether they really do or do not remember is a fruitless exercise. Instead, it is more effective to reverse incentives for dissociative habits of mind while creating incentives whereby remembering and taking responsibility will become more adaptive than forgetting and avoidance of affect. Reversal of amnesia may not happen in the first session, but the clinician can begin this process in the initial assessment phase. Having the young person achieve memory for her own recent behavior is a very important treatment goal, as the healthy mind must utilize all incoming information in order to plan, reorganize, and adapt. More in-depth discussion about reversing amnesia is provided in Chapter 8.

The list below describes some questions useful for the assessment of amnesia. Keep in mind that the most important amnesia to assess and reverse in the early assessment phase is amnesia regarding the child's or teen's recent behaviors. While gentle inquiry about traumatic events is appropriate, trying to reverse amnesia about traumatic events from the past is *not* part of the initial assessment phase. The protective mechanism of dissociative amnesia for traumatic events may continue to be adaptive farther into treatment.

Questions to Assess Amnesia

> *Do you forget things you should remember—what you did with friends, places you went, birthday parties?*
>
> *Do you sometimes forget what you did when you were angry? Let's try together to remember one of these.* (Make sure to emphasize that it is logical that they felt anger in order to destigmatize the child's shame associated with the events.)
>
> *Do your friends and family members report that you have done things that you cannot remember doing?*
>
> *Do you ever forget good things that happened to you?*
>
> *Could you remember this better if your grounding punishment was reduced after you remember?* (Try this out with the family's permission.)

ASSESSING SOMATIC SYMPTOMS

An initial assessment should include an analysis of the child's or teen's relationship to his or her body, as signs of trauma are often dramatically acted out on the body. Younger children may have symptoms of picking the skin, tearing at their nails, or injuring the body in other ways. Older children often use objects, including pencils or even razor blades, to cut or harm the body. Questions about the child or teen's relationship to pain can provide an opening into this area of assessment. For example, *"Do you find that you do not experience pain the way other children do?"* Many children who have endured trauma are proud to report that they do not feel pain, a skill they developed in response to repeated experiences of early physical pain. Talking about this as a skill rather than a deficit invites further discussion of dissociation as a coping tool.

Another area of inquiry involves questions about physical strengths or weaknesses that may shift. Many children and teens find that they have shifting access to physical strength, particularly noticing extreme increased strength when they are angry. One child told me he had an imaginary friend called "Adrenalin Man" who gave him strength when he was really angry. Less common, but sometimes reported, are shifting physical and cognitive disabilities. Conversion disorders and pain disorders without organic cause are also not uncommon among survivors of extreme trauma. I have had several patients with profound leg weakness attributable to physical and sexual abuse for which no organic causes could be found.

The following questions can assist with evaluating somatoform dissociation or dissociation manifest in the body. More information on this topic area is covered in Chapter 9.

Questions to Assess Somatic Symptoms

> *Do you notice that you do not experience pain the way other children do?*
> *Do you find yourself injuring your body in some way repeatedly? How does it feel after you do this?*
> *Do you have a pain or disability for which no medical reason can be found?*
> *Do you have unusual weakness in your body or unusual strength at times?*

RISKY BEHAVIORS

Children and adolescents with significant dissociation may display a variety of high-risk behaviors such as delinquency, suicide attempts, running away, self-mutilation, sexual promiscuity, sexual aggression (Burkman, Kisiel, & McLelland, 2008; Kissiel & Lyons, 2001; Liebowitz, Laser, & Burton, 2011), or drug abuse. It is important for the evaluator to be sensitive to all of these potential problems, some of which could have lethal outcomes. Some of the more risky behaviors, such as use of drugs, promiscuous sexuality, or self-harm, may be initiated during dissociative episodes and the clients may have limited memory for these events.

It is important during early assessment to ask children whether they have been told they engage in risky behaviors that they don't remember doing and to explore these thoroughly. Protocols for addressing specific problems, such as eating disorders or substance abuse, may need to be modified if there is a dissociative component, as it will be important to explore any hidden motivations contained in the dissociative parts of the self for treatment to be effective.

DEVELOPMENTAL DISABILITIES

I have found that dissociative symptoms or disorders can also co-occur in the population of children and adolescents with developmental disorders, such as Asperger's, or other children on the autism spectrum. Donna Williams (1992, 1994, 1999) wrote a series of books describing her life dealing with autism. She described what appear to be dissociative identities that helped her cope with early maltreatment and other traumatic experiences of her life. Her writings suggest that the sensation of sight and sound can be so overstimulating to an autistic person that these experiences can be traumatic, causing autistic individuals to develop dissociation as a coping tool. I have interviewed many autistic children with vivid imaginary friends who appear to have a dissociative process secondary to their difficulties in tolerating sensory stimulation.

One of my young dissociative clients who falls on the autistic spectrum would hide in a box in her classroom when the classroom became too loud. She described an imaginary friend she called "Snow" who helped her cover her eyes and ears so she was not "hurt" by yelling. In addition, children with disabilities and those with communications disorders are particularly vulnerable to being victimized, as perpetrators realize that these children will have difficulty telling about their experiences. Thus, careful assessment of all potential traumatic risks in the environment is essential with disabled children.

ASSESSMENT INSTRUMENTS

An interview can yield rich data, help you join with the child or adolescent in discovering the source of maladaptive behaviors, and can set the stage for developing a joint treatment plan. Assessment can be aided by the use of measurement tools specifically developed for assessing traumatized children and teens. The following are some of the tools that I have found to be the most useful.

The Trauma Symptom Checklist for Children (TSCC) and The Trauma Symptom Checklist for Young Children (TSCYC)

John Briere (1996, 2005) developed these instruments to aid in the assessment of trauma-related symptoms in children. The TSCC is a 54-item self-report scale designed for trauma symptoms related to sexual abuse and other traumatic events.

It is made up of two validity scales (indicating over- and underreporting of symptoms) and six clinical scales (Anxiety, Depression, Posttraumatic Stress, Sexual Concerns, Dissociation, and Anger). The TSCC allows children to rate on a scale from 0 to 3 how often they suffer from certain common symptoms of traumatic stress, including flashbacks, nightmares, sleep difficulties, anger outbursts, and preoccupations. In addition, the measure includes dissociative symptoms such as feeling like one's mind goes blank and feeling like one is in a fog. It takes a very short time to administer, and the scores can be easily graphed, providing a visual representation of the peaks and valleys of various symptom clusters.

The TSCYC is a 90-item caretaker-report instrument developed for the assessment of trauma-related symptoms in children ages 3 to 12. This measure assesses the types of hypoarousal and hyperarousal commonly seen in traumatized young children, in addition to dissociation. I have found this test particularly helpful when presenting the behaviors of nonverbal children to a judge who must make decisions about a child's life without the benefit of clear disclosures of traumatic events. The presence of posttraumatic symptoms, such as startling in response to loud noises, avoidance behaviors, or angry outbursts above expected norms for the child's age, can help judges understand how trauma can broadly affect children's functioning in measurable ways.

The Child Dissociative Checklist (CDC)

Since its development in 1981 by Frank Putnam, this checklist has become a standard tool for clinicians seeking to evaluate dissociative symptoms in young children (see online Appendix D). The CDC assesses 20 key behaviors commonly found in dissociative children on a scale from 0 to 2, and has been found to reliably distinguish a dissociative population of young children from a general population (Putnam, Helmers, & Trickett, 1993). The items assess dissociative symptoms, such as children referring to themselves with other names, having vivid imaginary friends, avoiding talking about known traumatic events, or denying observed behaviors. The questions also assess a variety of posttraumatic symptoms such as nightmares and sleep difficulties. I have found the CDC to be particularly useful when interviewing caregivers, as they often respond with numerous examples. Putnam's sample of dissociative children averaged a score of 23.3, while my own research sample of 30 dissociative children had an average score of 22 (Silberg, 1998c). Putnam (1997) considers scores above 12 to be cause for suspicion and scores above 19 to be strongly associated with dissociation in young children.

The Adolescent Dissociative Experiences Scale (A-DES)

This measure, developed by Armstrong et al. (1997; see online Appendix E), adapted items from the adult Dissociative Experiences Scale (DES) to make them applicable to young people age 11 and older. Dissociative experiences, such as feeling "there are walls in one's mind," "finding items that don't belong to you," or "feeling like there are different people inside me," are scored on a 10-point scale. Scores that average above 4 suggest significant dissociation. The A-DES has been widely used in research, to establish a relationship between dissociation and risk-taking in sexually abused youth (Kisiel & Lyons, 2001), investigate dissociation associated with medical trauma (Diseth, 2006), explore dissociation in adolescent sex offenders (Friedrich et al., 2001), and document disclosure patterns in abused adolescents (Bonanno et al., 2003). It has also been validated in a variety of languages and cultures (Nillson & Svedin, 2006; Shin, Jeong, & Chung, 2009; Soukup, Papežová, Kuběna, & Mikolajová, 2010; Zoruglu, Sar, Tuzun, Tutkun, & Savas, 2002).

I have found the A-DES to be particularly useful in encouraging discussion of dissociative phenomenon in adolescents who tend to be reticent. Once they have filled out the form, I use their answers as a basis for further conversation and exploration.

The Child Dissociative Experience Scale and Posttraumatic Stress Inventory (CDES/PTSI)

The CDES/PTSI was developed by Stolbach (1997) to identify dissociative and posttraumatic pathology in school-age children (see online Appendix F). Children are asked to rate on a 3-point scale their similarity to a variety of characters who evidence some dissociative or posttraumatics trait. For example, an item that assesses the symptom of talking aloud to oneself is: *Linda talks out loud to herself when she is alone, and Julie does not talk aloud to herself when she is alone.* The child is then asked whether she is more like Julie or more like Linda. The CDES/PTSI helps uncover dissociative pathology among children who may have a hard time describing their own experiences. The answers provided by the child provide a fruitful springboard for further discussion.

Traditional Psychological Testing

In 1998, I conducted a psychological study in which I looked at some of the features of psychological testing on children who had dissociative disorders, and discovered that both their behavior and their responses distinguished them from other children admitted to the Sheppard Pratt inpatient facility (Silberg, 1998c, 1998d). During individual psychological testing, the dissociative children often engaged in staring episodes, odd movements, and shifts in the developmental level of their language. In addition, dissociative children tended to emotionally overreact to seemingly neutral stimuli and report shifting somatic complaints. On projective testing, I noted that children with dissociative disorders tended to draw or perceive multiple images, such as an individual with two heads, four eyes, or

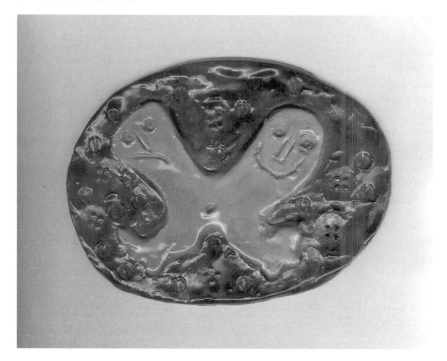

Figure 4.1 Six-year-old dissociative boy represents himself with two heads. Used with
permission.

other multiple body parts. These drawings or self-representations may be created spontaneously outside of a formal testing session as well. Figure 4.1 is a
clay plaque created by a 6-year-old boy with a history of dissociative symptoms,
depicting himself with two faces, clearly demonstrating his divided sense of self.

My research also found differences between dissociative children and other
children in psychiatric inpatient treatment in their responses to projective tests
such as the Thematic Apperception Test and the Rorschach. The dissociative children responded to projective testing with a high number of morbid images of
death, blood, and destruction, a feature also found on the psychological testing
of adults with dissociative disorders (Brand, Armstrong, & Loewenstein, 2006).

Dissociative children also reported images of what I term "magical transformation"—where a person shifts into an animal or an animal transforms in some way.
In projective stories, dissociative children often described images of good and
evil, and displayed reversals in emotional descriptions such as calling "happy"
"sad." In addition, they tended to use what I term "dissociative coping," that is,
the resolution of a problem by forgetting, sleeping, pretending, or denying. For
example, one child stated, "This is a story about a child who is being beaten every
day, but he forgets about it and so it does not bother him anymore." These stories

often provided dramatic examples of the use of dissociation coping to escape from traumatic experiences.

The assessment of dissociation through interview and assessment tools often provides a powerful entrée into a therapeutic relationship with new clients, as they may feel that their "strange" symptomatology is being understood for the first time. Like Cameron, who asked to see the "lady who knows about voices," your newly assessed dissociative clients will often feel a powerful bond that can help you through the sometimes stormy course of treatment. In the next chapter, we will explore some central tenets that will help guide the therapy with this challenging population.

5   Beginning the Treatment Journey

"You are the weirdest doctor I ever met. Are you sure you are really a doctor?" said Jennifer, a 14-year-old who was referred for evaluation of dissociative symptoms. According to Jennifer, every doctor she had previously seen thought she was crazy. "Did they tell you you were crazy?" I asked. "No," she replied. "They don't have to say it. I can just tell. I don't mind seeing you because I don't *feel crazy* when I am here." Jennifer was articulating that when she saw me, she felt free to be honest with me, and to work toward health because she knew I saw that as possible.

Clearly, the attitude of the therapist conveys to the young client multiple messages that can empower the child or teen toward their recovery. In this section, we will look at some of these messages that are conveyed implicitly or articulated to the client by the therapist's actions and approach.

TREATMENT PRINCIPLES

Principle 1: An Attitude of Deep Respect for the Wisdom of Individual Coping Techniques

The first principle underlying therapy with traumatized children involves communicating to the child that you have a deep respect for the coping techniques that they have developed. The therapist approaches the seemingly destructive behavior patterns of the traumatized children with an appreciation for the fact that these choices were likely their only viable option. Children are accustomed to being judged, reprimanded, and told they can do better. Rarely does anyone approach them with the kind of empathetic understanding of the therapeutic stance described here. Some children feel "stupid" or "crazy" because of their symptoms, particularly when dissociative behavior patterns lead them to forget what other children seem to remember, or lead them to engage in embarrassing destructive episodes. Helping them understand how their minds chose this manner of coping in order to avoid painful feelings is very welcome, as shame regarding their symptoms adds to their distress and hopelessness.

Early sessions can be spent helping the young people understand their hidden reasons for their behavior patterns. They may act out aggressively to retaliate for their past victimization; they may engage in self-harm to illustrate their sense of being victimized; or they may dissociate to protect themselves from awareness of pain. These explanations are case specific and emerge through discussions with the child about the purposes and wisdom of their choices. This opens the discussion to what new choices might make sense now, as hopefully their environment is safer and their lives less traumatic. Throughout this book, I present numerous psychoeducational strategies for helping children appreciate and understand their body's and mind's creativity in coping with traumatic events.

Principle 2: An Intense Belief in the Possibility to Heal and the Potential for Future Thriving

Children and teens can feel profoundly demoralized and trapped. Sometimes, envisioning a positive future is beyond their capacity. Demoralized children need to "borrow" a sense of hope from the therapist—someone who continually believes in them, no matter what setback or detour their life has taken. Sally was a 12-year-old who had suffered from severe neglect in a Romanian orphanage until adopted at age 6. Sally's recovery was thrown off course by the news that her adoptive parents were going to separate. She appeared nearly catatonic, with a blank, lifeless gaze, conveying the sense of the trapped helplessness that she felt. When I asked her to draw a picture of what "hope" might look like, she drew a tiny yellow sun in the far-left corner of a large poster-size paper. I told her I would keep "hope" with me in my office. Over the course of a six-year therapy, until she left home for college, she told me that that message of hope that I gave her stayed with her. Although she could not always believe that she had the strength to pull through and thrive, she knew that I deeply believed this, and derived energy from the hope that I never abandoned.

It is important to note that the hope that you have for your clients cannot be faked, as children and teens are very perceptive about insincerity. We must find a place in ourselves where we can deeply believe in the possibility of personal transformations for our clients and transformation of their life circumstances, even when the challenges seem overwhelming.

Principle 3: Utilize a Practical Approach to Symptom Management

Working with children and adolescents involves juggling the complexities of many sources of impact on their lives—schools, afterschool activities, families, peer relationships, pets, and so forth. Given these complexities, a child therapist must be practical and realistic, offering coping tools that children can integrate easily into their busy lives, and finding local resources that can assist them. Some traumatized children need flexible alternatives to conventional pathways that are not working for them. A large percentage of my traumatized and dissociative teens could not adjust well to public high school, so they left high school, took the GED (high school equivalency examination), and then went to community colleges. I have also gotten permission over the years for my clients to miss certain classes, be moved to other seats in school, arrive late to class to avoid triggering events, or to wear alternative clothing in gym class to hide self-inflicted injuries. Some clients may need home-teaching programs temporarily while serious school problems, such as bullying, are being addressed. Therapists need to reach out for resources in the community that can assist with the unique cultural or religious needs of the clients. Twelve-year-old David, attending Catholic school and highly devout, was convinced that the voice he heard in his mind was the devil himself. Having been involved in a car accident where a cousin had died, David blamed himself, as he had wished his cousin ill during a fight, and he thought his actions had caused the death of his cousin. Having limited credibility in my own right to address this religious conviction, I involved a priest in a series of sessions to help David understand the differences between his own self-torment, symbolized in this critical voice, and the potential influence of the "devil."

The therapist should prioritize symptoms that interfere with the child or teen's developmental trajectory. Children and teens really can't function when experiencing trance states or ongoing amnesia about their own behavior. Thus, recent amnestic episodes must be dealt with right away. If the therapist keeps in mind this principle of practicality and prioritization of acute symptoms, it will help provide a realistic child-friendly approach to the treatment.

Principle 4: Create a Relationship of Both Validation and Expectation

Marsha Linehan (1993) has provided us with many important insights through her innovative treatment approach known as Dialectical Behavior Therapy. One of these principles is the balancing of the two poles of validation and expectation. Linehan cautions that the therapist must strike a delicate balance between trying to push the patient into change, and honoring the barriers and impediments to change. Even from the point of view of cellular biology, these two processes define life and growth (Lipton, 2005). According to Bruce Lipton, cells can either accept signals or information from the outside and obtain nourishment and growth, or can enter the self-protection mode and defend against outside toxins that would inhibit growth. If these processes are not working effectively, the cells may accept toxins and reject nourishment, or build walls to protect against growth and nourishment. Lipton suggests that the cell membrane can be seen as an energy regulator equivalent to the human mind. Similarly, people can either be open to incoming information and grow through the process, or stay where they are, re-group, and build better walls.

Particularly after trauma, there is confusion about which of these two processes to engage in—building walls, or promoting growth. The art of psychotherapy involves knowing when to engage in each. Some trauma therapists have been criticized for indulging patient's regressions, while behavioral therapists have been criticized for expecting too much without validating feelings. Neither is right or wrong, but there is a time and a place both for validating, keeping the walls up, and a time for challenging and requiring change and growth. Challenging too much before validating will leave your client angry and questioning your alliance. Validating too much may leave your client stuck in self-defeating behavior patterns that are no longer adaptive.

A similar tension exists in parenting behaviors that promote either safety and security or exploration and growth. A therapeutic program for mothers that teaches them how to tune in empathically to their developing infants, Circle of Security, focuses on helping parents learn to distinguish how and when to engage in either of these polarity of behaviors—either soothing and comforting, or promoting exploration and play (Hoffman, Marvin, Cooper, & Powell, 2006). As a therapist, you will have to help your client's parents understand when to use each of these parenting strategies, no matter what age the child or teenager.

Principle 5: Recognize Traumatic Symptoms as Both Automatic and Learned

Disruptive symptoms that your client displays are multidetermined. These symptoms and behaviors have likely originated as adaptations to a traumatic environment that were reinforced over time. This is the principle of operant conditioning from basic learning theory—behaviors that are reinforced will continue and increase in strength. However, traumatic symptoms have their origins as well in classically conditioned responses that we know are much more resistant to change. For example, consider a child who enters a sudden dissociative shutdown state and is seemingly impervious to outside stimuli. The dissociative behavior is likely a conditioned and automatic response, learned over time, to a variety of triggers. Yet it is also likely reinforced by its consequences—for example, avoidance of uncomfortable situations or people. When approaching a symptom such as this, one must remember that it is likely multidetermined, as is most human behavior, and it would be wrong to assume that its origin is purely reactive or "classically conditioned," or purely "strategic" and reinforced by its consequences.

Sometimes, therapists from different theoretical schools will argue over whether the child is "doing it on purpose" and is "just manipulative" (the operant analysis). Other therapists will say the child "can't wake up" or "can't stop himself" because it is an automatic conditioned response. The dissociative behavior is probably sustained by both psychological principles. Consequently, treatment will involve desensitizing the client to automatic triggers, while also understanding the environmental contingencies that support disruptive behaviors. The rewards that sustain a traumatic symptom can be both internal rewards (avoidance of an unpleasant situation) and external rewards (parents reacting with increased attention and indulgence). All of these factors must be taken into account when addressing how to reverse problematic behaviors.

THE THERAPEUTIC RELATIONSHIP

The therapeutic relationship provides a context for the child to understand relationships in a new way—opportunities for empathic connection, reciprocity, and trust. The importance of the therapeutic relationship for the healing of trauma has been emphasized in the adult trauma literature (Chu, 1998; Courtois, 2010; Pearlman & Courtois, 2005; Pearlman & Saakvitne, 1995). This attachment to the therapist for child and adolescent patients is, hopefully, not the primary relationship in which attachment skills are learned, as one of the main goals of treatment is to help the family learn how to provide the safety and trust that the young client needs. However, for teens in institutional settings or whose parents or foster parents will never achieve the psychological skills to provide the unconditional love these children require, the relationship with the therapist may be their only opportunity to experience a relationship based on respect and nurturing. Traumatized children and teens expect the worst from relationships, seeing them in terms of inequality and objectification. Children's automatic internal working models will play out in the therapeutic relationship, as the children and teens question your motives, what you want for them, why you are trying to help them, or why you have been unsuccessful in helping them.

With children and teens struggling with dissociative states, these internal working models may be in conflict, and some parts of the child may find therapy fun, rewarding, and worthwhile, while at other times the children are resentful and avoidant. The astute therapist must notice these variations in mood, and embrace the whole shifting self of the client, acknowledging that therapy can be boring, and a waste of time, and be ready to apologize if sessions have not gone as well as hoped. Mastering the ability to apologize authentically to a client without defensiveness is a key skill a trauma therapist must learn (Dalenberg, 2000).

Traumatized children and teens are often highly sensitive to the moods of others, so therapists must be on their toes to honestly acknowledge their own feelings that arise in the sessions. If you have a headache, or stomach pain, you can be sure your young clients will notice and generally attribute it to themselves and your feelings about them. Therapists must model reciprocity by listening intently and offering compromises when the child's or teen's view differ from the therapist on plans, appointments, or techniques. Therapists must model the attunement that an attentive parent shows a developing infant by acknowledging and resonating with the client's feelings, highlighting these in nonjudgmental ways, and deeply and truly enjoying the client's strengths and abilities.

Despite the best intentions of the therapist, traumatized children and teens will inevitably react to the therapist based on what they learned in a traumatic early environment. Certain therapeutic stances can help to defeat the intensity of this traumatic transference toward the therapist. I have organized these therapeutic stances into sentences that embody the therapist's approach to the child or teen client (adapted from Silberg & Ferentz, 2002).

"I Can Accept You No Matter How Terrible You Think You Are"

The traumatized child, on some level, believes that he or she has deserved what happened, and therefore must be deeply flawed and repulsive in some way. The therapist must embody this radical acceptance of the child's or teen's actions, worst impulses, contradictory and maybe frightening dissociated states, and even the recesses of a sometimes gory imagination. In order for them to accept their own identity, the clients must believe that you, the therapist, can handle the full extent of who they are.

"I Deeply Want You to Get Well, but It Is Ultimately Completely Within Your Control"

The clients themselves must ultimately feel in control of the change that you are trying to promote in them. If they sense that you are more eager than they are for change, or that you feel yourself have the power to change them, then therapy may become a power struggle rather than an opportunity for growth. Similarly, if they sense their parents care more about the change than they do, the therapy may become a medium for disempowering their parents. Helping parents adopt a similar viewpoint will help your client develop the self-direction that is a primary treatment goal.

"I Can Accept Your Anger and Disappointment (Even in Me) and Not Reject You"

The therapist must model the acceptance of feelings of anger and disappointment without judgment, as these are a necessary part of the cementing of enduring relationships.

"You Can Abandon Me; I Can't/Won't Abandon You"

The therapist-child relationship reverses the power dynamic that the child survivor has previously experienced. In fact, the child or teen in some way has more power in the relationship than does the therapist, as the therapist is expendable—a relationship that can be discarded. Yet, the therapist's ethics, at least in outpatient practice, require that the therapist show enduring commitment, despite frustrations that may arise. I find it useful to explain this in some form to children who have felt powerless in previous relationships. For example, I might say, *"You know I work for you. I am like a teacher or coach to help you get through these difficult moments in your life, but I will not be here forever, and only you can judge whether what we are doing is helpful or successful. You will have the choice, after discussing with your parents, to try to find someone else if you find that what we are doing doesn't help as much as you hoped. But I really can't do that if I am frustrated. I will hang in here with you even if we both get frustrated. I am your therapist, and will try to stick with you."* Even in residential treatment centers, where therapists may shift, I think it is important in some way to embody this principle that the child has more control ultimately over the relationship than does the therapist.

"You Don't Have to Do Anything to Please Me. We Are Here for You"

Children and teens who have learned to accommodate others in trauma-based relationships may feel their job is to please you or to tell you what you want to hear. Particularly, children who enjoy coming to therapy, and like the attention and the toys, may think you will be happier with them if they just report things are fine, and then they can just play. It is important for them to know that when they are honest, you can help them the most, and that their feelings are much more important than are your feelings. I try to let the families call me ahead of time with important updates that I listen to on my answering machine before the child or teen arrives, so that I can gently point out to the clients the ways their own behavior may be interfering with their life. This illustrates that I am serious about their well-being, and the job of therapy is to deal with the reality of their life and help them make changes.

These principles of therapy are relevant to work with all traumatized children and provide an overarching framework for any interventions with this population. The dissociative children and teens in my practice require some specialized techniques as well, and those will be the focus of the next chapter as we begin to look at Dissociation-Focused Interventions. These interventions provide trauma therapists with additional tools to help children and teenagers with some of the most difficult symptoms traumatized children may present.

6 Educate and Motivate
Introducing the EDUCATE Model

Seven-year-old Cindi was quietly playing with Legos in a waiting area I share with Dr. Loewenstein, who directs the Sheppard Pratt Health System Trauma Disorders Program, an inpatient program for the treatment of traumatized and dissociative adults. "My adult patient waiting to see me was quite upset by your patient today," Dr. Loewenstein tells me. "Did she throw something, have a tantrum, wet her pants?" I wondered, though I had heard nothing unusual outside of my office that day. Before I had a chance to ask what caused the upset, Dr. Loewenstein explained, "She is getting help when she is only seven. My patient wants to know why no one helped her at that age. If only they had . . ."

The dissociative adults in Dr. Loewenstein's program are highly symptomatic, with recurrent flashbacks, self-harming behaviors, memory loss for their own behaviors, unregulated and sudden changes in affect, the inability to trust, and self-destructive and/or addictive behaviors. Many return to inpatient care multiple times during the stormy course of their protracted illnesses. Do we have any reason to believe that the "if only" wish of the adult patient is founded? Do children who receive help for dissociative symptoms and disorders when they are young avert the stormy course of the patients on the adult trauma disorders unit? My experience tells me yes, that we can interrupt the negative consequences of dissociative symptoms through early intervention. My successfully treated formerly dissociative teens and young children often write to me when they get married, graduate from high school or college, or have their own children. They report that they are successful nurses, teachers, doctors, and advocates. Their life successes affirm for me the power of early intervention with dissociative children suffering the effects of severe, early traumatic events.

Furthermore, I have had three clinical opportunities to observe the developmental course of dissociative processes left untreated. In all three of these cases, a preschool or school-age child presented with vivid imaginary friends, the feeling of being compelled to do things he or she did not wish to do, and hearing the sounds of conversations and conflicts between imaginary friends in his or her mind. None of these children qualified for a diagnosis of DID when younger, yet without treatment, all three later returned to my care as teenagers and at that point met the diagnostic criteria for DID. Without therapeutic intervention, these children's early manifestations of dissociation were reinforced over time and had solidified into discrete identity states. Unfortunately, these clients were more resistant to treatment as adolescents than they had been when they were younger.

One of these children, Steven, described in Silberg (2001c), had been taken out of therapy at age 5 by his mother, who was angry about a mandatory report that I had made to Child Protective Services. At the time I treated Steven, he had three imaginary friends: an angry dinosaur, a baby, and a calm and sweetly singing mother-like figure. These imaginary friends had helped him cope with physical and sexual abuse he had suffered while in the care of his father, who had kidnapped him. When found, dirty and hurt, he was returned to his mother's care and brought to treatment. When I suspected there was an unsafe caregiver in her home, I reported it, and she discontinued Steven's treatment. Steven returned to me at age 13, referred by a residential treatment center where he had been sent after breaking into a neighbor's home and stealing some money—an event Steven said he could not remember. I was able to determine in our first session that his imaginary friend, the dinosaur Dino, had developed over time into an identity state that harbored intense feelings of anger. This angry state would at times influence Steven to do things out of his awareness. In therapy, we were able to break down Steven's dissociative barriers, and Steven rapidly achieved an integrated sense of self.

The two other dissociative children whose treatment was interrupted and who later returned to my care followed a similar pattern—early vivid imaginary friends that controlled their behavior, disruption in treatment, and later confirmed diagnosis of DID. These cases vividly illustrated for me the natural course that dissociative processes can take when left untreated.

Research supports these clinical observations. Putnam et al. (1996) analyzed the symptoms of children with dissociative disorders across the age span, and found that the older children more closely resemble adults with features of DID, including more amnesia. It seems that Dr. Loewenstein's patient was correct in her wistful wondering of "If only I got treatment sooner . . ." This is empowering information for child therapists. Just as treating an infection in its beginning stages affords a better prognosis for a sick patient, treating dissociative children in the early stages of their symptoms provides the opportunity to make life-changing alterations in the course of their life trajectories.

DISSOCIATION-FOCUSED INTERVENTIONS: THE EDUCATE MODEL

Dissociative children in treatment provide many challenges and often seem unengaged. They may be impervious to things that you say and simple behavioral programs that work well in other contexts seem to have little effect. Parents and teachers often report that dissociative children seem oblivious to the naturalistic cause-and-effect learning about consequences that usually occurs in families and schools. Dissociative children have learned automatic response scripts appropriate to past traumatic contexts, which prevent flexible responses to current situations. Having learned to avoid the painful affect associated with interpersonal relationships, dissociative children may code your interaction with them as "irrelevant input," and your therapeutic input may then automatically bypass the decision-making portion of the brain (prefrontal cortex). However, when you can engage the whole mind in the therapeutic endeavor, you are more likely to have success and to establish a precedent that leads your clients to be more invested in treatment and allied with you as the therapist. The Dissociation-Focused Interventions help you establish this kind of alliance.

The acronym EDUCATE provides an organizing framework for the interventions utilized in treating dissociative children and teens. Each letter in EDUCATE represents a class of interventions that are utilized sequentially and that help to address dissociative symptoms and reverse dissociation-based resistance. While it is difficult to expect treatment to follow in a completely linear path, the acronym helps therapists plan and pace their work throughout the treatment process.

The acronym EDUCATE stands for the following classes of interventions:

E: Educate about dissociation and traumatic processes.

D: Dissociation motivation: Address and analyze the factors that keep the client tied to dissociative strategies.

U: Understand what is hidden: Unravel the secret pockets of automatically activated affect, identity, or behavioral repertoires that help the client bypass central awareness and engage in avoidance.

C: Claim as own these hidden aspects of the self: These interventions, which allow the client to embrace what had been dissociated, are the central objective of Dissociation-Focused Intervention.

A: Arousal Modulation/Affect Regulation/Attachment: Learning to regulate arousal and the ebb and flow of feelings in the context of loving relationships is the new learning central to defeating the dissociative habits.

T: Triggers and Trauma: Identifying precursors to automatic trauma-based responding, and processing associated traumatic memories helps the client move forward.

E: Ending Stage of Treatment: The final challenge in treatment is to help the client flexibly approach new situations without trauma-based responding. (See Appendix A, for a comprehensive list of EDUCATE interventions.)

In this chapter, I will address the "E" and "D" of the EDUCATE model. Interventions associated with each of the subsequent letters will be addressed in subsequent chapters.

E: EDUCATE

Education about dissociation and trauma is a necessary first step when beginning treatment, as it creates a shared language and provides for the development of shared expectations about the purpose of treatment and its expected course. Some children come into treatment having false ideas about dissociation, influenced through family conversations, books, or television. Some children have been told the purpose of treatment is to have their imaginary friends "go away," which frightens them.

There are five key psychoeducational principles that must be taught to children about dissociation during the beginning stage of treatment. These concepts help the child to understand the symptoms and the goals of treatment.

Concept 1: Trauma Causes Disconnections in the Mind

Trauma therapists for children are accustomed to explaining basic principles of trauma to young children—that trauma treatment is helpful, that their particular experience of trauma is not uncommon, and that trauma is associated with certain known effects of the mind and brain (Cohen et al., 2006). In addition to

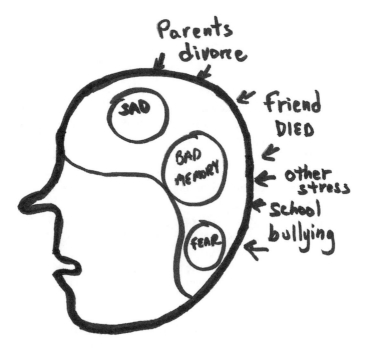

Figure 6.1 Picture of brain to depict effects of trauma to children. Used with permission.

this overall psychoeducation, I explain trauma-based dissociative processes in children. To convey this information in a way that children can understand, I find it helpful to draw a simple profile picture of a person with the brain outlined, as shown in Figure 6.1.

Once the child or teen has explained to me the sources of trauma or extreme stress in their environment in general ways—divorce of parents, death of friend— I write or draw a symbol of each major trauma outside of the picture of the brain. Then, I draw corresponding circles in the outline of the brain with walls around each circle. I explain, "*Regular everyday things are felt by the brain and under-stood and handled. However, when things happen that are really, really bad and hard to think about and remember, walls go up around the part of the brain that tried to deal with it, and the feelings and memories may be behind these walls. These walls protect the mind from having to remember, feel, and deal with these things, especially when there is not much that can be done about it. These walls can be a good thing at first to protect you so you don't have to think about it, but then can turn into a bad thing when they lead you into doing things you wish you did not do. We will be trying to understand what may be behind some of these walls.*" If children have already identified voices in the mind, dissociative identity states, imaginary friends, or isolated affects, I write the names they use when referring to these in the walled-off circles I drew inside the brain. This helps to prepare the child for the next part of the psychoeducational process.

Concept 2: A Healthy Mind Has the Most Connections

In this part of the psychoeducational process, I draw a picture of a neuron and show children how the neurons connect through axons and dendrites, and ex-plain that electrical impulses pass through from one brain cell to another. I tell children that growth in the brain involves building lots of connections throughout the whole brain so that it can work as one well-coordinated organ. I explain that, like in a school or a company, if one department does not know what the other department is doing, there can be a breakdown in communication and functioning.

I refer children back to the picture of their own brain with the islands of walled-off information and ask them what they think the solution should be. At this point, children immediately recognize that making connections between the walled-off islands is going to be the necessary treatment. In order to illustrate this process for them, I have children draw connections with arrows between the segregated islands in the picture of the brain we have created. We do this in a lighthearted and enthusiastic way, which shows them that the work we will be doing together is a joint project that can be enjoyable and even fun at times.

At the end of the session, when their parents come into the room, I have the children teach their parents what they have learned, and they invite their parents to add connections in the brain picture that we have developed. This exercise shows children that the therapy process does not involving "losing" but rather involves "gaining"—gaining more brain connections and improved capacity. Throughout the treatment, if the child or teen makes some special connection or accesses information that may have been previously hidden, I will comment with playful enthusiasm, *"I think I just heard a sizzle in your brain as the brain cells just connected with each other."* Although I do this playfully, this metaphorical depiction of what is being accomplished in therapy is consistent with our current neurobiological understanding of the deleterious effects of trauma on integrative functions, and the necessity of growing new neural pathways in order to recover.

Concept 3: The Whole Self Must Work Together

The concept of unity of the whole self can be illustrated with a variety of metaphors or toys. My colleague Frances Waters utilizes a toy caterpillar that has multiple segments connected by hinges. When the caterpillar works together, she explains, then it moves quickly, but when one part is not in line with the others, the caterpillar hobbles along (Waters & Silberg, 1998a). I have a bird's nest puppet with three little birds that share a nest, and a finger goes into each baby bird (see Figure 6.2). Using the puppet, I show the child the baby birds fighting, each demanding to have the mother's prized worm first, and then illustrate how the baby birds can get along and take turns. Similarly, I explain that if the "war" or

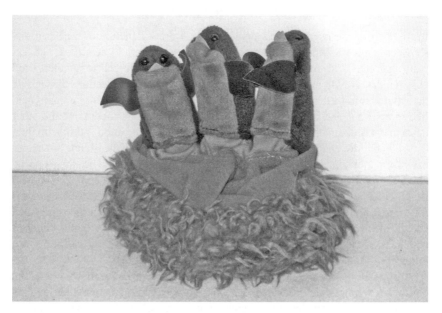

Figure 6.2 Baby bird hand-puppet showing parts working together. Used with permission.

"fight" in their mind could resolve, they too would have more energy and be better able to function.

With younger children, I sometimes make up poems or songs and add hand motions to illustrate the concepts that we are discussing. Six-year-old Stephanie had vivid imaginary friends that she perceived as the cause for her tantrums and aggression against her siblings. She felt controlled by these imaginary friends and sometimes lost memory for angry behavior displayed when interacting with them. I made up a song that we sang repeatedly: "All the little feelings inside of Stephanie's mind are going to come together, together, together." While we sang this song, we wiggled our fingers and then clasped our two hands together, showing all of the feelings merging as one. By providing this rhythm, movement, and acting out the integration physiologically, I helped her anchor the educational message of unity, both somatically and cognitively.

Sometimes it is important to illustrate that even when internal parts feel different emotions, they all share the same body. With young children, I might trace their hand on a piece of paper, or trace the entire body on large poster paper, and then retrace it multiple times with different colors for each of the imaginary friends or voices that they hear in their mind. This serves to provide the children with a concrete illustration showing them that the pattern of the hand or of the body is *the same* for each different part. Even when drawn in different colors, the same physical hand or body is displayed on the paper. I might ask the children to look at an object and then cover their eyes and ask if their imaginary friend can see the object with different eyes. Activities demonstrating the oneness of the physical self can help the child grasp the important concept that the consequences of the actions of parts of the self will always apply to the whole self.

Some children engaged in out-of-control behavior may attribute their misbehavior to "bad boy Joey," or "mean me," and believe that it is wrong for them to receive any consequences, since it is "not really me" that misbehaved. Psychoeducation in this first phase of therapy emphasizes to the child that, just as their whole body is one, consequences will always apply to the whole self. It is important to note that some children don't entirely realize that self-destructive acts carried out by one part of their mind will actually harm or kill their own body, or that if hospitalized for dangerous and out-of-control behavior, the entire self will have to go to the hospital. While this may seem obvious, many children with dissociative manifestations do not really realize this unless it is directly explained and emphasized.

Concept 4: Voices, Imaginary Friends, or Other Identity States Are Feelings, Reminders, or Signals

A major thrust of the psychoeducational work with dissociative children is helping them to understand what inner voices, vivid imaginary friends, or identities represent and why they are manifesting. Some children develop their own "scientific" explanations for these phenomena. One 10-year-old boy told me that he thought that his braces served as radio receivers, as he noticed that he began to hear the voices after he obtained braces. It is important to realize that despite the oddness of many of the theories that children develop to explain dissociative phenomena, they are not engaging in psychotic thinking; rather their explanations are the best theories they can derive when trying to understand why they hear what appear to be foreign voices in their own minds.

Some children assume that they are hearing ghosts or spirits, devils talking to them, angels, or God. The most frightening and destabilizing theory that the children have is that a perpetrator voice in their mind is really the actual perpetrator—either living in their mind or able to communicate with them from a distance. The belief that their perpetrator is always with them and they can never escape his or her presence causes children to feel perpetually unsafe and controlled. This belief can also lead children to engage in self-harm or act out aggressively, as they try to rid themselves of the sound. Reassurances by an adult that they are now safe must seem like a cruel joke to these children who constantly hear the sound of someone who abused them threatening to kill them, harm them, harm their loved ones, or harm other children.

Many children have already heard from therapists to ignore, push away, or not respond to the sound of an angry voice, or the voice of their abuser in their mind telling them to harm themselves or others. While children try to listen to this advice from well-meaning adults and therapists, it is virtually impossible to do so, as the threats to them that they hear in their mind tend to escalate the more these voices are ignored. Moreover, the mental effort required to push these voices away and to ignore the messages contained in them reinforces the process of dissociation, making it more likely for the child or teen to engage in behaviors without awareness or memory.

Affect theory as introduced in Chapter 2 provides tools to develop explanations for children about perplexing and often terrifying dissociative phenomena. As Tomkins (1962) explained, affects are learning tools for the self. Affects are the amplification of responses to lived experiences that help a person pay attention to salient events, either good or bad, so that they can remember the lessons of these experiences. Similarly, these internal voices are simply personified mediators of these affect states that serve to signal to the traumatized child survivor which actions to take, or avoidance strategies to engage in, so that painful affects are bypassed and warnings about impending danger are heeded quickly. In other words, these internal voices serve as guides to remind the children how to protect themselves and avoid potential harm in an environment in which surviving abuse may have been a daily struggle.

For example, a perpetrator's voice telling the child to harm himself may suddenly be heard when a child perceives rejection from a parental figure. The sequence may go something like this:

> The foster mother asks the child to put his dishes in the sink.
> The child does not react quickly.

The child sees an angry look in the face of the foster mother.

The angry look is a trigger, a learned signal that the child associates with beatings and abuse from his previous home.

That signal in the past was associated with the sound of his stepfather's voice, saying, "I'm going to get you."

The child now hears "I'm going to get you," which sounds like his stepfather, whom he had not lived with during the last two years. This is a warning of danger and a signal to hide or fight.

The child tries to manage the voice, now a substitute for the feeling of danger and fear, and may engage in self-harm in order to silence the voice, or attack the foster mother, or both.

While this process may appear complex, there are ways to make this understandable to even younger children. If the child has a theory about the voice, ask the child if she would be willing to consider another explanation. Children are often willing to hear your theories about what else could explain the voices, as they are usually mystified by the phenomenon and believe no one else experiences or knows anything about it.

Your conversation might go something like this, "*You know even though that voice in your mind sounds a lot like Victor, I think your mind may be playing a trick on you and it really isn't Victor at all. It may just be a 'Reminder Voice' helping you to remember how bad it really was when Victor was hurting you. Your mind may want to give you this 'Reminder Voice' to warn you when someone else might be hurting you. You could even thank the voice for trying to give you those reminders. Let's call it Reminder Voice instead of Victor, OK?*"

By subtly changing the name in this fashion, you are helping the child recognize the voice as something in the child's own mind that is functioning for the child's own benefit. This is the first step in giving the child back her power. If the child is reluctant to dispense with the name of the perpetrator, you can agree to call it the "memory of Josh voice," for example, and then over time drop the name and call it the "memory voice."

Sometimes the voices are more benign, and reframing them as feelings may make sense to the child. Here are some phrases to call voices that children can understand:

> *Your feelings talking to you.*
> *Your voice of scared feelings.*
> *Your signal voice.*
> *Your reminder of sadness voice.*
> *Your bad-feeling memory voice.*

By talking with children about what is happening when the voice comes, what it communicates to them or reminds them of, you can develop a descriptive name for that voice that is unique to each child's circumstances.

Seven-year-old Tina heard the sound of an abusive older stepbrother, Francis, who no longer lived with the family, saying, "Francis, Francis," in a deep growl. Her first belief was that this was the actual Francis somehow inside of her in order to scare her. After I explained to her that it was not the real Francis, Tina agreed to call the voice "the scary signal voice." She was proud of herself as she learned to identify the scary events that precipitated the signal. One day, she came in excited that she had heard "the scary signal voice" saying, "Francis, Francis" and understood why. She told me she had been sitting in the school cafeteria when a schoolmate told her you can get sent to the principal for not finishing your lunch quickly. Terrified of the principal, she heard "the scary signal voice," but this time she knew that she was afraid of the principal and not the real Francis. This incident represented a breakthrough in her understanding that this frightening symptom was actually giving her information she could use and understand. Once the child realizes that the voice can be seen as a part of her own mind giving her information, she can begin to find new ways to get this information without relying on the voice. Figure 6.3 shows the picture Tina drew of sitting in the cafeteria and hearing the voice in her mind. Drawing these internal experiences helps children feel less isolated and less afraid of these frightening aspects of their internal worlds.

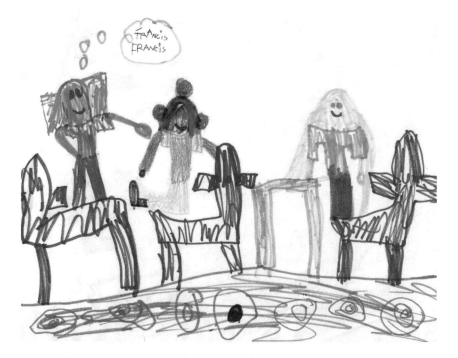

Figure 6.3 Tina's picture of the voice of Francis in her mind. Used with permission.

Concept 5: No Part of the Self Can Be Ignored or Dismissed

When some children hear that therapy is about the resolution of a war or fight in the mind, they think that means one side must kill off the other. Tension and conflict between warring parts of the self is what fuels dissociation. Consequently, the notion that some part of the self must be destroyed must be corrected immediately. Children must be helped to understand that no matter how negative, harmful, or destructive a part of their mind might seem, it has an original purpose that is helpful. Children find this notion surprising, as it is often contradictory to everything they have heard before. The creativity of the therapist is sometimes sorely tested as she is challenged to positively reframe these seemingly destructive voices, imaginary friends, or dissociative states.

Children's literature can be a helpful adjunct to this educational process. Many children's authors appear to have intuitively grasped the internal sense of struggle that many children feel, and have captured these struggles in poetic, child-friendly ways. For example, in *Where the Sidewalk Ends*, Shel Silverstein (1974) writes, "I will not play a Tug o' war, I'd rather play a Hug o' war, where everyone hugs instead of tugs, where everyone giggles and rolls on the rug, where everyone kisses and everyone grins and everyone cuddles and everyone wins." Utilizing this poem, the therapist can teach children why a "hug of war" will ultimately lead to more success than an internal "tug of war." In addition, reciting lines of this poem can become a cue during difficult times to help the child remember that the whole self must work together.

Dr. Seuss (1982) presents a similar theme in the book *Hunches in Bunches*. Dr. Seuss writes, "One of me could *never* do it, and quite suddenly I knew to get a job like that done would take more of me . . . like two." The child character in the book resolves the confusion between all of the versions of himself in the following way: "We all talked the hunches over, up and down, and through and through. We argued and we bargu-ed! We decided what to do." This story can be used to help describe the internal dialogue that children must engage in to resolve internal conflicts of warring voices or imaginary friends. "Arguing and bargu-ing" can become a funny name for their own internal process as they try to resolve conflicts using their whole mind. These entertaining and amusing books also help dissociative children recognize that their struggles are not so different from other children's internal experience.

One remarkable book called *(George)*, presciently written in 1979 by E. L. Konigsburg, describes a child named Ben with an imaginary inner voice named George. George advises Ben, and ultimately solves a mystery about an illegal drug ring at his high school. At the end of the story, Ben learns, "For the rest of his life, Ben will be mindful of his inner parts" (p. 152).

Unfortunately, even with child-sensitive education and an abundance of child-friendly toys, literature, and other resources, education alone is insufficient to move dissociative children into the self-acceptance and motivation required to move forward. In the next sections, I discuss how to address motivational problems by building on this initial educational information.

D: DISSOCIATION MOTIVATION

Engaging in dissociative avoidance strategies has become a habitual way of life for many traumatized children. Their forgetfulness, automatic behaviors, and shifting states keep others at arm's length, and allow them to keep themselves from really facing the results of their actions. Harnessing their motivation to find another way to cope is a huge challenge. This work on motivation for change occurs throughout the therapy, even at late stages of treatment when the child or teen may become fearful of the newfound responsibilities that increasing health brings. It is at the very early stages of therapy that this motivational factor must begin to be addressed squarely.

Build Some Future Awareness and Hope

The first step in evaluating the client's motivation is to engage in conversation about what the child or teen likes or dislikes and what he or she can visualize as a possible future. While many traumatized individuals cannot theorize easily about the future, I begin to require them to think about these things early in the treatment. I might ask if they know anyone with jobs or lives that they find impressive and how they see themselves in five years. I have found that without a concrete vision of what a potential future might look like, it is hard for children to stay motivated during challenging times. Discussing their future educational goals helps broach the subject of how important it will be for them to combat amnesia. They won't be able to become a veterinarian, forensic scientist, or cosmetologist if they have sudden amnesia during exams. Having a future necessitates engaging all of the capacities of their mind and not turning some of these off.

One technique for helping young people visualize a possible future is to have them imagine a conversation with an older version of themselves, maybe five or even ten years into the future. This imaginary older version of the self may have the future career they envision, a family or love interest, or whatever else they perceive as being ideal for them. Then the younger self can ask their imaginary older self, "What do I need to do to get to where you are?" Once this future successful self has been visualized, this idealized image of their future can be referred to throughout the therapy as the long-term goal that makes the hard work of therapy worthwhile.

Frank Discussions About the Child or Teen's Reliance on Dissociation

In order to assess clients' motivation for dispensing with dissociative strategies, we must first deeply understand why children continue to rely on dissociative defenses. What is it in their internal world of thoughts, memories, and feelings, or the external world of requirements, relationships, or circumstances, that might make the clients feel that change may not be worthwhile? Frank discussions of the pros and cons of learning a new way to organize their internal world should happen at this early part of treatment. There may be barriers to growing up, such as the fear of sexuality or fear of becoming like a parent who abused them. There may be a deep fear of breaking down amnestic barriers, as the child or teen may feel that he may be faced with intolerable knowledge about someone he relies on to take care of him. Children and teens can also become very attached to the loss of responsibility they experience when they have no memory for their out-of-control, angry behavior. Sometimes parents play into that escape from responsibility and agree with the child, that it was not he, as they know "he" would never do anything like that. At this early stage of treatment, setting up clear boundaries for what will happen when behavior is out of control will begin to propel the treatment in the right direction.

As the hidden motivations and environmental pressures that sustain dissociation are uncovered, it may be helpful to have children write out a pro-con list with all of the advantages and disadvantages of fully engaging in treatment. Some of the advantages of dissociation may be surprising to discover. Children may explain that they fear being lonely without the continuous chattering of internal voices, and they may enjoy the safe feeling of never having to face past behavior that is embarrassing. Sometimes the reason to keep the dissociation cannot be fully articulated, such as when the child or teen is still protecting an abuser and living in a dangerous environment that he or she has not revealed. These kinds of hidden motivations may become clearer as therapy progresses, and it is unrealistic to expect that everything will be revealed in these early sessions. Doing better in school work, not losing friends, and having the potential for a successful future are some of the advantages children may list in favor of working on decreasing dissociative symptoms. The discussion of advantages and disadvantages associated with dissociation begins a conversation that may be revisited repeatedly throughout the treatment.

Establish Firm Boundaries Based on Realistic Consequences and Central Responsibility

Generally, clients presenting with histories of chronic trauma and dissociation are engaging in symptoms that threaten their living arrangements, school placements, and their opportunities for increasing privileges like driving or dating. I have found that successful treatment involves some careful and firm discussions of the environmental what-ifs, not in a threatening way, but in an informative way at the beginning of treatment. The parents or foster parents must be engaged in this early part of treatment so that these clear what-ifs can be crafted together. If the child's behavior is so out of control that the parents or foster parents are considering an out-of-home placement, the child may perceive this, even if it has not been articulated. More commonly, the parents scream at moments of intense stress, saying something like, "Keep that attitude up and you'll get kicked out of here!" or some other threat that stimulates abandonment anxiety but without a clear-cut plan. I try to address these realities with very matter-of-fact discussion that provides a reality boundary of why work in treatment is so important. When framing these out-of-home living alternatives for out-of-control children, I phrase it not as the choice of the parent to abandon them, but rather as the requirements of a safe community.

Twelve-year-old Timothy experienced intense physical abuse from a biological grandfather with whom he no longer had contact. Timothy acted out his anger in violent ways against his mother and grandmother, with whom he was living. Both regularly received bruises and muscle strains from restraining him when he was out of control. Timothy had been hospitalized multiple times, and while in the hospital, he made empty promises about being safe, only to repeat the cycle of violent acting out when limits were set. Feeling guilty about having exposed Timothy to his grandfather's violence, his mother and grandmother had difficulty explaining the reality that they could not continue to parent him with his aggressive behavior. In times of argument or stress, they said things like, "You can't live here anymore," but then took him back after the hospitalization. From Timothy's viewpoint, the mother and grandmother were not really serious. As a result, he was not really facing the seriousness of his behavior and the reality that the existing cycle could not continue. To make matters worse, much of Timothy's angry behavior occurred in a dissociative state, which he identified as the behavior of "angry voice" that commanded him about how to fight when he was threatened and for which he had little memory.

Early in treatment, I explained to Timothy what was likely to happen if things continued the way they were going.

Did you know that when you leave bruises on your mom and your grandma, you are actually breaking the law? That may seem strange because no one took those laws seriously when your grandfather was leaving bruises on you. But that is called "assault." People are not allowed to do that to each other. We have these rules so people can live safely with one another. Your grandfather broke those rules, and he is not allowed to live with you ever again. The courts won't let him. People are not allowed to live with people who cause them harm; even if they say they want to. The harm you are doing to your mom and grandma is getting to be very serious and as much as they love you, they will not be allowed to let you live with them anymore if this keeps up. I know that you don't remember what you are doing a lot of the time, and it is "angry voice" that seems to make these things happen. Because you and the angry voice inside of you share the same body, the law makes no distinction between you. Whether you or "angry voice" is doing the harm, it is your own body that can't live in the house with your grandma and mom. This is very sad for them because they love you so much and wish you could be there. But our country and society has rules and laws, and when you keep breaking one of them, I, the social workers, and other people helping you are going to have to find another place for you to live. But I believe, even though it is going to be very, very hard to do this, that you can learn to share feelings with the angry voice inside of you and find ways to show anger without harming people. I will teach you how to do that and how to communicate with the angry voice inside of you so that you can continue to live at home with the mother and grandmother you love and who love you. I feel sure that you can do this because you are bright, you understand your past and why some of this is happening, and you want to stay living with your mom and grandmother.

Like Timothy, when children first come in to treatment, they often believe that the way they are managing their emotional world has been working. Even if they are creating chaos around them, they are maintaining an emotional equilibrium that seems to be effective for keeping traumatic content at bay, and avoiding feelings they fear. When you, the therapist, enter a dissociative child's world, you need to make it clear that the status quo is not ultimately functional for them.

Not all of the early "if-then" frames are as drastic as out-of-home placement. Often, teens who come to my practice very much want to learn how to drive and their parents are unwilling to let them begin this process because the teen's unpredictable dissociative episodes convince them that driving would be an unsafe activity. The desire to drive can become a prime motivator for treatment and can be explained by the therapist in clear-cut, matter-of-fact ways that help motivate dissociative teens to buy into treatment.

For example, I might say, "*I know you want me to tell your mom that you can drive, but I myself am worried about that. You know how you told me when you get really scared, you just shut down and stop talking or moving. Well, think about driving. What if something scary happens on the road? It would be really unsafe for you and other drivers if you just shut down and stopped driving. That could cause accidents. But I am sure if we work together, you can learn new ways to handle things when you are scared. When you are able to do this, I will definitely recommend to your parents that they let you drive.*" As therapist you can thus align with what motivates the teen and enlist her cooperation to get access to new privileges such as driving. Ultimately, my dissociative teen clients appear to be very good drivers as they learn to become very alert to both internal and external signals and take the responsibility very seriously.

The underlying message involved in establishing these early if-thens is that your client is responsible for everything she does, whether or not she has full awareness. Your client will come to believe as you do that she will get full awareness over time by investing in the work of therapy.

Evaluate and Work to Change Any Environmental Factor Sustaining Dissociation

The most significant environmental change requirement that may come to the therapist's attention is the need to remove a child from an unsafe environment where physical, sexual, or emotional abuse is occurring. When children are in an unsafe environment, addressing dissociative symptoms is inadvisable and generally impossible. When there is suspicion that the child comes to the session from an abusive home, the issue of dissociation must be approached cautiously. Directly dealing with the dissociation and frank discussions about its pros and cons will not be useful. If the therapist suspects ongoing abuse in the absence of a disclosure or clear-cut evidence, gentle commentary about the dissociation may help the child begin to trust that your office is a safe place to reveal the information. One clue that ongoing abuse may be an issue is when the child continually refers to a secret and lets you know that one of their imaginary friends or voices has a secret that cannot be shared. If such a comment is made, the therapist might say, *"I am the kind of doctor that can sometimes help children with scary secrets. And if I find out something that makes me think you are in danger for telling me the secret, I will work with all the adults I can think of to make sure you stay safe."*

Arnie, a 6-year-old boy with many dissociative symptoms, brought a plastic snake to every session and told me that Snappy the Snake had a big secret but yelled at Arnie constantly to "keep his mouth shut." In the session, his affect shifted dramatically and he talked to himself in different voices, often with aggressive and sexual content. Whenever I asked him questions about weekend events at his father's home, he told me that Snappy the Snake was telling me to "shut up." I turned to Snappy the Snake and "told" him that it must be very scary for him and I would do whatever I could to help him feel better and was sorry he had such a hard secret. At the beginning of each of his first seven sessions, Arnie told me that Snappy the Snake was going to tell me the secret, but at the end of the session said, "Next week." Finally, at the eighth session, when Snappy again "vetoed" what Arnie was about to tell, I suggested that Snappy the Snake wait outside with his mother and get all the comfort and care he could. Later in the session, with "Snappy" no longer present, Arnie shared a history of brutal physical and emotional abuse occurring on weekend visits to his father's house. A call to social services was made, and Arnie was protected after that session from future abuse. With young children such as Arnie, whose histories are unclear and the known facts do not support the intensity of dissociative symptoms observed, the objective is to safely glean information that will help protect the child.

It took six months for 8-year-old Adina to reveal to me the ongoing physical and sexual abuse she was subjected to during visitations with her father. During this time, I educated her about trauma and her dissociative symptoms, and explored the barriers that mentally divided experiences at mother's house and father's house. The real work on unity of the mind, however, was not possible until after Adina was able to tell her secret and be kept safe.

Often, there are milder impediments in the environment to dispensing with dissociative strategies. Family pressures, school pressures, or the pressures of legal visitation requirements can make children feel trapped, and they cope with these pressures through dissociation. Constantly feeling invalidated, some children must disconnect from their feelings to accommodate the environments that are stifling them. These more subtle pressures also need to be addressed for the child or teen to feel comfortable learning to dispense with dissociation. Adjunctive family work, to ease whatever pressures are uncovered, will facilitate the individual therapeutic work on dissociation. Throughout the book, you will encounter many examples where helping families, schools, and courts modify expectations of teens and children is an important part of the treatment.

The stage for treatment has been set by educating the child about trauma and dissociation and exploring the child's hidden motivations. It is now time to explore the hidden islets of dissociated feelings that may be contained in imaginary presences or voices that your young client may be secretly harboring.

7 Bridging the Selves
Healing Through Connections to What's Hidden

A few years ago, the Ad Council prepared a series of public service announcements encouraging parents to be careful about exposing children to frightening, aggressive, or sexual content on television. (See the "Boss of Slasher" and the "TVBoss. org" public service announcements, available on YouTube and other video sites.) In one of these service announcements, a mother answers the doorbell, to find two horrible monsters at her front door—one wielding an electric saw and the other with blood dripping down his face and scars all over his body. She invites them in with the kind voice any mother would use with children and offers them tea and cookies. Only after they are comfortable does she tell them in a sweet, high-pitched, motherly tone, "I am not going to be able to allow you to be here after 3 o'clock when my children come home, as you are a little too scary for them."

The commercial is jarring, as her tone of indulgence, support, and kindness appears shocking compared to their horrifying appearance, and her firm message at the end is delivered in the same kind and loving tone. This is a perfect characterization of the stance the therapist must take in order for children to approach their own inner demons without fear. The ads are funny and intriguing because they defy expectation, and similarly your young clients will find both intriguing and relieving your attitude of kind indulgence toward the parts of their minds that they fear. The inner monsters that children harbor, like the frightening monsters in the public service advertisement, respond to the kind, firm messages that you offer them. This stance allows them to relax internally and sets the stage for the curiosity needed to explore the mental contents they have metaphorically "banished" from consciousness.

These inner monsters may appear to the child as frightening as the bloody zombies in the Ad Council commercial. Figure 7.1 shows 13-year-old John's drawing of "Mr. Smiley," the frightening internal monster that led him to smash a neighbor's car window with a baseball bat. Mild-mannered John, pictured as the small, pony-tailed boy in the picture, would seem no match for "Mr. Smiley." Yet, "Mr. Smiley" responded with cooperation when I modeled for John acceptance of "Mr. Smiley's" anger as an understandable reaction to his history of harsh discipline at a former foster home. "Mr. Smiley," like the zombies in the Ad Council commercial, agreed to cooperate with an attentive and compassionate adult.

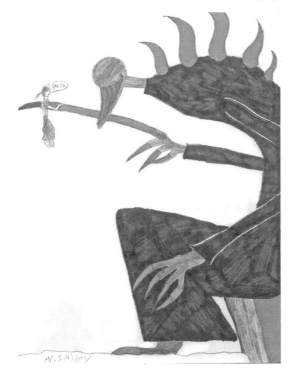

Figure 7.1 "Mr. Smiley." Used with permission.

The hidden islets of unprocessed traumatic memory, affect, voices, or imaginary selves dissociative children harbor and the self-induced barriers to revealing these hidden contents can be powerful. Balancing this reluctance is the fact that children and teens want to be known and accepted by adults, particularly if it is an adult who provides them with unconditional regard and validation. Thus, there is a kind of approach-avoidance conflict in dissociative children during the early stages of therapy between letting their private world be revealed and keeping it secret. The more the therapist can project an attitude of gentle, kind, nonjudgmental acceptance toward the guarded aspects of children's mind, the readier these clients will be to share this information with you.

"U" OF THE EDUCATE MODEL: UNDERSTANDING WHAT IS HIDDEN

The "U" of the EDUCATE Model covers techniques that can be used to help the children access hidden information. Child survivors may fear that you will judge them, or even punish them, if they express the real contents of the hidden, split-off parts of themselves. They may be hearing swear words, have homicidal ideas, or hear a running commentary telling them *not* to participate in the interview with you. They also may be scared to focus on material that they have been desperately trying to avoid. There are a number of techniques that can be used to help desensitize children to the contents of these split-off parts of their mind and to establish an environment in which sharing this content will feel safe.

The information dissociative children are hiding may be embarrassing, enraging, terrifying, or disgusting. The avoidance of traumatic memory and associated painful affect has often been generalized to the avoidance of these inner representations of the affects or memories associated with the trauma. The mental energy that is being spent to push away mental contents must be harnessed to develop an attitude of curiosity, kindness, and ultimately gratitude toward mental content that to this point has felt foreign and unknowable.

Let's look at a sample conversation during an initial interview with a 10-year-old girl, LaToya, referred for rage-filled attacks against her foster mother. I began by asking LaToya if she hears anyone or anything talking to her before she attacks her foster mother, telling her, "*Many children who have moved around from place to place hear the sound of someone they used to know talking to them during times of stress.*" Latoya told me she does hear a voice, but it is very, very bad; it sounds like the uncle that used to abuse her when she lived with her grandmother. I responded, "*How wonderful that you are able to tell me that you hear this. This will help us move forward with helping you.*" With this response, I have already challenged her expectation that I will jot down "psychotic" on my notepad, and respond with disappointment and worry. Then, I said, "*Hello, voice that sounds like LaToya's uncle, how are you doing? You must have seen a lot of scary stuff with all the places that LaToya has lived.*" LaToya looked confused and uncertain. "*Does he say something back?*" I asked.

She looked away embarrassed and hesitant. "*Oh,*" I responded, "*the voice must have said something rude and you don't want to let me know about it. That's ok; whatever he said is fine with me. I am just glad he is getting a chance to get some feelings out without hurting anyone. Did the voice call me names? It's ok, I don't mind.*" Reluctantly, LaToya shared that the voice had said, "Shut up, you bitch!" LaToya then assured me that she herself does not mean it. Again, I responded, without judgment, "*Wow, how wonderful you were able to tell me that—that must have been scary to tell. Would you tell the voice for me that I am not angry at the voice for its strong angry feelings because I know how hard your life has been. Having feelings that strong comes along with having a life filled with so many hard times.*"

LaToya then told me she has shared my thoughts, but the voice was telling her to stop talking to me. I responded, "*Yes, I know the voice has been kind of a secret for a really long time and that felt very safe. A lot of things about what happened to you have been a secret, too. I know it is scary to start to share some of that, and maybe we should thank that voice for being so brave for being willing to listen in here today. Tell him that I understand and I will try to help you and help the voice with all those strong feelings.*"

Within the course of these very few minutes, LaToya was able to tolerate conversations about something that was previously private and hidden, and able to hear me model a gentle, accepting, understanding tone that recognized that intense feelings are born from intense situations. Soon after beginning a conversation like this, LaToya, like most children, tried to argue with me about my outlook and said, "No, the voice is very bad, because it makes me hurt my foster mother or destroy things in the house." "*No,*" I responded, "*the voice is not bad, because the voice is part of you; it is your feelings talking to you. Maybe the voice is afraid of bad things happening again and fights before anyone has a chance to hurt you. Or maybe the voice thinks no one could ever like you and is testing them. But that is not bad; it is understandable. The voice is unsure of the best approach to take. Maybe the voice would be willing to get advice from you and from me about trying some other approaches.*"

By the end of my first 45-minute session with LaToya, we were able to develop an agreement with the voice to warn her about dangerous people in the environment, and then let LaToya plan how to respond, rather than fighting. We successfully separated the immediate procedural dissociative response of automatic aggression with a mediating step of thinking things through. By approaching her voice in this accepting and kind way, LaToya began to bridge a healing connection to what had previously been hidden and frightening.

Bridging these connections allowed LaToya to access her whole mind, including the prefrontal cortex planning centers, in order to engage in problem-solving and thus interrupt her automatic response of aggression. Simple modeling of acceptance and kindness profoundly shapes the child's experience of her internal landscape, allowing her to approach feelings in a new way and to examine behaviors that have previously been impervious to self-examination. Whether the hidden part of self is a voice as illustrated above, an imaginary friend, a transitional object that visits and commands, or a shifting identity state, this welcoming therapeutic stance can begin the process of the child becoming a validating witness to her own internal experiences.

Why I Don't Call out Alternate Selves or Ask for Identity Shifts

Many people have asked me if I ask to speak to the other selves, voices, or alternate identities, as is often done with adult DID clients. In fact, the definition of DID from the DSM-IV-TR requires that the mental health practitioner has encountered "two or more distinct identities that repeatedly assume control of the person's behavior" (APA, 2000, p. 526), suggesting that for diagnostic purposes one might try to observe a switch, an automatic nonconscious shift, to a different identity state. This is not my practice, as I view this as counter-therapeutic.

As you learned in Chapter 2, dissociation is conceptualized as a conditioned brain habit that has been over learned and now functions automatically to help the client avoid affect. The brain habit is practiced over time and becomes self-sustaining and reinforcing, as dissociative children become convinced that such avoidance is necessary for their survival. If the therapist asks for a different "identity" to emerge, or for a voice to talk directly to the therapist, the therapist is unwittingly giving the client more opportunities to practice the brain habit that they are attempting to extinguish. By allowing clients additional opportunities to practice dissociation, clinicians may reinforce the neural pathways that support dissociative coping. In younger children, the brain is still growing, pruning, and selecting the neural networks that will become most utilized as they grow into adults. Thus, it is contrary to my ultimate goal to instigate any more dissociative behavior than that which would occur naturally for the client.

Furthermore, by asking for switching, the automatic dissociative response of substituting one identity state for another, I believe that I would be giving a message that is inconsistent with my treatment goals. Our clients believe or demonstrate through their actions that dissociation is their only way to cope, that feelings would be too intolerable and overwhelming, and knowledge too frightening, if they were to accept the realities that are buried in their minds. I try to help them recognize that feelings are not the trauma—feelings can help navigate around, warn about, or prepare a response to trauma. This confusion between the feeling about the trauma and the actual trauma itself is one of the distorted viewpoints that therapy seeks to correct. If I were to ask clients to switch, it would be as if I were agreeing with the belief that the only way they have to get this information is through this dissociative strategy. Instead, I attempt to teach young people that it is preferable to build internal connections rather than practice a strategy of disconnection.

My overarching goal in working with dissociative children or teens is to encourage self-determination and self-regulation. Increased self-regulation stems from increased self-awareness. If I promote switching between identities, I am putting myself in the role of regulator of their functioning rather than the client as regulator of his or her own brain. Clients need to learn that they themselves can gain the ability to regulate state shifts and to notice that the onset of affects often precedes dissociative avoidance strategies. Responding to a therapist's signal to engage in this activity does not promote the child's learning to become sensitive to internal signals. Finally, asking for switching to alternate states might affirm rather than reduce the amnestic boundaries between the states. If the therapist becomes the only one who has the central information that your client requires, clients becomes increasingly dependent on the therapist for gaining information about themselves, rather than gaining this knowledge through forging internal connections.

I try to keep my responses, affect, and approach to the client consistent, regardless of their own shifting presentation. Our clients lack a sense of internal direction and often shift their internal state as an adaptive strategy to comply with shifting expectations. Our job is to keep the context as stable as possible, not unwittingly provoking automatic programmed reactions, so that the client is able to feel that wonderful sense of self-determination that defeats the powerlessness of their traumatic history. If a child or teen does appear to switch to another state spontaneously during a session, I try to continue as much as possible with whatever topic was being discussed at the moment of the shift. At the same time, I attempt to help the child or teen figure out what happened to provoke the shift. I ask the client to make the connections internally to explain what is stimulating the avoidance. Thus, I am working to avoid becoming part of the social environment that reciprocally reinforces and supports dissociative shifts.

Instead of learning about the hidden internal states through facilitating shifts, I seek to have young clients describe in words, pictures, or symbolic play their dissociated states, hidden voices, or imaginary friends. Symbolic ways of communicating through use of drawings, puppet shows, and plays are part of the normal tools of child therapists and are developmentally normative activities. For example, in working with John to acknowledge the feelings of "Mr. Smiley," I never had to "meet" "Mr. Smiley." The picture John drew was sufficient for me to acknowledge "Mr. Smiley's" presence. John did the work of accepting and understanding what he learned about "Mr. Smiley's" anger and was able to share these insights with me.

Listening In

Some dissociative children, who feel compelled to engage in behaviors they regret or don't remember, do not hear voices talking to them and have only a dim awareness that there is something besides their central consciousness influencing their behavior. If they are teenagers, their friends may have told them they have been places that they don't remember going, they may have trashed their own bedrooms without memory, or have gaps in their awareness of what happened during the school day. When confronted with these gaps in memory, they may act frightened and state, "It is better not to know." They may have some dim awareness that there is another part of themselves, but they do not want to know more and believe that accessing this information is impossible. These children's fear of learning about the things that are outside of their own awareness is countertherapeutic and will have to be overcome for therapy to progress. I want to help them see as quickly as possible that they can get access to this information and that it will not be dangerous or harmful to try.

In these cases where children's own behavior is a mystery to them, I ask them to take a moment and to "listen in" to their mind while asking a simple question to see whether there is something in their mind that can explain the mysterious gaps in time or strange behaviors they have been experiencing. I instruct them that this activity can only proceed with an attitude of acceptance, gratefulness, and self-love. If they approach what is in their own mind with fear or hate, it will cause their mind to separate more. I ask them to imagine hugging a young child who has been out of control, but really needs love to settle down, and then use this same kind of emotion toward themselves and their mind.

The first question I ask these children to consider is simply, "Is something there that will explain things?" I instruct them to ask this to their mind and then quietly listen for any answer that may come. The answer may come in pictures, feelings, or words. Some children just describe a sense of peace after this exercise and don't necessarily hear a response at this time. Usually, however, they do hear something. It may simply be the sound "Yes," or, often, an angry response saying, "What do you want?" Whatever happens, I praise them for the accomplishment of performing this difficult exercise, and starting the process of bridging toward hidden parts of the self.

I used this exercise with 14-year-old Angela, a client described in Silberg (2011). Angela was perplexed and upset by her friends' anger at her for rude behavior for which she had no memory. Angela was upset by similar reports by her mother, who said that she had talked back and refused to do her chores. I asked Angela if she could listen in to determine if there were some other part of her mind that knew about this information. Angela, at first, was extremely reluctant to engage in this exercise. She told me that if such a part was really there, "she was rude" and she wanted nothing to do with her. Fear of what she was going to discover was a large part of this reluctance. I told Angela that I thought these actions may not be rude, but an important form of self-defense against people who hurt her or took advantage of her.

Finally, with gentle insistence, Angela was willing to try the "listening in" exercise. She spent a few moments focusing inward while listening to my suggestions. Angela reported that she was able to hear the sound of "a rude voice" in her mind, answering her back. Together, we began to refer to this other part of the self as the "Other Angela." Angela's background included a history of severe abdominal pain that was undiagnosed for two years, causing her to miss significant amounts of school. She had spent weeks in her bedroom, disabled by excruciating pain. Eventually, the pain was diagnosed as severe gall bladder disease and surgery cured the physical difficulty, but the psychological effects remained.

By "listening in," Angela learned that the "Other Angela" had entered her consciousness as a way to help her deal with the excruciating pain she had endured. This "Other Angela" harbored significant anger toward her mother for not having found a way to help her sooner. The "Other Angela" also harbored anger against her friends, who seemed to be "fair-weather friends" who were only there for her when she was well. Finally, later in treatment, the "Other Angela" reported the secret of a sexual assault on a cruise ship at age 8 that led her to feel overwhelming shame, fear, and estrangement from her family. These ongoing internal dialogues with the "Other Angela" helped Angela learn to accept important aspects of her personality that had been pushed away—her legitimate anger, the fear and pain of her traumatic experiences, her profound disappointment in family and friends, and her need to take care of her physical health.

Symbolic Activities to Uncover What Is Hidden

Some children and teens feel most comfortable with drawing the hidden parts of the self, particularly if these feel more like imaginary friends or separate identity states. Through drawing, they can connect with their internal world and share it with the therapist, without direct eye contact or the intimacy of conversation. This provides some distance and safety. Through picking colors for the drawing and choosing the placement of the figures, the child is beginning the process of making the internal connections necessary to understand their inner world. Once these pictures are complete, the therapist can begin to ask about who the figures are, what they feel, and what they like to do. A very important question in this initial inquiry is asking the child to describe how each of the various figures drawn relates to their primary attachment figures. The relationship with a mother or foster mother is often a key arena in which a child in a dissociative state causes conflict and havoc. This is not surprising as the roots of dissociative pathology often lay in the conflicted attachment of a developing child.

Eight-year-old Marjorie had an early history of neglect before adoption from China at 3 years old. In drawing her first picture of what she called "the imagifairies," she depicted one with a scowling expression and red spiked hair. This one clearly looked different than the other three, who were calm looking and smiling. "Who is this one?" I asked, "She does not look very happy." Marjorie told me her name was "Sour." I asked her how "Sour" felt about living in the house with her mother, and she replied, "Ssssh, don't say that, the others will hear you; she hates my mother."

At this point early in our treatment, I could now identify a key target for our therapeutic work—"Sour's" feelings of anger toward her mother—feelings that needed to be explored, validated, and understood. Immediately, I worked to educate Marjorie about the work that we would be doing. "*I sure want to understand all of Sour's feelings about your mother, as she may have some very good points that are important for us to pay attention to. Maybe Sour has some ideas about what Mom could do differently to make your life happier at home. Maybe one day, Sour might be able to have a smile on her face too like all the other ones do.*"

Finding out about "Sour" provided an opening for understanding Marjorie's acting-out behaviors. I asked her, "*When you refuse to help your mom with chores around the house and run to your room and hide, does Sour have anything to do with that?*" "Yes," answered Marjorie, "Sour tells me to run away, 'cause no one can be the boss of me." I responded, "*How clever of Sour to know how important it is for you to make your own decisions. Sour's feelings are really important for us to understand better, as she seems to hold the key about how you might learn to get along better with your mom.*" In general, it is the most negative, angry, or hostile self-representation that I want to try to understand and ally with early on in treatment, as these hold the key to the destructive behaviors that often have led the child into treatment. In this early session, I begin to reframe and promote self-acceptance of the most challenging of the child's split-off feelings.

Some younger children prefer to act out symbolically the feelings and thoughts of dissociative states using puppets or dolls. Special dolls that can change expressions, have hidden compartments, or can transform into different shapes are useful tools for encouraging this kind of exploration. The therapist might ask the child, for example, which puppet or doll in the room could be used to show how his "angry voice" really feels. If the child is shy or hesitant about using a puppet, I might start the dialogue myself. Holding the puppet, and making a wolf-like gruff voice, I might state, "*I am really angry. Things around my house get me really, really mad. Want to know what?*" I then hand the puppet to the child who is usually eager at this point to participate in the conversation. This kind of play is common for children and does not stimulate the out-of-control feeling children often have during the involuntary changes of state that occur in switching between dissociative states. If the child is playing one role using the wolf-puppet, I might spontaneously pick up another puppet to represent the child and say, "*Now that I know how you feel, I can understand you better and you are not so scary.*" In that way, I begin the process of bridging the feelings between segregated states and the process of promoting self-acceptance.

Of course, many young children have an affinity for fantasy and easily engage in symbolic play, and these symbolic play activities are not necessarily a sign of pathological dissociation. As discussed in Chapter 4, there are important signs to indicate that this internal fantasy world is not completely normative. For example: Does the child feel that imaginary characters control his behavior without his knowledge or approval? Is the child confused about whether this is imaginary? Does the child wish the imaginary friend would go away or feel that there is a perpetual war going on in his mind? Is the child compelled to communicate with the imaginary characters even when engaged in real relationships or at school?

In some cases, the child appears to be so wrapped up in her fantasy world that it may feel counter-therapeutic to engage in symbolic fantasy play during therapy. In these cases, carefully tying what is discussed in the symbolic play to real behavior and events is important. Lydia was 8 years old when she was brought in to see me after having stolen a doll from a classmate—an action for which she claimed no memory. In our first session, Lydia revealed that she had "imaginary friends" that were named after characters in the Harry Potter books. She reported to me that "Draco Malfoy," the evil nemesis of Harry Potter, would sometimes make her do things in school that she did not remember. She further shared with me that she often doesn't pay attention in school as she is talking in her mind to Harry Potter and his friends, and listening in as they plan their next adventures. This over involvement in her fantasy world was clearly interfering with her school achievement and affecting her classroom behavior.

To bring Lydia's focus to the real world, I questioned her about what real things in her classroom might she or "Draco Malfoy" notice that make her angry. She was able to discuss her feelings about peer teasing and not getting enough praise or attention at school. At this point, I suggested we thank "Draco Malfoy" for pointing out what was upsetting her in the classroom. I recommended that we ask the other Harry Potter characters for ideas of ways she could handle her problems at school better. With cases such as Lydia, who are deeply invested in spending lots of time engaged in solitary involvement in a fantasy world, it is best to engage with the child in that fantasy world only to help with getting practical solutions to real-world problems. Children such as Lydia could spend an entire session telling stories about Harry Potter's adventures without ever approaching issues that brought them into therapy.

Sometimes it is important to help children with over developed fantasy worlds make a distinction between characters that are part of their fantasies and characters that they perceive as part of themselves. Lydia, in fact, had two versions of Draco Malfoy. She had the storybook Draco Malfoy who she imagined going through various adventures, and one that she felt inside of her to help her deal with peer conflicts. It is important to help children make these distinctions and ask them what they are referring to when they say something such as, "Draco Malfoy is getting ready for a war." For example, I might say, *"Do you mean the character in your stories, or the part of you that helps you solve school problems? Let's give the Draco Malfoy that solves school problems another name, Ok? We could call him 'Lydia's anger friend.' Now who is having a war?"* If the war is simply something she is playing in her imagination, it can be acknowledged briefly, and then the therapist can offer a quick bridge back to helping the child deal with their real-world problems. *"That is really a great story, and maybe you could draw a picture about that. Right now let's talk some more about the 'war' you are going through at school with the kids who tease you at recess."*

Encouraging children to draw or make storybooks about their imaginary worlds can be a good outlet for this kind of creative fantasizing. The characters in these creative projects can be distinguished from the imaginary selves of dissociative children, as these characters do not directly influence or affect the child's behaviors. While it may be informative to follow the themes and conflicts in the child's imaginative world, it is important that the child learns to make distinctions between the real world and the world of imagination, and between imaginary characters and their own sense of identity.

THE "C" IN THE EDUCATE MODEL: CLAIMING WHAT IS HIDDEN AS ONE'S OWN

Claiming what is hidden as one's own is the key to therapy with traumatized, dissociative children. This process continues throughout all of the stages of therapy. In order to accept themselves, accept their past, and move forward in an integrated way, children must find a way to embrace what their minds have tried to reject and avoid. The process of accepting feelings, memories, thoughts, or senses of self that feel foreign, hateful, enraging, or frightening, can be difficult but is essential if dissociative children are to develop central awareness and mastery of their behavior. The action of embracing what is hidden produces an immediate and powerful shift in the way the child or teen feels and experiences herself. Various exercises and techniques can encourage this process. The most important aspect of any of these interventions is the therapist modeling the acceptance, gratefulness, and attitude of fearlessness that the client needs to learn to develop.

Reframing the Negative Dissociated Content

Once I have explained to children the psychoeducational component of the treatment—that all identified aspects of their mind have a meaningful purpose and this purpose needs to be acknowledged—we can begin the process of reframing. Together, we talk about what purpose their dissociated anger, "fighting energy," or "rude voice" might serve.

I explain in a matter-of-fact manner that the voice in their mind might be there to help remind them that things are not the way they want them to be. For example, a voice that causes them to act rude might be helping them figure out a way of fighting back when they feel powerless. Even voices that tell them to hurt others can be reframed as holding feelings of the strength and power that helps them to fight back when they are being hurt. Angry voices might be a way of reminding them how angry they feel about things that happened in their past. If the dissociated voice that they are hearing has the name of the perpetrator, I will start to work on reframing this as the mind's way of remembering a painful part of their past and try to rename the voice in descriptive terms to help make this distinction. For example, I might say, *"Let's call that the 'Andrew reminder voice.' not Andrew."* As we talk together about what purpose these aspects of their mind have served, the process of desensitization to the emotions and traumatic content that those parts harbor may begin.

Self-destructive voices can be the most difficult kinds of voices to reframe. Identifying their positive aspect may take some time, but I have found that even the most recalcitrant and harmful voices or identity states can be reframed positively. Keep in mind that each reframing of a destructive or self-destructive voice, imaginary friend, or identity state must be uniquely suited to that child or teen's own history. Table 7.1 presents a list of possible ways to reframe a tormenting or self-destructive voice in a young child survivor.

Tracy, a 9-year-old anorexic girl, was sexually abused at the age of 7 by her grandfather, who babysat after school while her mother was at work. Tracy had a voice she called "Ted," which she said stood for "Tracy's Eating Disorder." "Ted" told Tracy to starve herself and this was painful and frightening to her. Tracy required hospitalization to restore her weight and naturally resisted my insistence that this voice might have a positive purpose. Tracy asked me to please make it stop and get rid of it. Sometimes Tracy would bang her head against the wall trying to silence the voice. She was terrified of the voice, and strongly resisted the idea that "Ted" could be anything but a sadistic and a dangerous presence within her. This fear of the voice was reinforced in her previous treatment where she had been told to fight the voice; to tell it she was stronger and would overcome it. This method did not work. The voice got stronger and stronger, and Tracy had more and more difficulty eating.

Despite her initial protests, I continued to gently insist that once we found out the good reason behind "Ted's" desire to starve her, we would be able to quiet this voice. I explored with her in detail the sensations associated with

Table 7.1 Ways to Reframe a Tormenting Inner Voice

Inner Voice	Reframe
Tells the child to attack	A body guard to protect from danger
	A way to help you feel your strength
	Your anger talking to you
Tells the child to harm the self	A reminder of how hurt you were and remind you what pain feels like
	A protection so you won't hurt others
	A way to distract you from painful feelings
Sounds like the perpetrator	A way to help you remember that there were some good things about your father
	A way to help you remember the nervousness you had when those things happened
	A way to remind you to always be on guard for dangerous people like him
	A way to keep you from doing things that might make others attack you
	A way to remind you not to tell because you were afraid your family might be hurt

hearing the voice of "Ted." She described feeling a strange nauseous feeling, and stomachache, and recounted a time she had thrown up in school and was very embarrassed because the other students had teased her. She remembered her stomach hurting in the same way while she waited for her mother to get home from work, and she remembered wishing her mother would come home sooner so that the abuse would stop. I suggested that "Ted" was her way of hearing her stomach say, "I am very nervous and might throw up because of my fear." In addition, the voice may be reminding her that she is scared and needs her mother. "Ted" might also be trying to prevent her from throwing up by telling her not to eat. She vehemently disagreed with my attempted reframe. Tracy told me that the "Ted" voice hated her mother, and so it could not be related to missing her mother.

Tracy's fear of abandonment and anger at her mother for placing her in the care of a child molester led to extreme separation anxiety and even difficulty attending a whole day of school. By relating the voice of "Ted" to this separation anxiety, Tracy was finally able to accept the "Ted" voice and begin to transform its power from destructive to therapeutic. I explained to Tracy and her mother in a family session that the voice of "Ted" was like a little child screaming "I hate you" during a tantrum, afraid of her mother leaving. "What would you do about this?" I asked Tracy's mother. Tracy's mother said she would hug the child and tell her she was sorry she was hurt and would love the child despite those words. With my prompting, Tracy's mother stated she could love even the "Ted" part of Tracy and knew that part of her probably felt hurt, lonely, and afraid.

With repeated gentle reframing from both her mother and me, Tracy finally began to accept that the voice of "Ted" was a signal of a nervous stomach talking to her because things in the environment scared her. I asked Tracy to keep a journal and write down any scared thoughts she was having whenever she heard "Ted's" voice. She was willing to do this, and noticed that the voice seemed to come when she was anxious about her schoolwork or fearful about separations. Finally, she no longer needed the journal and could identify the nervous thoughts she had every time she heard "Ted" yelling at her not to eat. She learned to say back gently to the voice, "I know I am nervous that mom might be late picking me up today, but I can still eat. Maybe I can ask the teacher if I can call her." Tracy began to understand the voice of "Ted" in a new way, a signal of nervousness learned at a terrifying time, warning her of potential dangers in her environment. Over the next few months, the "Ted" voice stopped ordering her not to eat. She began to hear it simply say, "You are nervous." Eventually, the voice stopped talking to her entirely. One and a half years after the onset of this symptom, Tracy told me "Ted" was simply the name she called "butterflies" in her stomach. Tracy's eating returned to normal, though she continued to have anxiety symptoms managed with antinausea medication and supportive therapy.

This case illustrates the importance of reframing negative dissociated content. What began as a treatment-resistant dissociative symptom that was life threatening evolved over time into simply the more normative experience of a nervous stomach that was reactive to stress. The purpose of the voice was redefined from a tormenting presence to one that warned her of environmental dangers. Ultimately, the voice went away as she learned new coping tools to deal with the experience of separation anxiety, and she began to feel the security of increasing safety with her grandfather no longer in the picture.

Gratefulness: The Thank-You Note Technique

Gratitude is a powerful emotion and has been identified as an antidote to depression and a key component of mental health (Seligman, Steen, Park, & Peterson, 2005). For the dissociative children and teens that I treat, the thank-you note exercise is usually one of my first interventions, and begins the process of claiming as one's own the hidden parts of the self that they have been using mental energy to reject (Silberg, 1998b). Once children have identified the aspect of their identity that leads to the most problematic behavior, such as "the angry voice," "mean Betty," "the rude one," or "Ted," and we have found a way to reframe it, I ask them if they would write a thank-you note to that dissociated part of their self. At first, they tend to be shocked and reject this idea, as it is the direct opposite of their customary way of handling this problematic aspect of their self. Yet, when I provide colorful markers, crayons, stickers, and construction paper, most children

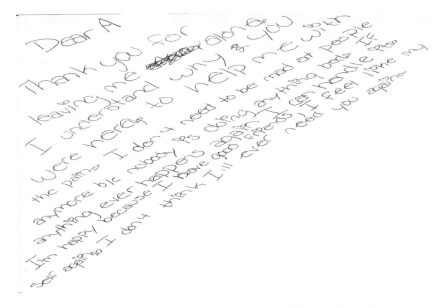

Figure 7.2 Angela's thank-you note to the "Other Angela." Used with permission.

or teens are willing to use the materials to indulge their therapist and will create this strange kind of thank-you note. A thank-you note from Angela to the "Other Angela" is provided in Figure 7.2, in which she acknowledges the "Other Angela's" role and tells her she won't "need her anymore." (The "Other Angela" remained for a considerable time after this first note.)

A thank-you note from a 7-year-old, with color names for her parts of self, is provided in Figure 7.3. Before leaving the hospital, Monica wrote this note from "Pink Monica" to "Black Monica," encouraging cooperation between the angry, "Black" part of herself, and the "Pink" or calm self.

The experience of writing these notes feels surprising and unfamiliar to the children and teens that I work with. If the mind is comprised of energy flow, as Daniel Siegel (2010) suggests, then one might conceive of this exercise as a way to change the internal flow of energy in the mind. The energy flow used toward avoidance and pushing out of awareness troubling mental contents is reversed during the process of writing this note. The child's energy now embraces and expresses gratitude for what had heretofore felt foreign and unacceptable. This produces a perceptible shift. Children and teens have described the feelings they experience after engaging in this process—a sudden calm, a feeling of peace, and a sense of hopefulness.

To get a sense of the insight such an exercise may provoke, try something similar yourself. Think of a character trait, a bad habit, or behavior you regret. Then imagine writing a thank-you note to this aspect of yourself. Are you unhappy with your weight? You might thank your overeating self for helping you realize

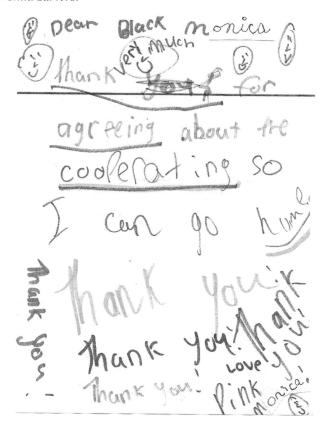

Figure 7.3 Monica's thank-you note to "Black Monica." Used with permission.

how much you deserve good food. Are you unhappy with your procrastination? You might thank that part of you for finding creative ways to avoid work. By acknowledging the part of yourself that you dislike the most, you can achieve some surprising insights about your own self-motivations that can lead to better insight and ultimately more centrally focused awareness that can lead you to engage your entire will in your decision making.

Regressive Voices, Imaginary Friends, or Identity States

Children with regressive identity states may talk in baby talk, hear babies crying in their mind, or even dramatically regress to the behavior of a much younger child when feeling the influence of these regressive pulls. Waters (2005b) described the difficulty clinicians may have in recognizing these dissociative shifts, particularly in younger children. These children may crawl, talk in single words, lose bladder control, and even have difficulty recognizing a new adoptive parent in these states. Regressive states are easier to reframe than are the negative ones described above, as children intuitively understand that there is a strong positive pull toward the lower expectations and unconditional nurturing attention to which babies and preschool children are accustomed. For some children who have been abused in infancy or the preschool period, these states involve traumatic reliving of the feared events. For those whose abuse occurred after the infant or preschool period, these regressions may reflect retreat to a period of time that was relatively stress-free and remembered as idyllic. For others, these regressions may be ways to engage their parents to have lower expectations for them.

Interventions to help children or teens accept their baby or younger states involve modeling love, caregiving, and safety—first by you as the therapist, then by the parents, and ultimately the child reinforcing these principles through extending care and compassion to the younger self. I use a baby doll to represent this younger aspect of the child. First, I hold the doll, and while the baby doll is rocked and cared for, I might say, "*You deserve all the love and safety you can get. I will take care of you and help you get stronger and grow up to be a strong and happy young man. Now you try it.*"

If the child has a problem with actively regressing to these younger states during inopportune times, such as at school or when the family is trying to get ready for an important event, the therapist can try to develop an agreement with the child to confine the expression of this regressive behavior to bedtime, when regressing in the form of needing mom's love and attention is more normative. Waters has had success using what she calls an "age progression" technique, having the child create and then rock a clay figurine that represents the baby self and mother. She then suggests that the baby within grows year by year until the baby reaches the true age of the child (Waters & Silberg, 1998a).

As with all automatic dissociative patterns, the moments preceding these regressions are important to highlight. The focus of attention is on the intolerable affects that lead to these automatic regressive pulls. What did the child feel right before she regressed? For example, right before the regression, did the child fear separation, feel rejection from the parent, feel abdominal pain, or experience anger at having to go to bed? Identifying the emotions at the transition moments before regression will ultimately help the child relearn how to negotiate those affects in more mature ways—through communicating his needs or appropriate self-soothing. Highlighting the transitional moments that lead to regression is key to the ultimate integration of this automatic conditioned regression.

Sexualized Voices, Imaginary Friends, or Identity States

One of the most perplexing problems facing child clinicians is children and teens who experience compulsive sexual symptoms, such as promiscuous sexual activities with peers or younger children, excessive masturbation, or acting inappropriately seductive with adults or older peers. Often, these compulsive activities are kept separate from central awareness and sequestered into split-off mental contents (Grimminck, 2011; Johnson, 2003; Waters & Silberg, 1998b) Dissociated sexualized behaviors are particularly resistant to treatment, as the child survivor claims little awareness for the activities and experiences high levels of shame when these behaviors are pointed out—causing further dissociative avoidance. As with other dissociative fragments that feel foreign or shameful, the therapist models acceptance and understanding to move the child toward reconciliation with the dissociated aspect of self.

Drawings that depict sexualized aspects of the self may help desensitize the child to talking about these experiences. The drawings themselves need not be sexual in nature. Waters describes using drawing in her work with a 7-year-old boy who was sexually acting out against younger children (Waters & Silberg, 1998b), reflecting the compulsive nature of his touching behavior. The boy drew the sexualized aspect of his identity as a figure with enormous hands.

Another important intervention with sexually acting-out children is helping them understand the sexual arousal they experience in an age-inappropriate way. Such a conversation may be something like this, "*God (or evolution for nonreligious families) made everyone so that they feel a funny tickle when their private parts are touched. This funny tickle gets even stronger as children get older, and when people grow up it helps them feel really close to people they love and it helps make more babies for God to love. But this is a private part of your body that you are the boss of, and no one else. Uncle Jonathan did the wrong thing when he touched your privates. Now your body learned from him about this and it makes you feel like doing it more and more. But this is something you need to save for when you are older. This feeling got turned on too soon, and I will need to help you turn it off for a while so that it can be there in the right way when you are older.*"

This may allow children to feel comfortable enough with the sexual part of their identity to talk to you more about the specific feelings they get when they are involved in sexually stimulating activities. For example, they may find these activities help them soothe themselves when they are angry or distressed, help them connect or bond to other children, or provoke adults into caring for them. Understanding how the sexual behavior is helping them allows them to reframe their behavior so that thank-you notes or other self-acceptance exercises can be used. Discussions then lead children to uncover some of the origins of these sexualized feelings, which can be processed in the trauma processing phase of treatment. By uncovering the motivations and goals of the sexualized dissociative mental contents of the child survivor, the therapist is prepared for the negotiating and bargaining that further helps to integrate your client's sense of self. At the same time that you are helping sexualized children to discuss and reframe their behaviors, you must also help set boundaries. Structure, limits, and careful observation and monitoring can limit and help redirect inappropriate behaviors.

Sometimes, younger children who have been sexualized at an early age engage in repetitive and compulsive masturbation. This behavior can result in injury or repeated urinary tract infections. By continuing to use this behavior as a means of coping with difficult feelings, the child survivor reinforces a self-soothing strategy that will cause more problems as he or she matures. Turning to sexual gratification to soothe hurt feelings may lead to promiscuity or sexual addiction as the child matures. Therefore, interrupting these compulsive patterns is important. I instruct the families to sit with the children at bedtime and provide substitute bedtime rituals of soothing that become new habits. For example, children can have their backs rubbed, listen to soothing music, and hug a stuffed animal as they drift into sleep. Rules that bedtime stuffed toys are for "above the waist hugging only" may need to be emphasized, as many children will use the stuffed toys as objects for masturbation. Newly placed foster children should be encouraged in these alternative habits so that the compulsive masturbation does not become their only tool for managing feelings. If the compulsive masturbation is occurring during the day, the parents can gently redirect and distract the child. While it is important not to shame the child for engaging in masturbation, it is also important that a child's development is not skewed by engaging in this behavior at the expense of time for learning, playing, and having happy relationships.

What If the Dissociated Part of Self Stays Hidden?

It is possible that despite all of these techniques, a child or teen still insists a behavior clearly observed is not his own, and claims no memory or responsibility for it. He or she may have no apparent imaginary friends, and deny hearing internal voices and any awareness of a dissociative state. The therapist can still talk about this aspect of themselves and name it something like "the mysterious Alan that others see steal things." The therapist can also ask the child to draw a picture of that "mysterious Alan." The quandary the child faces when her actions are observed by others, but she has no recollection of these actions, is squarely placed before the child—*"How difficult for you that you are being forced to take the heat for things you do that you can't even recall. What a bummer. That must feel totally unfair. I hope I will be able to help you figure a way out of this problem. Let's call that mysterious way you act, 'The angry Tammy.'"* The therapist can then refer to the behaviors in question without the child having to acknowledge memory for these events. The next chapter will provide further details about working with children with memory gaps for their own behavior.

Bridging the Gap Through "Arguing and Bargu-ing"

In Chapter 6, I introduced you to Dr. Seuss's (1982) book *Hunches and Bunches*, in which a boy resolves conflicting pulls in his mind through "arguing and bargu-ing." This is good terminology to describe the internal negotiations that can help dissociative children resolve the conflicting pulls in their minds. This process of negotiation provides a framework for early stabilization of out-of-control

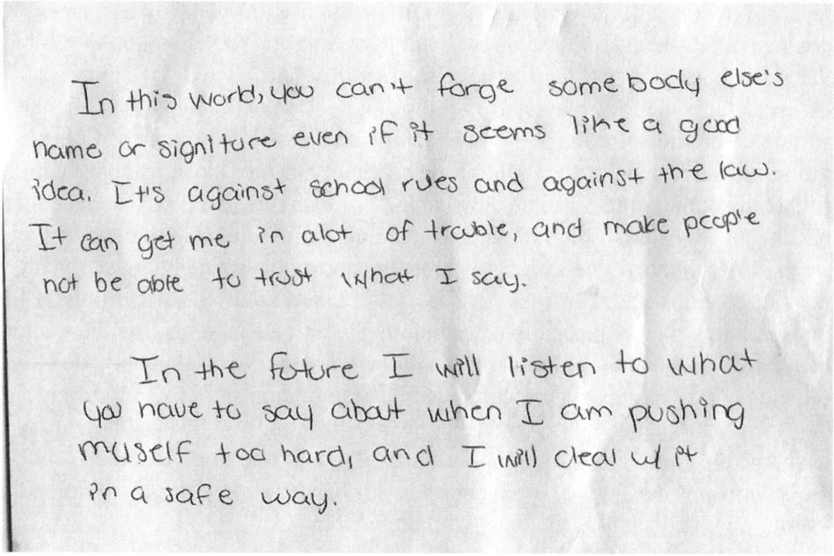

In this world, you can't forge some body else's
name or signiture even if it seems like a good
idea. It's against school rules and against the law.
It can get me in alot of trouble, and make people
not be able to trust what I say.

In the future I will listen to what
you have to say about when I am pushing
myself too hard, and I will deal w/ it
in a safe way.

Figure 7.4 Angela makes a deal with the "Other Angela." Used with permission.

symptoms. For example, I worked with a sexualized 10-year-old girl who reached puberty early and was having sexual contact with boys at school. The sexual part of the self agreed to be involved in helping her with tampon insertion, which we convinced her mother to let her use, in return for avoiding sexual contact with boys in the bathroom at her elementary school. Angry or aggressive parts can agree to serve as early warning systems of danger, offer help in writing angry letters, or participate in intense athletic activities in return for not directing aggression toward family members. Brand (2001) provides a good review of how these kinds of bargaining activities occur in the early phases of treatment with adults to minimize self-destructive behaviors. Although written for adults, the process of negotiation and quid pro quo is similar to the work with children and adolescents.

Figure 7.4 is a note written by Angela to her "Other Angela," which illustrates Angela's ability to recognize the "Other Angela's" role in stopping her from driving herself beyond her limits. In a dissociated state of the "Other Angela," Angela had written a note to her principal using her mother's signature to excuse her from a physical education class. In this note, Angela educates this other part of her mind about why forgery is wrong, and promises to try to pay more attention to her internal signals.

The "No Harm Deal" is an early agreement that the child and all parts of the child will not engage in destructive or self-destructive behavior "accidentally or on-purpose" (Waters & Silberg, 1998b). This can be a verbal agreement or a signed contract. Some children will sign these contracts with pictures, with multiple names, or with their own name, but state it includes all of the "invisible people" that they experience as inhabiting the nonconscious parts of their mind.

The bridging to hidden parts of the self is an ongoing challenge in therapy with dissociative children, and this stage of "claiming" these parts of the self continues throughout the therapy. In the next chapter, I will focus more specifically on the amnestic barriers that make it particularly hard for children to acknowledge these hidden parts of the self.

8 "I Try to Forget to Remember"
Reversing Amnesia

Frank was a model eighth grader at a special educational program where I consulted. He did his homework, never talked in class, and offered to help his teachers with copying materials and carrying supplies. His 9-year history of abuse and neglect by his birth mother, before his adoption to a loving middle-class couple, did not seem to affect his school behavior. His behavior at home, however, was a different story. He destroyed the hallway banister by scraping the polished mahogany surface with a pair of scissors; he cut holes in the Persian carpet; he broke treasured figurines displayed in the living room. When his parents returned from work and found the destruction in the house, Frank stated he could not remember anything about how it happened. They grounded him from television and phone use and docked his allowance, but the behaviors continued, along with his denial of any memory for his actions.

Frank's amnesia, if that is what it was, seemed severe and impenetrable. His school behavior continued to be so laudable that he earned the privilege of "honors" level, which let him eat in a special cafeteria, play ping-pong during recess, and he no longer had to carry a "point card" between classes showing that he was meeting school goals. In therapy, as at home, he continued to say "I don't remember" when asked anything about his destructive behavior at home. Therapy appeared to be at an impasse. Nevertheless, Frank seemed to be happy with the status quo—privileges and fun at school, destructiveness without bounds at home, and selective memory only for his successes.

Amnesia is a frightening word to use when describing child and adolescent memory. It seems so final and irreversible. Yet, amnesia seemed the best word to describe the rigid barrier that kept Frank from being able to recall his destructive behavior. This type of amnesia, presumed to be a result of psychological rather than physiological factors, is often termed "dissociative amnesia" or "psychogenic amnesia." Dissociative amnesia is a loss of autobiographical memory associated with chronic developmental trauma, Posttraumatic Stress Disorder, Dissociative Disorder Not Otherwise Specified, or Dissociative Identity Disorder. Dissociative amnesia is also a psychiatric disorder of its own, characterized by "an inability to recall important personal information usually of a traumatic or stressful nature too extensive to be explained by ordinary forgetfulness" (APA,

2000, p. 519). Dissociative amnesia as a separate disorder rarely occurs among children and adolescents. However, perplexing forgetfulness commonly occurs as a traumatic symptom in this age group. Child survivors may have amnesia for traumatic events they experienced and amnesia for important autobiographical information.

Amnesia in children, which usually has its roots in childhood trauma, has not been well described in the child development literature. At the same time, there is a level of public familiarity with these concepts, as amnesia is a frequent theme in television crime dramas featuring child witnesses who are too traumatized to recall violent events. Public recognition of dissociative amnesia following trauma has also been spurred by media coverage of sexual abuse cases involving Catholic priests. In the criminal trial for convicted former priest Paul Shanley, accused of molesting children in Boston, the jury accepted the victims' claims of dissociative amnesia and rejected the defense argument that such phenomena are not scientifically accepted. In a unanimous ruling, the Supreme Judicial Court upheld the Shanley conviction, affirming that repressed memory evidence could be used against Shanley (Ellement, 2010).

It is well established that adults can forget and later reaccess forgotten childhood traumatic memories (Brown, Scheflin, & Whitfield, 1999; Edwards, Fivush, Anda, Felitti, & Nordenberg, 2001). Among adolescents, some case studies have described global amnesia for documented traumas, and then spontaneous recovery of this memory (Corwin & Olafson, 1997; Duggal & Sroufe, 1998), and this type of amnesia has also been documented in case studies of dissociative children and teens (Cagiada, Camaido, & Pennan, 1997; Putnam, 1997; Silberg, 1998a; Waters, 2005b; Wieland, 2011b). Yet, the topic of amnesia for trauma in children and adolescents is only beginning to be studied in the developmental literature.

Freyd (1996) identified factors associated with the likelihood of forgetting a traumatic event that have been upheld in subsequent research (Freyd, DePrince, & Gleaves, 2007). These factors include: child maltreatment perpetrated by a parent, demands for secrecy, threats, lack of opportunity to discuss the events, younger age at onset of trauma, and isolation of the victim. Thus, a child sexually abused by a father during her elementary school years who is threatened with harm if she discloses is more likely to have a more robust amnesia for the event than would someone who is abused by a stranger when older.

Goodman et al. (2003) prospectively studied a prosecution sample of children whose abusers were convicted. They found that even among children whose maltreatment histories were discussed and made public, 12% did not report the events when later asked about their childhoods and two out of the 168 children reported no memory for the events. Lack of maternal support and dissociation were associated with more memory problems. Emerging research suggests that children with a high level of dissociation under certain stressful conditions are more likely to show memory impairments (Becker-Blease et al., 2004; Eisen, Goodman, Qin, Davis, & Crayton, 2007). Children asked to recount details of traumatic medical procedures have been found to have more memory problems when the events were more frequent or overwhelming (Kenardy et al., 2007). Similarly, children exposed to family violence have been shown to have difficulty recounting witnessed events and tend to be overly general in their descriptions (Greenhoot, Brunell, Curtis, & Beyer, 2008). These findings suggest that difficulties with memory may be part of a strategy that some children use to avoid the pain associated with traumatic events (Goodman, Qas, & Ogle, 2010).

How this memory failure occurs has been the subject of a series of laboratory experiments in which adult subjects are given instructions to forget certain content, or ignore information that is distracting (Anderson & Huddleston, 2012). These studies have repeatedly demonstrated that motivation plays a key role in memory, and that various cognitive mechanisms are engaged, some at the time of input, and others inhibiting the retrieval stage of memory. It is hypothesized that the active process of motivated forgetting engages specific brain structures that inhibit memory through practice over time in the same way that motor activities can be inhibited (Anderson & Huddleston, 2012). This course of motivated forgetting is described as a process: "Motivated forgetting is unlikely to be accomplished in a single cognitive act or even in a short time, particularly for complex events with emotional content. Rather, it may require sustained effort, particularly if a person is confronted with reminders. For these reasons, motivated forgetting may best be viewed as an ongoing process supported by adapting mechanisms that limit awareness of the experience" (p. 103).

In response to questions about his abuse, 6-year-old Billy described the process of motivated forgetting in the elegant words of a young child, "I try to forget to remember. It hurts to remember. It gives me bad dreams." Billy is aware that his mind has been working to avoid the information about abuse that I am asking about. He describes his clear motivation not to remember—the bad dreams and pain associated with the memory. According to Anderson and Huddleston (2012), "reminders do not merely fail to enhance memory, they actually trigger processes that impair retention of the suppressed memory" (p. 63). It is this active process of impairing retention—"trying to forget to remember"—that Billy seems to be describing in his statement. Eight-year-old Adina, returning from visits where she was abused, described the same process after it had become so automatic that the motivational roots were no longer evident—"It's like a brain seizure, your brain does this so you don't have thoughts and don't know what to think or feel." Actively helping children recover early traumatic memories that are not affecting their current safety is not therapeutically advisable, as these early memories surface progressively during carefully paced therapy at the time when the child is ready (see Chapter 13). However, recovering memory for a child's own recent behavior is a primary early goal of therapy because lack of ongoing autobiographical memory has such severe consequences for the child or teen's functioning at home, at school, and with peers. Sometimes, accessing the recent autobiographical memory will illuminate a hidden traumatic memory in a manner that feels healing and integrative, as illustrated with Sonya in Chapter 2.

Just as the development of amnesia for a traumatic event is envisioned as an ongoing process, so the recovery of autobiographical memory can be viewed as a process amenable to psychotherapeutic intervention. Anderson and Huddleston suggested that three factors could affect how memories once forgotten can be retrieved again—the presentation of context cues, practice trying to recall the memories, and simply the passage of time. The therapist, like the cognitive science researcher, can supply context cues, rehearsal, and motivation for the child survivor to recall autobiographical information central to their adaptive functioning.

RESTORING AUTOBIOGRAPHICAL MEMORY

Interventions to promote memory for the day-to-day activities that comprise a child or adolescent's life are key to restoring the child's ability to return to a normal developmental trajectory. As illustrated with Frank, inability to remember one's own behavior can strain relationships. Dissociative amnesia in traumatized children for day-to-day events tends to occur for behaviors involving aggression, violence, rudeness, or self-destructive acts—behaviors that children find embarrassing or would rather not remember. My clinical experience suggests that the factors affecting the severity of this type of amnesia include the aversiveness of the events themselves, the consequences of remembering, and the length of time that the children have practiced avoiding these types of memories.

You might wonder how one can distinguish between willful avoidance of acknowledging one's behavior, and real dissociative amnesia for one's own behavior. In order to effectively address this question, it is useful to conceive of amnesia as existing across a continuum. On one end of the continuum are cases of adult-like DID, where an individual seems completely oblivious to his or her own behavior in other identity states. Behaviors in an alternate self-state can seem completely out of character and foreign when dissociative clients are made aware of their behaviors. Dissociative individuals may be particularly skilled at "motivated forgetting" and with rehearsal and avoidance, learn to remove from awareness behaviors in themselves that they do not want to acknowledge. In addition, individuals with DID may have memories that are state-dependent, which can only be accessed when the individual enters certain states (Putnam, 1997). At the other end of the continuum are cases in which clients want to forget things they did that were embarrassing and claim they forgot to distract the interviewer and avoid the information. With gentle inquiry, these clients can remember or are willing to provide the details of what happened only moments later.

Children with dissociative symptoms fall somewhere in the middle of this continuum. Children are motivated to avoid remembering certain autobiographical information for a variety of reasons—fear of punishment, embarrassment about events, or the pain of confronting things about themselves that are discrepant with their self-view. Since we have described forgetting as a process that involves some degree of motivation, one could speculate that even momentary refusal to acknowledge a behavior could begin the subtle and elaborate process of motivated forgetting—if motivations to continue this avoidance are strong enough. Repeated avoidance of whole categories of one's own behavior, all angry episodes for example, could over time lead to selective memory in which children only remember events in which they were not angry.

Since amnesia found in dissociative children is often for behaviors for which they will likely receive some kind of negative consequence, children claiming they forgot are often perceived as manipulative and willfully avoiding consequences. It can seem strange for caregivers to look at amnesia as a continuum rather than a categorical phenomenon that is either there or not there. Caregivers often feel that acknowledging amnesia may give the child an excuse to avoid taking responsibility for misbehavior if they accept the child simply saying, "I forgot." Yet, amnesia is a subjective experience; as an outsider there is really no way to assess amnesia for personal information in a categorical way to determine if it is real. Moreover, entering into a disagreement with a client about whether they really don't remember, or just think they don't remember, or are just saying they don't remember, quickly becomes a useless exercise that evokes a power struggle that the therapist, teacher, or parent can never win. Thus, therapists and parents must walk the delicate line of sympathizing with the subjective feeling of memory loss, while encouraging and reinforcing all attempts of the child to develop increasing responsibility and awareness.

INCREASING MOTIVATION FOR MEMORY WITH ENVIRONMENTAL CONTINGENCIES

Armed with this theoretical understanding of autobiographical and traumatic amnesia, let's look at the intervention I used with Frank to help him gain access to memory for his destructive behavior at home. The method I employed can be applied to small momentary lapses of memory for recent behavior as well as severe dissociative episodes. First, I arranged with the school to put Frank on a behavioral reinforcement program. The goal of this program was to specifically address his difficulty with memory—*not* his behavior problems. According to the plan, each time Frank engaged in a destructive behavior at home, his parents were to call the school and the school would temporarily suspend Frank from the honors-level privileges that he had earned. As soon as Frank was able to remember the events in question and explain them and his own behavior, he could return to his honors-level privileges.

At first, Frank protested that since his behavior was fine at school, it was unfair to penalize him at school for behavior that occurred at home. The logic of our plan was explained to Frank in the following way, *"If you can't even remember your own behavior, it is not really safe to have you on the honors level at school, as we are counting on you to monitor yourself without staff watching you all the time. If you are not able to remember your actions, this level of freedom is not safe."*

Frank was also told that he would receive no increased punishment at home for remembering his behavior accurately; instead, in-home punishments would be reduced. Frank ultimately agreed to the plan. A week after this behavioral program was put in place, Frank's parents called the school to say that there was a deep knife scratch in the dining room table that Frank had denied memory for committing.

Many clinicians reading this will assume that once the plan was instituted Frank immediately started to remember his behavior at home. Unfortunately, Frank was adopted at age 9 from a traumatic environment where amnesia for his behaviors and the behaviors of his abusive caregivers was adaptive. Consequently, Frank's amnesia had been practiced and reinforced over many years. Even with the new motivational contingencies, Frank was unable to recall scratching the table. I did intensive therapy with Frank, working on identifying cues and associated emotions that might have triggered his behavior. I saw him three times a week for three weeks until Frank finally regained his memory.

Changing the contingencies provided the motivation for Frank to remember behavior he had previously been unmotivated to access. However, contingencies alone weren't enough. Frank also had to try and think about things he had spent his life avoiding and needed help to uncover the emotional triggers that led to his destructive acting out.

When working with children whose memory problems for recent behaviors are on the milder end of the continuum, it is still important that contingencies be put in place that reinforce remembering and responsibility. Even without memory for a given behavior, the family can impose consequences if the proof is indisputable that the child is the one who has engaged in the behavior or the child acknowledges it. Consequences for behaviors for which there is no proof and no memory will backfire, and probably *increase* rather than decrease memory barriers. With children who have behavior problems and associated amnesia, there are usually many incidents where families do have proof of the events. I recommend focusing on those events where there is a witness or hard evidence. The therapist might say, "*I know you don't remember doing this and it feels very unfair to you to receive this consequence. This is a very tough spot for you to be in and I would like to work with you to help you out of this unfair spot. Maybe the part of your mind that knows what happens can realize what an unfair bind you are being put in and can help you out of it.*"

When instituting consequences for disruptive behavior that the child can't remember, it is important that negative consequences are decreased once the behavior is remembered and described. For example, the therapist might explain, "*I know you don't remember breaking the garage door, and your parent will be so proud of you for working to get your memory back, that your community services at home will be one week less, if you can figure out with me how it happened.*" When imposing consequences for aggressive or destructive behavior with traumatized children, I prefer "community service" consequences that involve helping the family—helping clean the garage, raking the yard, sorting clothes—rather than depriving children of activities they enjoy. Traumatized children have not had enough time to enjoy their lives and be children, and so I don't like depriving them of growth-enhancing opportunities that outside activities often provide. Helping the family out with additional chores helps promote the kind of prosocial behaviors we are seeking to reinforce and also builds self-esteem. The family can then lessen the consequence once the child has regained his memory.

DESTIGMATIZING THE FORGOTTEN BEHAVIORS AND ASSOCIATED FEELINGS

Removing the motivational barriers to dissociative amnesia involves sensitivity not only to environmental contingencies, but also attention to the internal motivators that perpetuate amnesia, such as feelings of shame, humiliation, and self-disgust associated with self-awareness. Validating and highlighting the feelings associated with a forgotten event and destigmatizing them by noting how normal such feelings are can help to erode amnesia. The therapist can also help the child see that the behaviors make sense based on the feelings they were experiencing. By joining with young clients and telling them what they did was understandable, maybe even necessary, and by reinforcing every successful memory attempt, you can counter avoidance and reverse amnestic processes that may be in an early stage of development.

The following exchange illustrates how to destigmatize feelings and behaviors in clients with less severe amnesia than Frank. Alan, an 11-year-old foster child, destroyed things in his bedroom and claimed no memory for what happened.

Therapist: *Your mom tells me your whole room was wrecked and even your new video games trashed.*

Alan: Yeah, I know. I am so pissed. I don't remember doing it. She says I did it, but I really don't remember.

Therapist: *How awful for you, to have your whole room destroyed like that and not to even know how it happened.* [The therapist validates the stuck place of the client with no memory.]

Alan: Yeah, it's really bad.

Therapist: *I imagine for someone to trash your room like that they must have felt pretty angry and upset.* [The therapist associates feelings with the actions in abstract, without confronting or accusing.]

Alan: I guess so.

Therapist: *If you did it yourself, you must have been really mad, maybe even mad at yourself. Those were some strong feelings.* [The therapist highlights and validates feelings.]

Alan: I know. I don't remember.

Therapist: *Did you ever trash your room before? Do you remember how you felt a previous time you might have done that?* [The therapist tries to connect this behavior to previous feelings or events.]

Alan: I did it once at my group home after they wouldn't let me have a sign-out.

Therapist: *How wonderful that you can remember that you did it and why. You must have been really angry at not having the sign-out.* [The therapist reinforces even small steps in memory retrieval.]

Alan: Yes, it was very unfair. I earned it, but the other kids were acting out and they took privileges away from all of us.

Therapist: *That is really unfair. When things are so unfair, that level of anger is natural. I bet something really unfair is happening at your house now and that might give us a clue about what happened. What's unfair now?* [The therapist uses the child's words to make a bridge to possible feelings now.]

Alan: What's unfair is my bedtime. I am old enough to stay up until 10 o'clock. Also what's unfair is that my brother can play video games until 11 o'clock. He is only two years older.

Therapist: *So maybe it feels like it's hardly even worth playing video games when you have such a short time. Did you and your mom have a fight about this recently?*

Alan: Well, not a fight. She told me if I didn't turn off my video games, I would not be allowed to go to my baseball practice the next day and I was just asked to be catcher. They need me. I had to go; they were counting on me. It was so unfair.

Therapist: *Just like the group home, not being allowed to do something you really wanted to do was really unfair. How did you feel?*

Alan: Mad, I guess, I don't remember.

Therapist: *What did you do after your mom told you that?*

Alan: I don't know. I think I started kicking the door.

Therapist: *Wow. You are remembering. That is fantastic. What happened then?* [The therapist offers reinforcement for a small step in Alan remembering his own behavior.]

Alan: Then my mom said I definitely couldn't go to baseball. That was so unfair.

Therapist: *I don't blame you for being mad. You were counting on playing baseball and you were showing how angry you were, and then were punished for that.* [Therapist highlights the feeling.]

Alan: It's like I couldn't win.

Therapist: *You couldn't win. No video games, no baseball, no fun. A trap. It would make sense if you showed how trapped you felt.* [Therapist further amplifying and highlighting feelings.]

Alan: Yeah. What am I, an animal? That's how she treats me.

Therapist: *I can see why you say that because when you were little, the way your stepfather treated you was like you were an animal. No one should do that to you.* [Therapist makes bridge between present feelings and memory for past events that may relate to the child's feelings.]

Alan: I remember feeling really mad at my stepfather and my mom, too.

Therapist.   *That's wonderful that your memory is coming back.* [More reinforcement for memory.]

Alan: I might have thrown the covers off my bed then.

Therapist: *When you had no way to get your feelings out; you just found whatever you could to throw around.* [The therapist moves to the probable next step in his acting out his rage.]

Alan: Yeah, when I get that way, whatever is in my path is dead meat.

Therapist: *Even things that are special to you.* [Therapist validates and bridges to other things in the room.]

Alan: Even my own video games.

Therapist: *I can see how that could happen.* [Further validation.]

Alan: Yeah, I guess I did do it.

Therapist: *You had a good reason it seems. But now you've lost things you really care about. We should work on this.* [Therapist tries to instill motivation for change into the child.]

This technique of validating feelings and destigmatizing associated behaviors to promote autobiographical memory is also useful for children and teens who engage in sexual behavior for which they are amnestic. Destigmatizing the sexual activity involves validating feelings such as wanting closeness, wanting to feel desirable, wanting to feel loved, or even wanting to feel powerful in their sexual encounters. If the ways you reframe and destigmatize the experiences are accurate to the client, your interpretations will resonate with their experience. They will then be more likely to remember the experience and share how they were feeling when it happened.

With Frank, destigmatization was accomplished through psychoeducation about the value his anger may have served in his previous environment, and how anger is a valid and necessary self-protective feeling. The positive rewards for memory and reduction of negative consequences for memory retrieval also illustrated for Frank that his behaviors were not being labeled "bad," but were viewed as important clues to feelings that needed to be understood.

HIGHLIGHTING FEELINGS THROUGH ROLE PLAYING

Because arousal of affect is what initiates the dissociative avoidance, discovery of the precipitating affect can help restore awareness for forgotten events. The vignette with Alan illustrated how a therapist can try to suggest feelings that might have been associated with the type of behavior the child denies, and then use those feelings as a bridge for memory. For Frank, this was one of the most important techniques used to retrieve his memory. As with Alan, I emphasized feelings of anger to Frank, as Frank's destructive behaviors seemed clearly aimed at the things most precious to his adoptive mother. I also wanted Frank to begin to explore how people might feel if their precious objects were broken, and asked him to think about how he would feel if someone ripped up his precious baseball card collection. By helping Frank develop empathy for how people might feel if their things were broken, I was hoping to create an affective bridge to help him approach similar feelings in himself that might have provoked the behavior in question.

I played the role of Frank in an imaginary scenario of coming home from school and finding his baseball card collection destroyed. I asked him to play the role of someone who destroyed it. I said, *"How could you do that to my precious collection? I am so mad at you I could scream. Don't you have any respect for me?"* Frank role-played someone having initiated this hypothetical assault on his property and stated, "You deserved it. You don't love me." It seemed clear that Frank was getting closer to his own affective experience that might have led to the behavior for which he was amnestic. The memory of his behavior still did not surface after this intervention, but we were getting closer.

IMAGINE TOGETHER

Once emotions have been identified that seem to be associated with the missing block of time and the child survivor still can't access the appropriate autobiographical memory, the child and therapist might "imagine together" what might have transpired, and try to fill in any associated feelings or remembered events. For example, I said to Frank, *"So, Frank, let's say you might have felt angry when you came home from school, because you remembered the chores you were supposed to do when you got home and didn't feel like doing them. Can you imagine what you might have done?"* Even without the memory, the client can speculate about probable behaviors they know they *might* do in similar circumstances.

Frank said sometimes he would turn on the TV and just forget about things, or maybe slam the door to the house really hard. I asked Frank to imagine himself coming home angry and watching himself slam the door hard. I then asked him to imagine what he feels in his body, what he hears as he listens to the sound of the door, and what he thinks he might feel like doing next. The practice of imagining his own behavior when angry allows his mind to start approaching the forbidden material and may serve as a powerful cue to prompt retrieval of the actual memories. Please note, however, that this technique of having your own client imagine feeling a certain way, or imagine doing a destructive behavior he has wished to do, is completely inappropriate to use with attempting to recover traumatic memories of maltreatment involving someone else's behavior. Imagining events is a technique to use only to restore autobiographical memory for one's own behavior.

Through this technique, Frank was able to recall the smell of something cooking in a crockpot when he returned from school on the day the dining room table was scratched. He remembered he had slammed the door to the house when he walked in, and he remembered that the cat had been frightened. Frank then recalled looking at the dishwasher and feeling annoyed that it had to be emptied. He still could not recall scratching the table, but slowly we were making progress.

The technique of imagining together was also used with 13-year-old Steven (introduced in Chapter 6), who was brought by a worker in the juvenile detention center where he was being held for breaking and entering into his neighbor's home. Steven claimed no memory for this act and the treatment center wanted him evaluated for a dissociative disorder. Through "imagining together" what he might have done, what he might have seen, and where he might have found money in his neighbor's house, Steven was ultimately able to remember what had actually happened that day. Throughout the process, I reinforced Steven for how brave he was for working with me, hoping to combat Steven's own need to criticize and condemn himself for his behavior.

COLLECTING DATA AND DOCUMENTING CONTEXT CUES

When I work with dissociative children, the ongoing uncovering of hidden memory is framed as an important mission that we are working to accomplish together. This mission takes effort, and much of this effort must come from the client. Survivors of childhood trauma often have difficulty with goal-directed behavior and engaging in these efforts helps children understand that successful living involves effort, planning, and the identification of important goals to pursue. One way I enlist children in this goal-directed behavior toward memory retrieval is framing the missing information as a "mystery" that needs to be solved, and then enlist the child's skills as a junior detective.

Frank loved the Hardy Boys mystery series, and we used the metaphor of the amateur detective to help Frank become the detective on his own case. We set up a "case file" with questions such as "who?" "where?" "when?" and "why?" We filled in answers to these questions as we gathered clues. One of the clues, for example, was that Frank noticed that his cat was very jumpy when he first arrived home from school the day the table was scratched. He knows his cat gets jumpy from loud noises. Frank then deduced that he might have slammed the door, and wrote this down on our list of clues. We narrowed the time of the mysterious event by noting that the usual time he came home from school was 4 pm and the time his parents came home to discover the damage was 5:30 pm. Since Frank said he always watches a TV show from 4 pm to 4:30 pm, we deduced that the likely time the event occurred was between 4:30 and 5:30 pm. By focusing on these slowly accumulating clues, I helped Frank practice directing his attention toward the forgotten event. In effect, we were rehearsing retrieval skills directed at regaining his autobiographical memory.

I have used this technique on inpatient and residential units with teens who have a lack of memory for destructive or regressed behaviors they have engaged in. When working with dissociative teens, I first ask them to keep a notebook of any events they don't remember but in which they clearly played a role. I then ask them to interview staff members or peers, asking these observers to describe what they saw, along with any events that seemed to precipitate the client's behaviors.

Through this activity, I am enlisting the clients' self-observational skills and asking them to play an active role in focusing their awareness on their own behaviors. Once clients are required to take this much responsibility for self-observation, the frequency of switching between self-states usually decreases rapidly.

The notebook technique can also be used with families when a child or teen is unable to remember incidents that occur in their family life. I ask the child to keep a notebook in a central place and to record events that have happened. I ask everyone in the family to write down what happened based on their own point of view. The child or teen is motivated to write in the notebook as they want to describe anything that justified their own reactions, particularly when families have opportunities to comment on their own points of view, which are discrepant from the child's views. The child's self-observational skills improve as they practice focusing attention on their own behaviors and associated feelings.

LOOKING FOR HIDDEN DISSOCIATIVE STATES

After changing motivational contingencies, validating feelings, destigmatizing the events in question, and helping the client find clues to support memory retrieval, it is still possible that your client claims no memory for an observed behavior. In this case, it is possible that a hidden dissociative state may need to be accessed for full awareness. In these cases, the "listening in" skills described in Chapter 7 may need to be utilized, in conjunction with these other techniques. By asking the child to listen inside to any part of the mind that may have some information about the event in question, your client is likely to hear something or learn something helpful.

It was this "listening in" exercise that finally allowed Frank to discover what had happened at home the day the table was scratched. After several weeks of trying many of the techniques described here, Frank told me he heard something in his mind that called itself "Deep Anger." Frank told me that the voice of "Deep Anger" told him to "fight back" against his adoptive mother, who loved her "things" more than she loved him. "Deep Anger" was finally able to communicate internally to Frank and describe the whole story of how the dining room table was scratched.

Frank explained that the day of the incident, there was an afternoon special on TV that he was eager to watch. He knew if he didn't do the chores his mother had given him, he would be in trouble, and Frank didn't think there was time for both the chores and the television show. Feeling trapped by this bind, Frank slammed the door shut when he entered the house and frightened the cat, who growled and hid in a corner. The "Deep Anger" part of Frank's mind was angry at the cat for not showing him affection when he came home. He began to feel a sense of being unloved and unwanted, even by the cat. Remembering the chore he was supposed to do, the "Deep Anger" part of Frank's mind remembered the stern expressions on his adoptive mother's face when he failed to complete his chores. These stern expressions reminded him of how he was abused by his biological mother prior to his adoption. "How important could emptying the dishwasher really be?" Frank wondered. Was this more important than the TV show he wanted to watch? With "Deep Anger's" ongoing commentary in his mind, Frank remembered that he began to unload the dishwasher and took out a knife. Instead of putting it away, he went to the dining room and scratched the table, thinking, "That will teach her not to love her things so much! I should be what matters, not the things!" "Deep Anger's" name appeared to be quite descriptive of the feelings underlying Frank's destructive behavior.

Once this hidden state was discovered, Frank was open to helping "Deep Anger" to learn the differences between his birth home and his adoptive home, in order to help resolve lingering feelings of betrayal. The discovery of "Deep Anger" led to some important family work, where I helped Frank's new mother understand the hurt and betrayal Frank had felt with his biological mother and how some of these feelings were spilling over onto her. Frank's adoptive mother was able to reassure him that, indeed, *he* mattered more than her things; still, her things did matter to her, just as his things mattered to him.

Often, the discovery of a hidden state such as "Deep Anger" produces rapid therapeutic movement as the client and therapist can now "bargain" with the hidden dissociative state. For example, they can work to acknowledge the pain this part holds or offer other reassurances in return for cessation of the acting-out behavior. It was several months after the discovery of "Deep Anger" that Frank's destructive behavior at home completely stopped. In the interim, Frank got progressively better at accessing memories about his behaviors at home—from three weeks of intensive therapy, to two weeks, then one week. Eventually, Frank would page me the day after he had engaged in destructive activities, and say, "Get over here, Dr. Joy, I want therapy right away, so I can remember and get back on honors."

Finally, his own neural connections caught up with his motivation to remember, and Frank was able to maintain central awareness and refrain from the acting-out behaviors. Instead of acting out, Frank learned to write down what was making him angry and talk about it in our family sessions. I worked with Frank to develop a list of cue sentences to help him calm down when he got angry. This list included sentences such as, "My mom is different from the mom I left." "Things aren't people, but they matter, too." "Being angry is allowed, destroying things is not." This list of cueing sentences helped "Deep Anger" to remember his bargain to keep safe, and helped ground Frank by providing a link to our work in therapy. In addition, Frank was instructed to call my answering machine when he got home from school, just to hear my voice and to remind himself of the deals and contracts about safety that he had made with me. Frank's memory for autobiographical recent behavior continued to improve and by the time he was ready to graduate from his special school, he no longer showed any indication of a dissociative disorder.

Even if the "listening in" exercise is not productive, the therapist should not give up. The therapist can also work with the child to begin to develop clues, create safe contexts for remembering, identify the feelings underlying the behavior, and continue to explore with the client until he is able to fill in the missing details. If despite all of these techniques, the dissociative child continues to remain mystified about his own behavior, the therapist can describe the missing information as "the mysterious day," the "way you act, when you're like a zombie," or anything else descriptive. For example, I might describe the mysterious behavior as "the Jonathan who stole mom's kitchen knife." I will then ask, *"If there were such a Jonathan, how would he feel? What would he think? Why might he have done this, as surely he had a good reason?"* As you can see, the child claiming no memory has little reprieve in my office. I am determined to help the child find his central awareness, despite the many resistances that may be aroused in the process.

CAUTIONS

Some children and teens fear accessing memory for their own recent behavior as they fear that state-dependent memories of trauma will be aroused if they do remember. For example, a teenager who switches into a younger child state might fear activating terrifying memories of earlier abuse, which could be destabilizing and overwhelming. I have found that most clients utilizing the techniques described herein remember only the traumatic memories that are specifically related to the behaviors in question, and rather than feel overwhelmed by this knowledge are comforted that their behaviors have some inner logic. If they fear that they will be overwhelmed with old traumatic memories from remembering a recent behavior, the therapist should utilize imagery techniques to contain the traumatic content (described in Chapters 9 and 13), tucking them away in imaginary vaults until a future time when they can be understood and dealt with. Concerns about activating traumatic content should not derail efforts to help the client achieve integrated consciousness and memory about current behavior. It is extremely important for children to have consistently available autobiographical memory, as their functioning at home, school, and with friends is severely compromised without this. Thus, no matter how challenging it may seem, reversing amnesia for current behaviors must be a top priority.

OTHER CAUSES OF AMNESIA

When evaluating for the possibility of dissociative amnesia, it is important to always ask whether alcohol or other substances were involved. Use of substances, particularly alcohol, can produce "blackouts" where children and teens may engage in aggressive or sexual behaviors without memory. If the memory problem is a result of alcohol abuse, techniques for reversing amnesia will not be effective. Instead, involving the teen in an age-appropriate substance abuse treatment program may be necessary. When use of alcohol has progressed to the level that the child or teen is experiencing memory loss, the problem has likely reached a level of serious abuse.

Another increasingly common reason for memory loss, particularly at teen parties, is someone secretly spiking drinks with Rohypnol (flunitrazepam), GHB (gamma hydroxybutyric), Ketamine, or even Klonopin (clonazapam). A client who experiences memory loss after having a drink that was "spiked" usually describes missing from 4–24 hours of time, and not remembering anything about what transpired. Often, they will find their clothes in some state of disarray, and feel uncomfortable body sensations that suggest to them they were assaulted. These memories rarely return, but impressionistic feelings about what occurred and associated feelings of disgust and anger are common. If memory loss is atypical for your client, and occurred after consuming a drink where others were present, especially at a party with unfamiliar people, this type of drugging may be the explanation for what occurred. Teach your clients the importance of getting their own drinks from unopened bottles—particularly when they are in public areas or private parties where there are people with whom they are unfamiliar.

Another reason that you may be called upon to evaluate a child for amnesia is when the child fails to remember doing something that others presume they did. I evaluated a 12-year-old girl accused of harming a 4-year-old boy she was babysitting. The boy subsequently died from head injuries. The girl recalled him falling off the bed, but said that he didn't land on his head and could not remember anything that might have caused his death. A careful inquiry into the facts revealed that the young boy was showing clear signs of neurological compromise during the entire time she was caring for him. Ultimately, another perpetrator, the boyfriend of the mother, was identified as the real murderer. The boyfriend had struck the young boy in the head the day before. The girl who I evaluated had consistent memory for her time with the child, but was so fearful that something she had done had caused the boy's death that she accepted the idea that she had amnesia for the assault on the boy.

It is important to be skeptical, open-minded, and careful as an interviewer when questions of dissociative amnesia arise in a clinical setting. An attitude of acceptance and gentle inquiry will lead you to the truth if you are patient and validating, but relentless in pursuit of the real facts.

GLOBAL FORGETFULNESS

Sometimes, dissociative habits are practiced so often that clients develop a kind of generalized forgetfulness about everyday life. They may tell you that they have "a really bad memory" and can't remember simple things like whether they went to school the day before, what they had for lunch, or even basic math facts. These children are often diagnosed with AD/HD; however, inability to concentrate on activities of daily living can be a traumatic adaptation to a previous environment in which they felt perpetually helpless, ineffective, and traumatized. In these cases, not remembering has become an important survival skill, as everyday information could cue traumatic reminders. Knowing what was going to happen, or what had already happened, would only arouse feelings of helplessness and re-traumatization. Consequently, global forgetfulness has become the best strategy.

For these child survivors, I help provide the young person with abundant cues and practice in remembering. Rehabilitation is similar to that of brain-impaired clients who need external aids to cue memory, such as special organizing notebooks, buddies to remind them of assignments, daily e-mails home to caregivers with homework reminders, reliance on calculators or math fact tables, or classroom aides as they work in therapy to adjust to an environment where it is safe to remember. Appendix G provides a checklist to refer to when treating autobiographical amnesia.

Having addressed the disconnected awareness that leads to memory difficulties, it is time to focus our attention on disconnected awareness of the body itself. In the next chapter, I will address how to enhance somatic awareness, and deal with the hyperarousal typical of many chronically traumatized children.

9 Befriending the Body
Somatic Considerations for the Child Survivor

Tears streamed down Ellen's face during a consult while she talked about the family conflict that had led to a previous hospital admission. When I gently asked her what was wrong, she replied, "My face is wet." Ellen was so disconnected from her emotional world and its association with physical manifestations that she could not connect her wet face with the experience of emotion, and thus perceived the physical sensation without its associated emotional basis.

This chapter introduces techniques useful during the "A" phase of the EDU-CATE model, which promote the regulation of arousal and affect in the context of attachment. Many child survivors are estranged from the physical meaning of their body's signals. Some do not perceive the body signals at all, or misinterpret the sensations. Often, they perceive the signals of their body as unnecessary intrusions or threats that they try to silence through self-harm or avoidance. In other cases, children may feel sensations of pain unrelated to any current physical problem. Instead, their pain is based on somatic experiences from their past. Their bodies may be in a constant state of posttraumatic hyperarousal, with rapid heart rate and a frenetic intensity to their behavior, as if perpetually in flight from an enemy. A child with these types of somatic issues needs to learn to view his or her body as an ally and read its signals—attending to somatic signals that are relevant to the present, while calming ones that relate to a distant past. This is an ongoing process throughout all stages of therapy, but early attention to these issues may help your clients gain skills that will serve them well throughout treatment.

THE HYPERAROUSED CHILD

A person exposed to threat immediately experiences increased activity of the sympathetic nervous system, with associated increased heart rate and respiration, increased muscle tone, availability of sugar for energy to the muscles, and a narrowing of focus in awareness (Perry et al., 1995). This reaction to threat has wide-ranging implications for the entire body, as many bodily systems are impacted by the activation of the stress response, including brain regions that affect attention, motor activity, impulsivity, the startle response, sleep regulation, and even learning abilities and the immune responses (Ford, 2009; Perry et al., 1995).

With repeated activation, the threat response system becomes sensitized over time and can be set in motion by an increasing variety of minor stimuli. A state of hyperarousal becomes an enduring "trait" that comes to typify the child's behavior, even when threat is no longer present (Perry et al., 1995). Perry and colleagues contrast this hyperarousal response to threat with the hypoarousal response, which can also become a typical response pattern over time, even when threat is no longer present. This hypoarousal pattern is described in the following chapter, with an in-depth look at dissociative shutdown states.

Many children in my practice alternate between a hyperaroused style, with periods of extreme activation, and a hypoaroused style with periods of unresponsivity. As therapists, our clinical goal is to provide children with new tools for modulating the hyperarousal response without resorting to self-induced shutdowns, where they are impervious to all stimulation. Many of the teenagers I see who did not have access to therapy when they were younger have perfected these dissociative shutdown responses. The gradual shift from continuous hyperarousal to a state of hypoarousal may have a physiological basis rooted in the dysregulation of cortisol that is a consequence of trauma. Trickett et al. (2011) found that during childhood, the cortisol levels of abused girls were higher than in the control group. However, in adulthood, this pattern was reversed and abuse survivors had *lower* cortisol levels than controls. These findings suggest that children experiencing the developmental trauma of sexual abuse may have long-standing abnormalities in modulating their level of arousal.

Many of the hyperaroused children in my practice are young preschool children who have been recently removed from their families of origin where they were subjected to physical abuse, sexual abuse, and/or neglect. The first thing I notice clinically is their furtive moments. Unable to settle on any one toy in my office even briefly, they pick up toy after toy and then carelessly toss them aside as they search for the next one. Sometimes these children will briefly engage in posttraumatic doll play, throwing a baby doll down and saying "bad baby." At other times, they may become momentarily engrossed in a longer play scenario where a baby doll or its symbolic mother end up in danger or death, which then abruptly ends with another furtive movement or brief self-harming behavior like picking the skin, or banging the head. It is as if they are being flooded by a constant barrage of danger signals evoked both by the external world and their internal responses, and they dart frantically in an avoidance dance, as if dodging bullets. In this hyperaroused state, all of the necessary developmental tasks for their age will be sacrificed for the elusive goal of safety. In a state of perpetual hyperarousal, these children are unable to learn new things, play cooperatively with age-mates, or develop feelings of attachment and security with their new, safe caregiver. How do we calm down this fearful avoidance dance and get the child to a more optimal level of arousal?

Connecting on a Symbolic or Verbal Level and Reinforcing Safety

I have found that one way to calm down this type of frantic hyperarousal response is to gently and calmly use words to connect to the meaning of the child's behaviors and present my office and my presence as an end to the feared threat. These traumatized children are not used to someone tuning in to them accurately and empathically, and can't seem to believe that someone might know of or understand the frightening sounds and images of danger that are present in their minds. The children will suddenly stop their frantic movements, make eye contact with me, and pay attention to my words, as I comment on their fear and need for safety. New adoptive or foster parents watching are surprised by the sophistication and maturity these children can show when they feel that their experience has been understood and represented accurately. For example, if a child suddenly hits himself in the head, I gently hold the child's hand, and I say, *"When you just hit your head like that, I wonder if you heard someone say something scary in your head. I am going to keep you safe in here even from any scary things you might hear or see. No one gets hurt in here."* If the child acknowledges that they did hear something, I will immediately ask them to draw it or tell me about it. Using whatever name or description the child offers, I will gently invite even a "scary monster man" to help me find ways to make Johnny feel safe and loved. I say, *"I hope that scary monster man voice in your mind will work with me to learn about feeling safe. Maybe one day he will learn to relax, too, and say good-bye to the scary stuff."*

If a child is showing a baby doll hurt, and says "bad baby," I will gently respond, *"Maybe that baby feels bad because she keeps getting hurt, but no babies are really bad, let's try to help her feel better. I wonder if she knows that she could find a safe place one day."* Commenting in some way on the theme of danger as displayed by the child's behavior, and bringing up the idea and promise of safety with words and a reassuring tone of voice, is often helpful in the early stages of working with a hyperaroused preschool child. In my experience, these verbal interventions are very calming to these young children. Just as we talk to babies before they can fully understand all of the meanings of the words, verbal and symbolic interventions, even when they are not processed or understood completely, can help create an environment where young children can feel safer and calmer. The child responds to the tone of reassurance in my voice, the empathy I show toward the child's experiences, and my willingness to be present with them and their experiences. The importance of the nonsemantic aspects of verbal communication, including tone of voice to modulate a child's level of arousal, is described by Yehuda (2011), a speech pathologist who regulates and stabilizes traumatized children through nonverbal as well as verbal aspects of communication.

REGULATING AROUSAL THROUGH SENSORIMOTOR ACTIVITIES

Kindergarten teachers know that using songs and associated clapping movements can signal children to enter a calmer state; they will often use these rituals of claps and "sit-down time" songs before circle time in a classroom. According to Perry's Neurosequential Model of Therapeutics (2006), rhythmic experiences help to stimulate subcortical areas of the brain that may have been compromised during early developmental trauma. In my work with children, I often use songs, or repetitive poems, that reassure a child that safety and calm can replace chronic states of hyperarousal.

Tracy, who you met in Chapter 7, had been abused by a grandfather at the age of 7 while her mother was at work. At 9, severe separation anxiety would overwhelm her at school. Tracy would find herself unable to breathe and become preoccupied with worry about her mother. As part of her arsenal of calm-down strategies, I taught her to recite a brief poem as she looked at a picture of her mother.

> I know I can calm down today,
> Because my mom is here to stay.
> I may not see her in this room,
> But she will be here very soon!!

I instructed Tracy to recite these words while she used alternate hands to tap her knees, thus activating her brain bilaterally as recommended in Eye Movement Desensitization Reprocessing (Adler-Tapia & Settle, 2008). The creation of the poem, along with creating accompanying decorations and illustrations, and rhythmic recitation of the poem, helped counter Tracy's hyperaroused state, both at the level of cortical processing (creating art and processing the semantic meaning of the words) and subcortically (the soothing aspects of the rhyme and rhythm).

Children can be taught to slow down and regulate their breathing by placing a pillow on the abdomen and watching it move up and down as they slowly breathe to a standard count (Cohen et al., 2006). Generally, if I am teaching breathing techniques, I will accompany this with some auditory stimulation as well, using a sound machine that has a choice of sounds—waves, birds in a forest, wind, or rain. I ask children or teens to pick the sound that is most calming to them.

The sensation of touching a soft toy or fuzzy blanket can also help calm arousal. My office has many plush stuffed animals, pillows, and a blanket that children and teens can utilize to get themselves into a comfortable position. Rocking with a soft and cuddly stuffed animal may provide both rhythmic and sensory stimulation that can be calming. Even some adolescent boys are willing to attain comfort in this manner when the opportunity is available.

Most latency-age and adolescent boys prefer calming-down activities that involve controlled sensorimotor activation along with focus and concentration, such as supplied by video games, building materials such as Legos, or games such as pick-up sticks or Jenga (also called Timberrr, a building game where the object is removal of a block without causing the tower to fall). The effort used to control motor movements in these activities seems to channel children's hyperarousal, and the instantaneous reward of getting points, avoiding touching a pick-up stick, or avoiding making a tower fall, provides reinforcement for staying motorically calm to maximize achievement. I include activities like these during sessions to help hyperaroused clients calm themselves, particularly if intense and emotionally loaded material has been discussed. I also explain to parents that allowing their child to spend some time playing nonviolent, challenge-oriented video games at home can serve as a stress reliever for trau-matized and hyperaroused latency age and teen boys. Sometimes, deprivation of video games as a source of punishment will plunge these boys into full-blown rage reactions. The deprivation of the fun of these activities is not the only rea-son for this extreme response. Children often report that focused sensorimotor activities like video games are their main source of calming and self-regulation. While this outlet for stress relief can become addictive and overused, if the games are chosen carefully so as not to simulate interpersonal violence, and they are not the sole activity of the young person, they can play a role as one of the tools in the arsenal of calm-down activities.

In the children's inpatient unit of the Sheppard Pratt Health System where I consult, there are sensorimotor rooms with a variety of calming activities to help regulate the extreme arousal often found among our hospitalized children. Weighted blankets provide a sense of security by simulating the experience of holding and swaddling of an infant, and this can be profoundly calming on a subcortical level. Also available in the sensorimotor room are tilting and twirling seats in the shape of bowls that provide proprioceptive stimulation, large balls on which children can bounce that provide rhythmic stimulation, and soft chairs that mold to the child's body. Trauma therapists are increasingly recognizing the importance of these sup-plementary sensorimotor activities. In fact, some therapies for traumatized children, such as the Sensory Motor Arousal Regulation Treatment (SMART) program, have been developed specifically to regulate arousal through sensorimotor interventions (Zelechoski, Warner, Emerson, & van der Kolk, 2011).

IMAGERY

One of the primary modalities I use to help modulate arousal is safe-place imag-ery. I ask children or teens to tell me of a place that they remember feeling calm or at peace such as beach vacations, boating experiences, or camping in the woods. When envisioning their safe place, I try to get clients to think of somewhere re-moved from their everyday experiences so that no new associations in real life can taint the imagined safety of their image. Some children have not experienced a place that they consider safe and we create an imagined safe place together. An imaginary safe place can be anywhere, even on the moon or under the sea, as long as it is associated with peace and tranquility. However, it is important that the therapist can describe and reinforce sensory details about the imagined experience of being in the safe place, so you should not use a place like the moon as a safe place if the child will be upset that he or she cannot breathe there.

Once the children have identified and described an image of a safe place, I have her draw, or paint a picture of it. Having the child draw the safe place helps the therapist learn which details are salient to the child and these details can then be expanded upon during the imagery installation. The picture the child draws can then be hung in her bedroom to help remind her of it when trying to relax or fall asleep.

Imagery installation involves vivid suggestion of the safe place, after first inducing a relaxed state in the child with counting backwards, a magic elevator that takes you somewhere special, imagining a special flower-garden, or other induction techniques that appeal to children (see, e.g., Kluft, 1991; Wester II, 1991; Williams & Velasquez, 1996). These relaxation and imagery exercises are not formal hypnosis, but knowledge of hypnotic techniques used with children can help the therapist master the skill of inducing relaxation and suggesting vivid sensory details. The sensory details suggested during these exercises—such as feeling a cool wind on the face, warm sand between the toes, hot sun on the face, cool water all around—should be pleasant and easy for the child to imagine. This vivid sensory imagery helps to reestablish feeling sensation and bodily awareness as a positive experience rather than one associated only with overwhelming sensation and pain. The goal is to develop safe places that children can access in times of increased arousal. Other imagery techniques that can be adapted for children involve ego-strengthening exercises that emphasize the inner strength and internal coping resources that the child or teen has within (Phillips & Frederick, 1995; Wieland, 1998; Williams & Velasquez, 1996).

WHEN THE BODY IS NUMB

Traumatized children may be proud of their insensitivity to pain, sometimes bragging that they are able to withstand attacks from peers or endure painful illnesses or injuries without suffering. It is easy to see how numbing the body to pain is an adaptive strategy for children who have endured uncontrollable pain. Dissociation is employed as a strategy for coping with pain, not only by those suffering from childhood maltreatment, but also by those suffering from medical problems, such as burn injuries (Stolbach, 2005), chronic abdominal pain (Silberg, 2011), or the effects of painful medical procedures (Diseth, 2006).

While numbing may be adaptive in the face of unrelenting pain, insensitivity to body sensation can lead to problems in everyday management of bowel and bladder function. Insensitivity in this area is particularly common among children who have been victims of sexual abuse. Sexually abused children may have problems with involuntary urination or defecation as a reaction to even moderate stress, and they may lack the sensory awareness needed to work toward reversing these problems. There are several discrete reasons why problems with defecation and urination may be sequelae of sexual abuse for children. One reason is that relaxation of the bowel is a component of the fear response, as excessive adrenaline from sympathetic nervous system activation may shut down digestive organs, thus relaxing the intestines so that more energy is available to the muscles. At the same time, parasympathetic activation during severe stress may stimulate peristalsis. Thus a combination of decreased sphincter tone and increased peristalsis may result in stool escaping from the anus in an involuntary way. Similar muscles are involved in urination, and involuntary urination can result from overwhelming fear.

A second reason for dyscontrol in urination and defecation among sexual abuse survivors is the history of stimulation of the anus or urethra that is common during sexual abuse and becomes associated with fear. This fear generalizes to benign or normative stimulation of the anus or urethra during the process of evacuation or urination. As a result, the abused child may have an uncontrollable conditioned response of involuntary defecation or urination when confronted with something frightening, or a trigger reminding the child of events associated with abuse. Over time, continued involuntary activation of urination or defecation can lead to the progressive desensitization of sensation in the anogenital areas. Finally, perceptual sensitivity is further reduced by dissociative processes as the child learns to avoid awareness of the anogenital area in order to avoid triggers associated with any anogenital stimulation. The awareness of normal sensations of having to go to the bathroom is thereby compromised, which can lead to incontinence of urine or feces. Sometimes, these initially involuntary processes become organized around imaginary characters or identity states that are perceived by the child as responsible for the accidents (Waters, 2011).

Involuntary urination or defecation is an embarrassing problem that can take on a life of its own and spin the family in circles. Often, caregivers believe that the child has some degree of control over the symptom, as it happens more commonly at home than at school. Parents frequently react in anger when clothes are ruined, carpets are stained, and life is seemingly turned upside down by these symptoms. In fact, the family's extreme reactions to the problem can set a cycle in motion as the child or teen fights for some control within the family—even negative control. In these cases, any control the child does have over bowel and bladder elimination may be used to punish the family by having "accidents" on purpose. Because elimination problems in dissociative children tend to be multidetermined and complex, they can be very difficult to treat.

To reverse the cycle of negative reinforcement that easily can sustain these symptoms, the therapist must first destigmatize the behaviors through explaining that they are a natural and common effect of the kind of experiences that the child has suffered. The therapist must work with the child to find ways to reward and expand on small islands of successful mastery of feeling sensation and bodily control.

Samantha was a 10-year-old girl adopted at age 4 from a family in which she suffered physical and sexual abuse. She had made an initial positive adjustment in her new placement with a single mother, but had nighttime enuresis that would come and go over the years. When she experienced some problems with bullying in starting a new school in fifth grade, her nighttime wetting symptom spilled over to daytime, as well. She ended up having to leave school repeatedly with wet clothes, which led to more peer teasing upon her return. However, the symptom was reinforced as Samantha got to leave school whenever this occurred. Samantha reported to the therapist that she had no feeling when she had to urinate, but would suddenly just feel warmth and wetness trickling down her pants, and then she would run out of the classroom.

Immediately, I reinforced Samantha for being able to feel the "warmth and wetness." I asked her to describe it in detail and to draw a picture of what this sensation felt like. Even though this was the sensation that came *after* the involuntary urination, I wanted to help Samantha highlight the sensations that she did feel, as this would encourage her to focus inward on her body's sensations. I asked her to pay close attention the next time she has the "warmth and wetness" and jot down some notes in her journal about how the sensations felt and what thoughts she was having immediately preceding the involuntary urination. I encouraged her mother to back off the expectancy of having her regain control immediately, and with the school's permission, have Samantha attend a shorter day of school that minimized contact with the lunch bullies that she feared the most. The next time Samantha saw me, she reported that she had gotten better at controlling her urine, and that it had only happened two times. She reported that she noticed she had scary thoughts right before she wet herself that sounded like "a mean girl" saying "you deserve it."

When I asked her whose voice the "mean girl" sounded like, she said it sounded a little like her biological aunt who used to yell at her before her adoption. Thus, it was clear that Samantha's involuntary urination was associated with traumatic memories from the past as well as the present trauma of being bullied by "mean girls" at school. Together, we wrote a letter to the "mean girl" in her mind. We asked for her help in helping Samantha learn to "feel her pee coming out" and we explained why we thought Samantha did not really "deserve" the bad things that happened, either in the past or now. Because she seemed to know so much, we also asked the voice to help Samantha with learning how to "pee with more control." Samantha reported feeling that the voice "felt better." I encouraged Samantha to continue to tune in to the feelings she had before and after an episode of involuntary urination, but also to tune in carefully to the times she was able to go to the bathroom by choice and describe those feelings as well. Samantha's involuntary urination resolved relatively quickly after that; the voice of the "mean girl" that Samantha reported hearing never came to the forefront again in the therapy.

The "mean girl" seemed to represent a short-lived dissociative fragment that related specifically to the involuntary urination and traumatic activation of fear that the peer bullying aroused in Samantha because of her traumatic past. This symptom was resolved through a five-step process: (1) addressing the current trauma through reducing exposure to the bullies, and ultimately a change in schools; (2) destigmatizing the symptom; (3) reducing its power in the family to begin a cycle of negative reinforcement; (4) engaging the dissociative voice as an ally; and (5) helping Samantha tune into her body sensations more effectively by reinforcing small steps in this process.

Problems with bowel incontinence can be addressed similarly. With encorpresis, the colon becomes chronically distended from constipation and stool leaks around a hard mass of collected stools in the colon. This leaking stool causes staining of the underwear without accompanying sensation. The distended bowel causes the colon to lose sensation, which compounds the lack of sensitivity resulting from dissociation and a history of abuse. It is important to work alongside a medical practitioner in these cases, as the child may need to be on laxatives to reduce the bowel distention that aggravates this problem. Waters (2011) describes a dissociative child with encopresis whose symptoms were resolved through identifying all hidden states, nonverbally processing memories of abuse, and encouraging the whole self to work together. It is also important not to assume that all encopresis is trauma-related, as this is a fairly common pediatric problem that often arises without a specific trauma history. Refer to Appendix H for a therapist checklist to manage urinary and bowel incontinence.

Lack of sensitivity to body sensations can affect eating behaviors as well, as child survivors may undereat because they may not be aware of feelings of hunger, or overeat because they do not experience the sensation of fullness. Sometimes, children experience hunger in several different states of awareness. These children may have no memory that they have just eaten, and ask for a meal again. This symptom is more common in children who have come from neglectful homes where they were not fed on a regular basis, and normal cues of satiety and hunger have not developed adequately. As with other somatic symptoms, the therapist can help the child tune into body sensations, name them, draw them and describe them. When multiple dissociative states are competing for food and the child is amnestic for his behavior, the therapist should try bargaining and working on cooperation, as described in Chapter 6.

HURTING THE BODY

One of the most alarming adaptations that children may develop to cope with trauma is the habit of self-harm. This may include hair-pulling, picking nails or skin, head banging, and cutting or stabbing themselves using razor blades or other dangerous objects.

It is not surprising that survivors of painful trauma will try to achieve a sense of control over their bodies by inflicting pain to themselves. They find some comfort in inducing familiar sensations. In addition, self-inflicted harm is powerfully reinforced by stimulating the body to release endorphins, which are internal opiates that can have a drug-like effect. Self-harm can radically interrupt an uncomfortable affect state, which children feel they have no other way of regulating (Yates, 2004). Self-harm may also serve as a symbolic demonstration of their plight, as if to communicate to observers a powerful message about what they feel they are worth, or how they perceive themselves being treated.

Ferentz (2012) compiled a comprehensive checklist of 29 different reasons people may engage in self-harm. I have adapted her checklist for children and adolescents and it is included in online Appendix I. This self-injury checklist may offer a springboard for discussion about reasons children may harm themselves. Teens may identify multiple reasons for self-harming behaviors, including communication of their pain, regulating mood, punishing themselves, or inhibiting aggression toward others. On the other hand, younger children are often completely unable to articulate why they engage in repetitive self-harming behaviors.

When addressing self-harm, it can be helpful to explain to children that there are powerful physiological processes that sustain the behavior. I usually start with explaining that the body has its own way of handling pain by releasing its own drug that combats the pain. I ask them to remember the last time they had a sore in their mouth and to recall whether they took their tongue and touched the sore repeatedly even though it was painful to do so. I explain that the reason our tongue goes there, even though it is painful, is because unbeknown to us, touching the sore releases this internal drug. I explain that it is almost as if touching the sore in your mouth can become a momentary addiction. This explanation helps children and teens understand the physiologically based compulsion they feel to engage in the behavior, the power of which is often mysterious and inexplicable before they hear this explanation.

It is much easier to treat self-harming behaviors before they have become habitual and ritualized. Helping to motivate children to stop self-harm is key to successful treatment. However, as Ferentz (2012) points out, many teens will not feel ready to deal with this symptom if they are not convinced that another "life vest" for managing feelings is available to them. One source of motivation to work in therapy to stop self-harming behaviors is concern about others seeing their cuts or scars. For example, some clients are concerned about how their body may appear when summer comes and the harm inflicted on their body will be more visible. Other motivations to work with the therapist may be fear of their parents discovering it or knowledge that it feels and looks "gross." It is a good sign when children express embarrassment about showing their body to their friends, as it suggests the behavior is not really ego-syntonic. Younger teens and children are easier to motivate than are older teens, as the latter tend to retain discomfort about the behavior. With older teens, the therapist must be cautious not to reinforce shaming negative self-cognitions about their self-destructive behavior (Ferentz, 2012). With children or teens that have internal voices, imaginary friends, or dissociative states that encourage self-harm, the therapist must try to bring that dissociative state into alliance with the child, and reframe their usually negative motivations in more positive ways.

Once children or teens have been educated about the physiology of self-harm, and their motivation to work with the therapist has been established, the therapist can work with them to identify "danger times," when the desire to hurt the self is aroused. These "danger times" may be times of extreme emotional arousal, often during conflicts in interpersonal relationships, such as during family fights, being picked on by other children, or talking with an old boyfriend. The desire to self-harm, such as picking the skin or pulling hair, can even be aroused when the child or teen describes being bored, such as when they are mindlessly playing on the computer or studying.

Once danger periods are identified, the therapist should work with children and teens to identify a variety of alternative behaviors that they can engage in when the urge to self-harm occurs. Ferentz (2012) described a series of substitute behaviors that the client can engage in to replace the self-harm; these behaviors follow the acronym CARESS. The client is asked to agree to "Communicate Alternatively" by creating a picture or other description of the desired behavior, "Release Endorphins" though active exercise, and lastly, "Self-Soothe" by doing something positive for the self, such as a bath. I usually encourage children to seek some communication with a caregiver who can assist with supporting the alternate behaviors during identified "danger" times. Young children readily understand the concept of "danger" times and are usually able to identify these and seek help from the parent.

With younger children engaged in picking their skin or nails, picking sores, or hair-pulling, I advise the parents to gently redirect them by substituting a planned alternative, like petting a rabbit's foot or squeezing a stress ball. One young child who engaged in hair-pulling was able to substitute pulling on the elastic "hairs" of a "koosh" ball. For young children, it is important to build in concrete rewards, such as stickers or options to see movies or go on outings, for successfully replacing the self-harming behavior with new behaviors.

HEAD-BANGING

Sudden onset of head-banging behavior—punching the head, or banging the head on a wall—is a symptom of acute distress, and is generally associated with some inescapable bind or harmful experience that the child is enduring and unable to report. Head-banging in traumatized children is generally associated with a child trying to silence or inhibit direct communication about some current danger. These children may be hearing a voice in their mind telling them to harm themselves, or may be violently stopping themselves from talking about something frightening that may be happening to them. Violently hitting the head is a way to deal with the impulse to tell, especially if the child has been threatened. Clinicians should take head-banging very seriously and investigate where harm in the environment may be coming from, or what internal impulse or voice the child is fighting. Hospitalization may be necessary to fully evaluate the traumatic source of this behavior.

On the other hand, chronic head-banging at bedtime, particularly in children with developmental disabilities or early neglect, may be part of a self-soothing night-time ritual, and is not as serious as its sudden onset in the day.

Six-year-old Estie tried to jump out of her second-story window directly before a visitation with her father. The visits were being supervised after Estie disclosed that her father had abused her. On initial evaluation, Estie began hitting her head and running out of the room when asked about her visits with her father. Careful interviewing finally revealed that Estie heard the voice of her father talking to her in her mind, calling her and her mother abusive names. Even though the domestic violence had stopped with father out of the home, when Estie was in close proximity to her father, she experienced flashbacks of her father's abusive language. At age 6, Estie was unable to distinguish between the voice in her mind during flashbacks and the actual voice of her father. Therefore, even in the supervised setting, she experienced her father as actively disparaging her and her mother. After a short hospitalization, Estie was stabilized, and the family court judge was convinced that Estie would be further psychiatrically harmed by continued visitations. The judge wisely gave Estie time to heal in therapy from her posttraumatic stress before requiring further visitation. Unfortunately, many judges cannot appreciate that supervised visits with abusers can provoke flashbacks that to young children can feel just as vivid as the actual abuse they experienced.

SOMATOFORM PAIN AND CONVERSION SYMPTOMS

Dissociative children may experience a wide range of somatic symptoms with no apparent physical cause that appear to be related to past traumas. Nijenhuis (2004) has termed this somatic reexperiencing "somatoform dissociation." As Nijenhuis points out, recognizing somatic symptoms as dissociative symptoms is consistent with the writings of Pierre Janet, on whose insights much of the contemporary dissociation literature is based.

One of the most surprising symptoms that child survivors may show is somatic reexperiencing of injuries, often at the site of some original injury. Waters and Silberg (1998b) described a boy who reported feeling a cold spot on his back, for which there was no explanation. His older brother reported that, as a baby, the boy had been placed in a freezer by their abusive parents, for which the younger child had no conscious memory. Other children report unexplained pain that coincides with places they have been injured in previous placements.

One of the ways I frame these sites of pain for children is to tell them that it is their body's way of asking questions such as: "Am I safe yet?" "Can I relax and feel better now?" Then I ask the child if they might like to ask those questions to their new, safe caregiver. In family sessions, we may playact the body asking these questions to the caregivers, who then can answer with reassuring statements about their safety, and provide soothing massage, or application of imaginary "magic love potions" at the site of the pain.

For older children and teens, I use imagery such as entering magic healing pools, or other magical pain-relieving images as the client is encouraged to imagine a healthy, pain-free body. I also ask children if they perceive any blockades to healing the pain. If there are, I ask them to bring these blockages into central awareness so we can address them. Children and teens who enter dissociative states frequently experience severe headaches, accompanying the shifts in state or upon arousal from these states. Whatever their cause, these headaches are amenable to imagery techniques about "tight helmets" getting looser, or other images that capture the child or teen's perception of what the pain feels like.

Some children or teens present with perplexing physical disabilities, such as an inability to walk or use one of their arms. These can be severely disabling and result in missing school or inability to participate in normal activities. Some have argued for the inclusion of these "conversion symptoms" under the rubric of dissociation in the DSM diagnostic scheme (Bowman, 2006; Brown, Cardeña, Nijenhuis, Sar, & Van der Hart, 2007). I have found that the first step in helping children who experience conversion symptoms is to honor the child's perception of being unable to function, while at the same time instilling hope that they will find a new path out of their dilemma. For example, to a child who suddenly finds that he cannot move his legs due to pain, I might say, "*I realize that no matter how hard you try, you cannot move your legs. That must be scary for you and feel strange. Your body is clearly telling you through that pain that it is unsafe to move your legs, and I would believe your body when it tells you that. I am quite sure when your body feels that it is safe again to move your legs, you will be able to. I am not sure what it will take, but I will work with you until your body is able to feel safe moving your legs again.*" Framing it this way makes it clear to the client that you are accepting that the pain might be either physical or psychological, and plants the suggestion that there will be a time when there will be a recovery of function. Along with a nonjudgmental approach about the conversion symptom, I encourage clients to attend physical therapy programs and other physically supportive programs, without judgment over whether the pain is physical or psychological.

Mandy, a 15-year-old girl, presented with sudden onset of pain in her hips, pain so disabling that Mandy could not bend at the waist and was unable to use the bathroom without assistance. A medical evaluation determined that there was no physiological explanation for the incapacitating pain. The pain began when a new boyfriend of the mother had moved into the house, and Mandy's activities had become more and more limited. She stopped attending school and was spending most of her days confined to bed, and was ultimately admitted to a psychiatric floor in a medical hospital. At the hospital, an occupational therapist provided Mandy with a cane to walk and provided an assistive device so that she could use the bathroom independently.

Given the space from her mother, in individual therapy Mandy was able to talk openly about her early history, during which her mother had had many different boyfriends, which had been confusing to Mandy. Whenever she began to talk about one particular boyfriend, Mandy became panicky and reported that her pain escalated, and she needed to go back to her bed. I commented that the pain seemed to relate to this man and I suggested it might be very frightening to think about him, but reminded her that she was safe at the hospital. Ultimately, Mandy remembered that the man had sexually abused her and threatened that if she told, her mother would be hurt. Mandy remembered a time that she had bumped her hip on her bed frame and was allowed to stay home from school, and her mother had stayed home from work and cared for her. Thus the pain in Mandy's hip had indirectly protected her from being abused by the boyfriend who used to babysit for her after school while her mother was at work.

When her mother's latest boyfriend moved in, it rekindled Mandy's fear and memory associated with this past abuse. Mandy felt trapped in the current situation and was afraid to tell her mother about the past abuse because of the history of threats. Her memory of this event, the fear of the new man in the house, and the sense of being trapped found expression in Mandy's hip pain. The pain helped Mandy feel "protected" from her mother's new boyfriend and the memory of the old boyfriend, and symbolically expressed her sense of being trapped. Although Mandy felt unable to disclose her past abuse and her fears of it happening again, her body found a way to "tell" nonverbally that she was "stuck" and could not move. After a series of intense sessions in which Mandy processed the abuse, and expressed her anger and sense of betrayal to her mother, the pain dwindled and eventually faded away. In family sessions, Mandy's mother also heard Mandy's fears about the new man in mother's life, and plans were made that Mandy would not ever have to be alone with him after school. After discharge, Mandy continued to improve and continued with individual therapy and family therapy. Official reports were made to the social service department in the town in which Mandy and her mother had been living when the abuse occurred, and an investigation began about the whereabouts of the man she remembered abusing her.

EMBODIED MASTERY

There has been a burgeoning development in the field of Sensorimotor Therapy for adults (Ogden & Minton, 2000; Rothschild, 2000). This therapy approach is based on the idea that motor responses to fight or flee at the time of threat are often blocked during overwhelming trauma, and these unprocessed, incomplete actions are the source of many of the somatic symptoms that traumatized people display (Levine, 1997). Sensorimotor therapy involves helping the client remember the sensorimotor reactions the client experienced during the time of trauma and processing these while in a state of optimal arousal. The client is encouraged during the therapy session to complete the blocked action by moving the muscles that were frozen during the time of original trauma (Ogden & Minton, 2000; Ogden, Pain, Minton, & Fisher, 2005). This approach helps clients learn to become more aware of their body sensations and can reverse the numbness and disconnection that some trauma survivors experience.

The concept of completing actions that the body wanted to take, but couldn't complete during trauma can be helpful when working with children. During trauma, the sympathetic nervous system is activated, preparing the body for fight or flight. However, in young children, these options are rarely available to them. They are too small to fight and often too overpowered to flee, and thus their bodies tend to freeze. Using therapy props—toys, sandtrays, clay, and art supplies—or activities with their bodies, children and teens can be encouraged to actively resolve traumatic scenarios in action. I call therapeutic activities in which the children restage symbolic resolution to traumatic events "embodied mastery." For young children who have been traumatized, we may practice together running as fast as we can to get away from "bad people"—set up symbolically with toys that recreate a scenario similar to their own traumatic experience. I will sometimes run down the hall with a child, or outside on a nice day, pairing the running response with the imagined escape from the traumatic event. This activity works well for developmentally disabled young people as well who enjoy the powerful feeling of "running away" and validation of their feelings of having wanted to escape.

Ernie was a 5-year-old boy who had been abused by a 14-year-old cousin who worked as his babysitter. We placed a doll representing his cousin on a chair in the therapy room, and Ernie giggled with glee as we repeatedly practiced running away from the doll while saying, "You are not allowed to do that to little boys; I am running to tell my mommy." This reinforced both the escape response that was blocked at the time of trauma as well as rehearsed an important child safety rule—inform a caring adult when you are hurt. Even teens can enjoy behavioral reenactments that give them new sources of strength in combating a remembered trauma. This rehearsal of physically empowering responses to trauma can also be done with imagery, which is described in more detail in Chapter 13.

As children and teens practice a variety of motor responses to past traumatic events, the therapist can help teach them how posture and the way they carry themselves is associated with confidence, fear, or depression. Sometimes, I demonstrate this by exaggerating the body posture associated with certain feelings and create dances or exercises to display how the whole body is engaged in an emotion. I worked with a child who had trouble saying "No" to the inappropriate requests of friends. We practiced a "No" dance, with good posture, a smile, and marching movements. The "Yes" dance of acquiescing, on the other hand, involved stooped shoulders, dragging feet, and lowered head. Thus, the dances symbolized either the power of appropriate boundaries or the demoralization of complying with something inappropriate—an important lesson for survivors of interpersonal trauma.

Sometimes the effect of traumatic experiences compromises the body to such an extreme that it seems the body has entered a state of profound collapse. In the next chapter, you will meet children and teens whose modulation of arousal is so impaired that they may enter extreme states of hypoarousal in which they are impervious to environmental stimuli.

10 Staying Awake

Reversing Dissociative Shutdown

She was not responsive to my voice or gentle touch. Her face was pale and her body limp. Her breathing was rhythmic and shallow. Do I call the medics? I wondered, or have her mother carry her out? Luckily, she was my last client for the day so I had time to process the dilemma of how to physically end my session with this unresponsive teen. I was seeing dissociation in its most extreme form—the body shutting down in a position of "freeze," similar to the way animals respond when a predator has caught up with them. What in my session did 17-year-old Jennifer perceive as predatory? There had been a casual conversation about college plans and a boyfriend. There had been no talk of abuse memories or frightening experiences. How did she get into this sleep-like state? I wondered, more importantly, how do I wake her up?

Jennifer was demonstrating the other pole in the arousal continuum—a state of stress-induced hypoarousal. Sudden dissociative shutdown may have multiple pathways. One common reason for sudden blackouts is the vasovagal reflex, which causes a reduction of blood and oxygen to the brain, accompanied by a drop in heart rate and blood pressure, slowing of respiration, and relaxation of skeletal muscles, resulting in a temporary loss of consciousness commonly referred to as "fainting" or "syncope." This reflex can be precipitated by a variety of physiological triggers, such as standing up too quickly, or by emotional factors, such as suddenly hearing overwhelming news. Fainting can also be precipitated by triggers that remind one of an emotional event, particularly in vulnerable individuals with a history of trauma whose brains have been conditioned to respond to emotional triggers with dissociative states. In Jennifer's case, the vasovagal reflex causing syncope may have been only one small part of the picture. Usually, with syncope, the restoration of blood supply to the brain when the individual goes into a reclining position causes her to wake up. In this case, Jennifer stayed in an apparent unconscious state, despite being in a reclining position.

Jennifer's resistance to waking up even after reclining was probably mediated by another section of the vagus nerve in reaction to stress. The vagus nerve regulates heart rate, respiration, and digestion, and is a key player in the parasympathetic branch of the autonomic nervous system, the branch of the nervous system generally associated with resting or restorative states. Porges's (2003) Polyvagal

Theory posits that the two branches of the vagus nerve perform different functions. The dorsal or back branch of the nerve, stemming from our primitive evolutionary roots, regulates escape from threat; while the ventral or front branch of the vagus nerve fosters and regulates social emotional engagement. The more primitive branch of the vagus nerve takes over functioning in situations of inescapable threat, where it is adaptive for the organism to withdraw from the outside world and conserve body function. This immobilization of the body stimulated by this primitive vagal response causes slowing of heart rate, slowing of respiration, and loss of muscle tone, and also the release of endogenous opioids that dull pain sensation.

Bruce Perry (2002) emphasizes this internal release of endogenous opioids—self-calming and self-soothing hormones that dull pain sensation—as a central feature of this kind of psychological shutdown. According to Perry et al. (1995), these kinds of episodes are best understood as sensitization and dysregulation of the central nervous system's opioid systems that have been repeatedly activated due to extreme stress. This activation and reactivation becomes an enduring "trait," so that small reminders of trauma can stimulate profound reactions where traumatized children have sudden alterations in consciousness. Perry points out that medical professionals are often puzzled by this type of shutdown and may diagnose them as "syncope of unknown origin," "conversion reactions," or "catatonia." Perry has had success reversing these states in children using the drug naltrexone, which directly blocks the opioid receptors (Perry, 2002).

In the literature on dissociative children, unexplained physiological manifestations involving odd motor movements and other behavioral signs along with absence from awareness have been termed "somatoform dissociation" or "night spells" (Waters, 2011). When brought to neurologists, these children are often diagnosed as having psychogenic nonepileptic seizures (PNES), formerly referred to as pseudoseizures. In the DSM-IV, these psychogenic seizures would be classified as "conversion disorder" or "somatization disorder," which "can be characterized by the presence of symptoms or deficits affecting voluntary motor or sensory function" and include apparent seizure-like activity (APA, 2000, pp. 492–493). Based on her experience with 800 patients with conversion seizures, Bowman (2006) argued that PNES is best understood as a dissociative disorder. Up to two thirds of adult dissociative patients have some conversion symptoms (Bowman, 2006).

Nijenhuis, Vanderlinden, and Spinhoven (1998) have pointed out that animals in the wild display a freeze and submission response, which may be the evolutionary root of the dissociative response we see in humans subject to extreme terror. The tonic immobility or "playing dead" that animals display, associated with analgesia, prepares an animal for its fate of becoming prey, or may fool the predator into finding another victim. This tonic immobility in the face of terrifying attack is an involuntary response in humans, as well. One study shows that up to 37% of rape victims go into a freeze mode, which actually leads to increased self-blame and increased posttraumatic stress symptoms when the attack is over (Galliano,

Noble, Travis, & Puechl, 1993). Newer brain imaging studies have demonstrated that the physical analgesia found in animals that freeze in response to a predator is a documented phenomenon in patients during dissociative states (Ludäscher et al., 2010). Older theorists termed the submissive response of animals to a predator "animal hypnosis" (Ratner, 1967). This terminology foreshadows the next phenomenon that we will explore that may explain Jennifer's reaction in my office.

So far, we can surmise that Jennifer may have suddenly lost consciousness due to loss of blood to her brain as a result of fainting from an emotional trigger, may have had a dorsal-vagal response to threat involving slowed heart rate, breathing, and poor muscle tone, and that her body may have released endogenous opioids, an analgesic, to dull her body from expected pain, showing the tonic immobility of an animal facing its prey. Does that explain everything? Is Jennifer simply reacting as a terrified animal in threat?

I would suggest that there is at least one more brain pathway to consider in accounting for Jennifer's unresponsiveness—the phenomenon of hypnosis. This last physiological explanation of Jennifer's dissociative state is one that is mediated through the higher centers of the brain. It is regulated by the cerebral cortex, unlike the fainting and freeze responses described earlier, which originate in lower, subcortical brain centers.

So what do we know about hypnosis? It is a state of altered consciousness involving intense focus, which can lead to some documented physiological changes, many of them similar to the ones evoked by the vasovagal response and the prey submission response. These changes include slowed breathing, slowed heart rate and blood pressure (Diamond, Davis, & Howe, 2008), and even unique patterns of neural activity (Barnier, Cox, & Savage, 2008). Brain imaging studies described by Barnier et al. (2008) have recently demonstrated that hypnosis is indeed a unique physiological state, involving specific brain activity that cannot be simulated by unhypnotized people. New neuroscientific findings suggest that these hypnotic states are physiologically similar to dissociative states in that both involve similar patterns of prefrontal neural activation (Bell, Oakley, Halligan, & Deely, 2011).

The similarities in physiological processes between the vasovagal response (syncope), the dorsal-vagal mediated prey submission response, and hypnosis suggest a possible pathway for the development of dissociative responses. My theory of dissociative shutdown posits both a conscious component of dissociative responses and a more primitive nonconscious one. A child faced with a repeated frightening event—such as repeated rape by a caregiver, from which there is no escape—may respond at first with a primitive fear response involving fainting or freezing. Over time, this response may generalize to associated stimuli as thoughts and feelings about an impending visit with their perpetrator can lead to the shutdown state. During this state, the child might perceive herself as having left her body and created an imaginary world that she retreats to where bad things are not happening. Although the body is immobilized, the mind remains active and can invent solutions. With time and practice, the ability to escape to this other world may become automatic. The mere thought of needing to escape a situation may now trigger a self-induced hypnotic retreat along with the associated nonconscious and more primitive freezing response.

In my proposed model of the development of a dissociative response style, the child soon learns to anticipate the freezing response and learns to "go away in their head," inducing this state as needed in preparation for anticipated harm. Thus, dissociative disorders may evolve as the developing child's mind finds ways to regulate the automatic physiologic responses to fear and organize them into escape fantasies through autohypnotic suggestion. These processes may, in turn, become subject to automatic conditioning by traumatic triggers.

The dual component of these processes, both conscious and nonconscious, becomes important as we talk about intervention. Treatment involves finding ways to make nonconscious escape processes, which appear to take on an increasingly autonomous life, back under the control of the individual. Hypnotic processes thus may provide a therapeutic bridge for helping clients to gain more control over dissociative states.

Theory goes only so far when a child is lying limply on your couch, with no indication of achieving consciousness any time soon. I asked Jennifer's mother to come into the room and she gently shook her daughter, saying, "Jennifer, session is over," in a calm motherly tone. No response. I suggested to Jennifer in a hypnotic tone that she would find herself getting more and more awake, ready to face hard roadblocks in her life. No response. Together, Jennifer's mother and I decided to call 911. Jennifer's mother was surprisingly calm, apparently accustomed to the strange behaviors we had come to expect from Jennifer. The medics took Jennifer to the local emergency room, and I thought as they transferred her to the stretcher and then the ambulance she would wake up. She did not.

Two hours later, my cell phone rang. "Dr. Soybean" (her playful name for me), Jennifer implored, "tell the hospital doctor that I do not need psychiatric admission, and that I am not crazy!" Relieved as I was to know that Jennifer had woken up from her dissociative slumber, I saw a great opportunity to move her forward therapeutically. I asked Jennifer to come to my office first thing in the morning and if she could successfully explain what happened in the exact moment preceding her dissociative shutdown, I told her we could avoid the hospitalization. If, however, she was unable to uncover the feelings that led to this self-defensive reaction, I thought it would make sense for her to go the hospital after our session. Jennifer agreed to this, and I told the ER doctor that she would be fine and we would process her reaction in the morning and help her learn how to avoid reactions like this in the future.

The next session involved the kind of "fishing expedition" that is often required with dissociative patients. Blocked from the feelings that usually help people string together a coherent narration of events, memories, and sequences, the dissociative client's reactions and responses often appear as mysterious to themselves as they do to others. Jennifer remembered we had talked about her high school science project, her ambition of being a biochemist, and a boyfriend she was outgrowing. She had come very far from the early years of therapy immediately following a sexual assault from a neighborhood boy, when her dissociative reactions were often this severe. I suggested that something in our conversation had awakened for her the old feelings of being trapped, helpless, frozen, and unable to move forward. As Jennifer got in touch with this feeling, she suddenly remembered what in our conversation aroused this feeling in her. When we talked about college, Jennifer remembered that her father had threatened to withdraw college funding for her chosen school if she did not agree to overnight visits at his house. Jennifer's parents were divorced with joint custody. Her father lived 40 miles away and as she had gotten older, she often had plans that made it inconvenient for her to visit him. While the court no longer enforced these visits due to her age, her father had found a new way to force her to visit him.

Interestingly, never in the course of our seemingly casual therapy session that day did this threat from her father emerge enough for her to explain it. Instead, her mind remembered the feeling of being trapped and hopeless, and responded with the same dissociative response she had used as a younger child experiencing repeated sexual assaults and observing domestic violence in her home. Her body remembered the feelings and acted accordingly, presumably without the full engagement of her prefrontal cortex. She responded to the feeling of threat with her automatic well-practiced conditioned response—her dissociative shutdown state—a complex physiologic combination of the vaso-vagal reflex, the dorsal-vagal submission response, and practiced autohypnotic responses to these triggers. The bind of being unable to have the freedom she needed and being held hostage by her father's money appeared to her to be an inescapable dilemma; so inescapable, that processing it, figuring something out, even telling her therapist, were all solutions that were eliminated nonconsciously.

In our therapy the next day, we were able to bring her dilemma to consciousness and talk about her options. I agreed to serve as intermediary to negotiate with her father, with whom I had maintained a good relationship. I had a conversation with her father in a subsequent session, in which he promised to never use this threat again. Jennifer, for her part, never showed that degree of dissociative shutdown again, as she became more confident that direct communication could be effective, even with her parents.

Most children who have difficulties with the regulation of their consciousness do not have as little control as Jennifer evidenced in this session. In addition to blackouts, dissociative shutdowns can also manifest as lapses in attention, or even momentary avoidance of eye contact with no memory, staring into space for several moments while appearing to be in a daze, or repeated episodes of fainting-like spells that are short-lived.

Let's look at why, at certain times, it is adaptive for the child to lose focus or awareness. Some stimulus, either internal or external, has triggered a "danger message" and avoidance of that danger feels to the nonconcious mind like the child's very life depends upon avoiding that stimulus. Not being aware of what is going on may work when you are trapped with a predator, or when you are helpless to escape the inescapable. While the child feels that at that moment not knowing is key to psychological survival, as a therapist you know survival and thriving depends on awareness and the choice of what to avoid and what to approach.

The problem is that "choice" is a murky thing. The dissociative traumatized child lives in the no-man's land between "can't" and "won't." Behaviorally oriented therapists will argue that Jennifer had been reinforced for not following through with active problem-solving; her family had likely encouraged regression, and her avoidance strategy was simply a learned behavior that she could choose to stop—the "won't" side of the equation. The psychodynamically oriented therapist who believes in hidden motivation would argue that she "can't" wake up, no matter what the reinforcements from her environment. Her behavior is predetermined by forces outside of her control.

They both are partially correct. It is true that Jennifer's past history has taught her that dilemmas in her life are often inescapable, and she is helpless to change them. It is also true that her physiology has encoded that experiential history in conditioned responses over which she has little apparent control. Yet, consciousness is in a state of continually being created. As therapists, we enter into that exciting domain where things previously not under conscious control can become choices—planned or willed. In Jennifer's case the problem was solvable, though difficult, and the inescapable bind she felt was really escapable after all. Her choice to go to college and not go to her father's house for visits was ultimately honored.

STRATEGIES FOR REVERSING DISSOCIATIVE SHUTDOWN

The example of Jennifer largely illustrates all of the major components in working with children and adolescents who have these episodes of inconsistent awareness, dissociative states that appear to derail a cohesive sense of self.

These strategies involve:

1. Arousing the child from the state
2. Identifying the triggering moment and precursors
3. Unraveling the hidden traps and dilemmas that keep patients reliant on these avoidant strategies
4. Changing the environment to release the child from traps
5. Practicing a "re-do" of the moment
6. Rehearsing "staying connected" strategies
7. Honoring motivations to stay dissociative
8. Rewarding awareness and connection.

Although Jennifer's symptom was dramatic, her level of attachment to her family allowed rapid resolution of the symptoms without hospitalization. Fifteen-year-old

Bonnie, on the other hand, had much more severe early childhood trauma and losses and required more intense interventions to treat her dissociative shutdown states and accompanying symptomatology. In the rest of this chapter, I will discuss techniques for reversing dissociative shutdown states using case examples to illustrate each of the eight approaches I have listed.

Bonnie's aunt, who served as her guardian, called me feeling overwhelmed and helpless. Her 15-year-old adopted niece was having what she termed "seizures," but no neurological reason could be found. Bonnie would suddenly fall, lose consciousness, and wake up from 15 minutes to an hour later with repeated vomiting and severe headache. The episodes had increased in frequency, from once a week to several times a day. Bonnie was currently unable to go to school and was sleeping on a mattress on the floor so she wouldn't hurt herself by falling out of bed. Bonnie's history included sexual and physical abuse by multiple perpetrators before her adoption by the aunt at age 3. Particularly traumatic was that, prior to adoption, Bonnie had "good-bye" visits with her birth mother, a sporadic user of crack and cocaine who would disappear from the Bonnie's life for months at a time. Bonnie's mother used the "good-bye" visits to try to ensure that Bonnie would never attach to her aunt and uncle, telling her things like, "Always remember they are not your real parents. They can't really love you like I do."

Despite Bonnie's traumatic history and after a stormy few years with uncontrollable temper tantrums and oppositional behavior as a preschooler, she settled down into becoming a good student and seemed to function well through elementary school. In middle school, Bonnie began having problems—eating disorder symptoms, depression, and self-cutting behavior—apparently stimulated by peer rejection. Therapy in middle school focused on behavioral management of her eating and learning social skills.

As Bonnie entered high school, long-standing marital problems between her aunt and uncle came to a head and they began a trial separation, with Bonnie visiting her uncle every other weekend. Bonnie's first "seizure" followed the first visit to her uncle's new home. The frequency of the "seizures" quickly escalated over the next three weeks to the crisis point at which her aunt called me. Due to the severity of the symptoms, I arranged a residential placement at a treatment center, where I consult.

During the initial evaluation in my office, I suggested we sit on the floor for the interview, with pillows surrounding us, so that if anything we talked about stimulated a "seizure," Bonnie would not have far to fall. My intervention with the pillows was my way of letting Bonnie know that I took her safety seriously, but was not afraid of her symptoms. Instead, I was expecting, even welcoming, them. If a therapist reacts with fear or too much concern regarding "seizures," "blackouts," or other dissociative shutdown states, it instills a message of fear in the child that may further promote dissociation. In contrast, I let the children know that nothing about them is so frightening that I cannot handle it or work with them to resolve it. Bonnie, in fact, did have a "seizure" episode in our first session. We were talking about her future ambition to be a veterinarian, when I saw Bonnie's eyes dart sideways, her eyelids flutter and close, and then she keeled over on the pillows I had arranged around her. Bonnie was "out" for five minutes while I gently talked to her. I told her that she was safe, and we were going to figure out what was going on. Bonnie woke up with a headache and began uncontrollable retching. As noted previously, the vagus nerve is hypothesized to be involved in shutdown states and is also involved in the regulation of digestion and vomiting; thus, it was not surprising that retching accompanied the dissociative shutdown state. I was supportive as Bonnie vomited into the trashcan in my office. I gave Bonnie some water, and talked with her about what had just occurred.

Bonnie's dissociative shutdown states disappeared by the end of her three-week placement. While Bonnie was treated at a residential facility due to the seriousness of her presenting symptoms, the eight techniques that I used with her can be effective no matter what the level of severity of the symptoms.

Arousing the Child

Parents and clinicians alike can find it terrifying when a child lapses out of consciousness in front of them. Many children who go into these kinds of dissociative states are initially diagnosed with seizure disorders and sometimes put on anticonvulsants. When the children fail to respond to the medication and the neurological work-up is normal, these children tend to be diagnosed with psychogenic nonepileptic seizure (PNES). Approximately 20% of children referred for seizure evaluation end up with the PNES diagnosis (Benbadis, O'Neill, Tatum, & Heriaud, 2004). Aside from normal EEG findings, psychogenic seizures often present differently than seizures associated with abnormal brain activity. Patients with psychogenic seizure tend to thrust the pelvis in sexual-like movements, show bicycle-like movement of the legs, or thrash about in chaotic movements (Gates, Ramani, Whalen, & Loewenson, 1985). Psychogenic episodes also tend to last longer than do neurological seizures, and when the patients awaken, they are more clear-headed, not showing the lethargy and confusion that follows EEG-documented seizures (Luther, McNamara, Carwile, Miller, & Hope, 1982).

Still, children who enter dissociative states certainly look like they are experiencing a profound neurological episode of some kind. I have seen children lie limp on the floor of my office with jerky movements of their bodies, sometimes accompanied by vomiting, which to a nonneurologist looks like grand mal seizures. Frequently, these children report headaches when arousing from these episodes. Sometimes dissociative shutdown episodes resemble a self-induced trance state rather than seizures, as the child or teen falls back limply in the chair while breathing in a steady, rhythmical fashion. Sometimes the psychogenic seizure episodes are not as dramatic, but consist of simple motor movements with an accompanying dazed state. While these episodes may be frightening to watch, if the child has received a neurological work-up before coming to see me, I reassure myself first that these processes are a manifestation of the intensity of the emotions and conditioned neurological reactions that promote escape from traumatic reminders or overwhelming affect. The therapist's calm manner, without frantic worry or expressed alarm, is part of the peaceful environment that the child needs to feel safe enough to return to a normal waking state.

When faced with a child who seems to be in a dissociative state and is nonresponsive, I first check to see that he is in a comfortable position that does not restrict blood flow, and gently adjust his body as necessary. I softly call his name and make remarks that he is in a safe environment and no one is going to harm him. I describe in gentle language that he is in my office, that he came for an appointment, and that I am his therapist.

If I see the child start to stir, I am encouraging: *"It is ok to come back. I am here, I will keep you safe."* As pointed out by Perry (2006), the child evidencing a traumatic reaction has entered a precortical traumatic reaction, where activation of the lower brain centers has occurred and calming the body is necessary before any higher processing can occur. If the child is not calmed and awakened by the sound of my voice and the memory of the safety provided by me and our relationship, I may use imagery—preferably imagery that we have already created together. For example, I suggest that she may see herself in a peaceful meadow, or on a lovely tropical island surrounded by clear, turquoise water. I suggest something that captures the rhythm of breathing, like the lull of ocean waves. Then I use imagery to help wake the child up from the trance state that she is in. For example, I might state, *"As you are looking out at the waves, you see a huge flock of pelicans flying overhead, and they land right near you on the beach. You feel yourself eager to open your eyes and you feel your body able to be more and more awake. You will keep the sense of peace that you have right now when you feel ready to open your eyes. As I count backwards from ten, you will find yourself more and more ready to open your eyes. 10—9—feeling more alert—8—7—6, eyes may start to flutter, 5—4—3, starting to feel more awake, 2—."* Then I clap my hands. If you have paced your imagery with the body movements and breathing, the child or teen usually wakes up at this point. Then it is time to gently explore what happened that led to the dissociative shutdown.

Sometimes, the dissociative trance state is more violent and appears to be a reenactment of a traumatic memory. There can be some shouting of "no" or "stop," accompanied by violent arm or leg movements. In these cases, I have also been successful in creating an image that captures the movements in the body and then move the child into more controlled and peaceful movements. For example, if I observe the child kicking frantically, I have used the following imagery: *"As you kick away that person who has no right to be there, you find your legs getting stronger and stronger and stronger. You find that you are able to kick him far out of the room, and then you realize that you can use that wonderful leg strength on your favorite bicycle path. You find yourself on your favorite path, alongside the beach, and you are pedaling very, very fast using every bit of leg strength that you have. You find yourself soaring fast along the path with the feeling of wind in your hair and on your face. You continue to pedal, and realize you have built up so much speed that you can begin to glide. You find yourself not needing to pedal as fast and as your legs slow down, you realize that you are feeling more and more relaxed and more and more peaceful . . ."*

Using imagery like this, you can eventually slow down the legs, restore the body to a peaceful place, and arouse the client. When using this kind of trans-formative imagery, it is important to start with the flashback imagery and help the client to combat or overcome whatever he or she is struggling against. You can then transform the imagery from that mastery experience into something more calming. It is important not to rush this process. I find that in about 20 minutes, a client can be moved out of a dissociative flashback state into a calmer state, and then aroused. Because headaches are so common upon arousal, it is useful to use suggestions to combat headaches. For example, I will say the following: *"You will find your head begins to feel lighter and relaxed. All tension is leaving your head, so that your head lets all the headache tension be relieved, and you can feel strong and confident when you wake up."* If nausea tends to be present on awakening, you can incorporate suggestions to combat feeling nauseous.

Sometimes after an apparent trance-like state, children or teens emerge into a seemingly different self-state. If they appear to be reenacting a memory from the past in this state, entering what appears to be a flashback, I will use a similar technique to move them out of the flashback. If they see someone trying to attack them, I might tell them that their older self will help give them the strength to punch away the perpetrator, and then I try to quickly move them into the present. If instead of simply reenacting an abusive event, a new self-state has emerged that is talking calmly—perhaps in a childlike or other voice—I listen with curiosity and gentleness to what children have to say in that state while orienting them to the current time and place. I also encourage them to offer any new information that might be useful in helping them get well.

Ultimately, control of the waking must be given back to the child. The regu-lation of their own consciousness is an important skill for children and teens, and it is dangerous for children to begin to feel that only someone else can wake them from a dissociative state. To help place the rousing process in the control of the client, you can say things like: *"You will find a way to wake yourself up. When you are ready, you will find a way."* These were the words used that helped Bonnie restore herself to consciousness during her episodes in my office.

Having clients harness that indescribable and elusive "will" helps to reverse the helplessness associated with trauma. Cue words that appear to train the child to respond to commands of the therapist may be counterproductive, as they re-instill the helplessness that is the stance of victimization and place too much power and authority in the hands of the therapist. Our goal is for dissociative clients to learn the regulation of their own state of consciousness. Even if it takes time, we need to be patient to help children and teens find the way and time that feels safe enough to be present.

Identifying the Triggering Moment and Precursors

Generally, the onset of dissociative shutdowns or psychogenic seizure episodes is related to a specific environmental stressor that triggers a sequestered traumatic memory. The reactivation of this dissociated memory can generate profound symptomatology that is generally short-lived, though intense. The environmental trigger might be a hurtful comment from a new boyfriend, a change in the work schedule of the parent, parental fighting, or failure in a school subject. There are many events in a young person's life where feelings of helplessness, fear, ineffectuality, or fear of abandonment can be stimulated. Even the experience of sexual arousal can become a trigger for the onset of a previously hidden and dissociated traumatic memory to move to consciousness and temporarily cause the disruptive symptoms described here.

This is perhaps the most important principle for all work with traumatized people. The discontinuity in consciousness that may create a shutdown state, a flashback, a lapse in attention, an episode of acting out, a switch to a new behavioral repertoire, is triggered by some specific stimulus—thought, sensory experience, affect, tone of voice—that brings up memories and feelings associated with a traumatic event. However, sometimes it is difficult to discern the precipitants to these state changes. As many parents report, "He started acting crazy. It came out of nowhere." It is important to realize that children's behavior never comes "out of nowhere." While the parent, teacher, or client may not be able to discern the precipitant, there is always one there, even if it is internal or subtle. One high school student became mute and unresponsive during English class while the class was watching a movie. "It was out of nowhere," said the teacher. Later in therapy, the student reported a scene in the movie that contained a large, open meadow, similar to the place she had been raped.

Identifying the precipitant is easier when the client is with you in the office and you can observe for yourself what just happened, and what may have precipitated the change. But even when observing the client directly, the therapist often can't discern what happened. For example, in the case of Jennifer, nothing in the conversation clued me in to the difficult bind her father had put her in when we discussed her college plans. Asking the client in the moment, *"What just happened, then? Where did you go?"* is the best way to try to call attention to the precipitant. Then, follow up with asking, *"I wonder what I just said or you just said that made you leave us just now."*

When I was able to arouse Bonnie after her psychogenic seizure and vomiting, I gently explored with her what she thought had happened right before this episode. I was aware that we had been talking about her future plans when it happened. I asked her if another thought had come to her mind right before she lost consciousness, and she told me that she had heard the sound of her birth mother's voice saying, "You won't ever be anything." This was the first time she had disclosed to anyone that preceding these episodes she heard this voice of her birth mother talking to her. As we talked further, it became clear that the current separation of her aunt and uncle and the difficulty of her high school curriculum had stimulated her abandonment fears—fears that she might turn out like her mother, and fears that her aunt and uncle would no longer be there for her. The feelings from her "every other weekend" schedule she had had with her birth mother before the adoption were now being triggered by the alternating visits with her aunt and uncle, and the hostility between the parents evident to her on these visits. Having experienced this split schedule once before, as a 3-year-old prior to adoption, the current separation of her parents rekindled the old traumatic memories and fears of abandonment as well as strong needs for consistent attachment. Was it not safe to love these people as her mother had warned? Which one should she love and which should she abandon? Her early history had taught her you could not have both.

Besides exploring some of these thoughts, I asked Bonnie to explore the physiological precursors of the dissociative episode. She was able to tell me that she felt a tingly feeling above her eyebrows and a sense of pressure in the back of her head. I told her I noticed a shaking of her right hand and she agreed that also tended to accompany these episodes. Knowing these physiological precursors could provide an early warning signal before a state-change happened. In fact, by feeling the precursor, Bonnie learned to predict her "seizures" and she was able to notify the residential treatment staff. They would then bring her pillows and let her sit on the floor to prevent injury during these episodes. Eventually, Bonnie learned to avert the dissociative state by noticing the physiological precursors, and processing the triggering event with a staff person before the shutdown state.

Identifying a triggering moment is possible for younger children, as well. In the beginning of treatment, I introduce children to the idea that children can shift between moods, activity levels, or states of awareness. Early in therapy, I introduce children to dolls that demonstrate shifting emotional states, with expressions that change, different heads, or malleable parts. If children go into trance states, I may use a turtle doll that retracts its head inside its shell to illustrate a "hiding" reaction. I tell my clients that sometimes people change one way of acting into another way, which is fine as long as they are choosing to change for a reason. I tell them that we will work together to find out when changes happen and what the reasons are. This sets the stage for us to dig deeper when evidence of dissociative trance states or lapsed attention occurs.

When the triggering moment that we are trying to process occurs outside of therapy, it may take many sessions before a client is able to reveal the source of the difficulty. For example, Sally, a 12-year-old adopted from Romania and new to her middle school, told me she was never going back to history class again. She did not know why, but she felt her stomach go "weird" when she entered the classroom on her second day of class and then she fainted. Sally was terrified to return. Because I did not want her body to rehearse the "fainting response," which can become conditioned, I recommended that she not return to the classroom until we figured things out. The private school agreed to let her do work in the guidance office until then. In therapy, Sally and I painstakingly reviewed all the stimuli leading up to her fainting. Session after session, we discussed how the classroom looked, how her teacher looked, who her teacher reminded her of, and which moment she considered the worst one. Finally, Sally remembered that the teacher had told her, "You look just like your sister." As a late-adopted child with a preverbal trauma history and whose adopted sibling was biological, this statement stirred up so many mixed emotions of jealousy and abandonment anxiety that Sally was not able to cope with the intense feelings; she went into this dissociative shutdown mode. Sally did not really know or understand her reaction until the detective work that eventually uncovered the precipitant of her fainting. While this process is not an easy one, the moments that trigger dissociative reactions must be uncovered or they become hidden reinforcers to dissociative processes that strengthen over time.

Unraveling the Hidden Traps or Dilemmas

Once the precipitant is uncovered, it is important to clarify why that particular event, statement, internal thought, discussion topic, or perception reminded the child of a bind so apparently irresolvable that the child's body chose to shut down rather than face this information.

Elena was a 14-year-old girl with a history of multiple foster placements who was being recommended for return to her biological home, from which she was removed after disclosing that her mother had sexually abused her. When asked about the upcoming court date, Elena's pupils moved under her eyelids momentarily, and she appeared not to be mentally present for several minutes. When I finally got her attention back, I asked her, "Elena, do you know what we were talking about?" "Court?" she answered meekly. Her lips mouthed the words, "I'm going to tell the judge to move me back with my mother," while her face looked drawn and terrified. Elena was faced with an irresolvable dilemma in which she felt trapped. She had to choose between abandoning her siblings, who remained at home in her mother's care, or the possibility of enduring further abuse. Unable to come up with another solution, she "chose" to not be present mentally and let her mouth commit to what her heart could not. Elena's dissociation could not be resolved until the entities controlling her future—social services, her biological mother, her lawyer—found a way to empower her to give her true choice about her future—to keep her sibling relationships while avoiding further traumatization from her mother. That leads us to the next step in resolving these dilemmas, trying to effect environmental changes that help traumatized children out of hidden traps and dilemmas.

For Bonnie, her aunt and uncle's breakup brought on every fear she had from her early childhood that she had pushed away from consciousness. Her birth mother had told her that her aunt and uncle could never really love her. This appeared now to be true, as her new parents had broken up her home and seemed to be forever squabbling about who would take her. While she had begun to believe that they would be able to keep her safe after her early years of trauma, their breakup confirmed her worst fears. Bonnie began to believe that more trauma was inevitable. Bonnie wondered if she would be returned to her birth mother, or if she should choose to move back in with her birth mother so that she would not be such a burden to her family. Many of these thoughts were hints of ideas that she was not able to fully process or express. However, her mind expressed the deep trap she felt through an internal voice that sounded like her birth mother telling her that "You won't ever be anything." Bonnie's body then shut down into the frozen state that it remembered from her early years of abuse.

Escaping this pattern of shutdown involves finding ways to change the environment to release the child from some of these traps and binds. The traumatic reminders create a feeling of hopelessness and inevitability of trauma in the life of the child. Traumatic reminders are internal warnings that may be seen as evolutionary adaptive mechanisms to help traumatized individuals predict and avoid more traumatic events. Clients must learn that these dissociative responses are dramatic symbols of those events, serving a survival function by warning the individual of potential danger. However, before the toxic associations from past traumas can be metabolized and then detoxified, the client must see that escape is possible. There must be an escape plan, a strategy to get out of the current dilemma. Thus, planning on how to release the child from these traps is an essential part of the therapy approach.

Changing the Environment

Trauma survivors' lives are filled with minefields, traps, unfair expectations, and conflicting demands that make it very difficult for them to overcome their life of trauma without your help. To the extent that you have power to influence court decisions, school placement decisions, or parenting practices, you should try to do so. Children really are powerless, and traumatized children are doubly so. Many of the interventions that help children out of the binds that cause dissociative shutdown are naturally part of a therapist's practice—such as family meetings, or calling school counselors. Others may feel difficult, such as testifying in court proceedings, or even working on getting policy changes when a policy prevents a child from access to some needed service, opportunity, or individual that can be helpful.

The helpless passivity of dissociative shutdown states may become a way of life for traumatized children, a helplessness rooted in trauma but often reinforced by inflexible systems of care, often impervious to their needs. The helplessness pervades their views of what is changeable in their environment. Learning that they can effect change in their environment, often with their therapist's help, becomes a powerful lesson in mastery that counters the helpless feelings.

Unfortunately, the systems that dissociative children interact with often fail to afford them flexible responses. Eleven-year-old Hannah went into deep dissociative shutdown states every morning while getting ready to attend her fifth-grade class at her new middle school. As Hannah lay on the bedroom floor limply, her mother was unable to rouse her, sometimes for up to 45 minutes. Hannah's mother felt lucky to have her back, as Hannah had lived for two years with her biological father, who had sexually abused Hannah and kept her from contact with her mother. Her mother had fought hard to get Hannah back. She had finally succeeded in moving the case to a new jurisdiction where she finally got a visit with her daughter, and Hannah told the court about the abuse. Now, safe in her mother's custody, Hannah had intense fears of separation from her mother and fear of school, as the transfer of custody to her father had occurred directly from school. Hannah reported that she heard voices arguing in her mind before she went into a dissociative shutdown state. One would say, "If you leave your mother now, you will never see her again." The other voice, which sounded like her father, yelled at her to go to school. Faced with these warring voices, and feeling helpless and confused, Hannah's body would shut down.

When Hannah woke up, often after 45 minutes of her mother's cajoling her, Hannah would not go to school, as the school's tardiness policy required that any student arriving late needed to meet with the principal before returning to class. Hannah found this humiliating, and consequently avoided school completely for several weeks. In this case, I arranged with the school to bend their policy so that when Hannah was late, she could enter class inconspicuously, while we worked in therapy on the problems of the conflicting voices.

For Bonnie, escaping the bind of her dissociative shutdown state required me to work with the aunt and uncle to help them manage their conflict out of her presence. It also required a new living arrangement with an older cousin who lived close to her aunt's home. Living with her cousin felt safer to Bonnie, as her cousin had more time for her than did her aunt, and her house was close to Bonnie's school and after-school activities. In addition, Bonnie felt safer living without the emotional pull she had felt between her aunt and uncle during their stormy separation.

Practicing a Redo of the Moment

Even if the life problems have achieved resolution with the "activist" therapist strategies of the previous section, the dissociative shutdown states may persist. The conditioned avoidance responses have been practiced in the brain, and the brain mechanism of "kindling" predisposes the brain to reengage in patterned sequences that have occurred before. Thus, the client gets better and better at automatically moving into a dissociative shutdown. This automaticity must be reversed if the client is to get well.

The way to combat a behaviorally ingrained pattern is to practice a new one. This painstaking process involves identifying the moment that triggered the automatic sequence, and practicing responding differently to the same trigger. For Bonnie, this involved identifying every feeling she experienced, voice she heard, or sentence that she said to herself preceding a break in consciousness, and then identifying another way to respond to it. Bonnie was required to have a small notebook with her at all times in the residential living space for recording these episodes. As soon as she lost consciousness, a staff person stayed with her, and upon awakening, Bonnie was required to process what thoughts, ideas, or feelings she had preceding the event, and to write the thoughts or feelings down in her notebook with a counter thought. For example, if before her dissociative episode, Bonnie felt, "I will never get better," she was instructed to think of ways to counter that negative thought with hopeful thoughts about her future.

The notebook was brought to therapy for further processing of these thoughts and feelings that provoked her dissociative episode. Immediate processing counters the client's phobic response to the stimulus, and illustrates to the client that no thought, feeling, or image is too overwhelming to handle. The therapist's (and in Bonnie's case, the staff's) calm readiness to engage is one of the key interventions for countering phobic avoidance. By doing this quickly, there is a strengthening of the association between the stimulus and a new behavioral response pattern that interrupts the brain's habit of automatically moving into a dissociative shutdown state. Once a counter thought, a new idea, or a new solution is illustrated and developed, I may even walk the patient through the exact steps and actions she was involved with before the episode. Thus, there is not only rehearsal of a new way to handle the previously taboo stimulus, but also practice of a new sequence of behavior in which the unacceptable stimulus is detoxified.

Even without observing the triggering event to a dissociative shutdown state, the therapist can help rehearse new behaviors to counter the sequence that has previously led to the shutdown state. For example, Miranda was worked up for a seizure disorder at a local hospital after episodes of losing consciousness associated with jerking arm movements. When no seizure disorder was found, she was referred to me for ongoing therapy. I was struck by Miranda's inability when describing painful personal experiences to ever acknowledge any feelings of anger. When she described the repeated tapping of a pencil by a classmate as being annoying, I tapped a pencil on a table in my office and rehearsed with her how to ask me to stop. Miranda appeared paralyzed. She could not utter the word "stop," and began to describe the feelings of pain in the back of her head and tingling of the fingers that often preceded one of her dissociative episodes. Her history revealed that she had been sexually abused in a preschool by a teacher. When she asked the teacher to "stop," she had been threatened with having her whole family killed. For Miranda, even uttering the word "stop," or expressing appropriate anger became a trigger for her dissociative shutdown state. She reported that her father's eating habits at the dinner table "annoyed" her and she had wanted to tell him to "stop" but could not. We practiced with carefully crafted exercises and role-played how to say "stop," while processing her frightening belief that saying "stop" would result in death of her loved ones.

Similarly, Jennifer was able to overcome her shutdown reaction by learning to talk about her feelings about her father and college. The safety of my presence and my office, combined with her motivation to avoid hospitalization, allowed her to process her thoughts and fears, and to trust that I could help her solve this as we had solved other seemingly irresolvable problems in the past. The feeling of being in a safe place and in the presence of the therapist helps to combat the automaticity of the dissociative shutdown state during the practicing of "redo moments."

Rehearsing "Staying Connected" Strategies

Once children or teens have been able to identify some of the precursors that predispose them to dissociative shutdown states and handle these conflicts in new ways, they will often identify prodromal feelings that precede these states. These feelings can include headaches, tingling of the fingers, burning sensations, or dizziness. By tuning into these sensations, the client may be better able to notice what is upsetting him or her and practice ways to stay present. These are often called "grounding techniques" and generally involve heightening sensory awareness of the present to counter the draw to retreat into a dissociative world. Any of the senses can be used as the primary grounding stimulus.

Music works well, particularly with iPods preprogrammed with songs that help a youngster stay focused. When music is unavailable, children can be taught to sing their favorite songs in their mind. Also useful are tactile experiences, including feeling one's feet as they stamp on the ground, or feeling, scratching, or rubbing on some part of the body. Touching very cold objects, such as ice cubes, can serve the grounding function. Special necklaces, bracelets, or pins can also serve as a grounding object. I will help the client associate the feeling of the weight of the object on their wrist or neck with the feeling of staying focused and present using suggestions such as the following: "*Every time you feel the braided band of your bracelet on your wrist, you will realize that this bracelet connects you to your present life, a life you can stay in and feel in charge of. It is a pleasant feeling, a reminder, connecting you deeply with your dreams for yourself and your ability to pursue them.*"

Younger children or developmentally disabled children may carry favorite dolls or stuffed animals that can serve as grounding objects. Younger children can also be grounded with rehearsed songs such as, "It looks like things aren't going my way, but I am choosing to have a good day." Other children prefer cognitive techniques for grounding. I like to have children practice affirmations that counter their worst fears as a grounding technique. For example, "Each day I will be more and more in charge of my life and future," is a favorite affirming sentence of many of my clients. I explain to children that staying connected with the present will give them more options to ultimately be in charge of their future.

Bonnie became expert at noticing the odd body sensations that preceded her dissociative shutdown states. When she noticed these prodromal symptoms, she was taught to sit on the ground and focus on the sentence, "I am going to be fine whether or not I dissociate." Fear of dissociation had sometimes prompted her episodes and became a self-fulfilling prophecy. Thus, honoring the possibility that it might happen without the associated fear served a preventive function.

Some younger children respond better to visual cues, rather than verbal cues, when learning to anticipate and abort a dissociative shutdown state. Hand gestures such as moving the hands slowly downward in a calming lowering motion (Yehuda, 2011), or clasping two hands together symbolizing the self "working together," can also help younger children ground themselves.

Honoring Motivations to Stay Dissociative

Sometimes, despite my best efforts to move the client through the steps outlined, there is resistance and a lack of progress. You can throw out every life preserver you have, but if the drowning swimmer believes it is unsafe to grab onto it, he or she will not. While clients may tell you verbally that they want to get better, and while they may attend your sessions diligently, motivation to dispense with dissociative coping tools is a difficult and challenging commitment to make. Generally, the lack of progress indicates that there is an ongoing threat in the environment that has not yet been identified. In other cases, the fear of progress is in itself too great, because the client has identified barriers in the environment, either perceived or actual, that make recovery feel unsafe.

Rewarding Awareness and Connection

Sometimes we expect that a client's progress will be self-sustaining, believing that health and progress should be a reward in and of itself. Unfortunately, progress is accompanied by many challenges that may lead your client to doubt whether all of this change is really worth it. Thus, rewarding your young client's efforts through explicit comment and even behavioral programs that you develop conjointly may help them mark their progress, and take pride and pleasure in their accomplishments.

As a therapist, I am constantly taking note and commenting on even the smallest movement toward making progress. I laughingly comment that I hear the brain cells in their head "sizzle" as they make an important connection, or reverse a previously learned brain habit. Most importantly, when they *don't* use a familiar response of dissociative shutdown in response to stimuli that usually trigger them, I emphasize how amazing their accomplishment is. Each time the client successfully avoids the dissociative shutdown response, new brain pathways are being strengthened. These are key moments to praise clients' efforts and progress, and to rehearse with them what went on in their mind and how they can accomplish this again.

As noted previously, Bonnie got to the point that she would sit on a pillow when she felt the familiar prodromal feelings, identify the thought that was troubling her, and ask for help in countering it before shutting down. This became a time for the staff to praise her, to comment on how well she was doing, and to offer her the opportunity to engage in field trips off grounds. It was clearly too dangerous for her to go to the gym to play basketball while these dissociative shutdown states were frequent and disruptive. By proving her success in avoiding them, she earned fun activities, which were made possible for her by her new achievements. Thus, Bonnie's success in managing her dissociative states earned her tangible benefits.

The behavioral programs set up to reward these moments are different from conventional behavioral programs in several important ways. First, what is being rewarded both concretely and through praise is not simply the avoidance of a disruptive or inappropriate behavior. Instead, what is being rewarded is the child's courage, skill, and ability to counter an overlearned "brain habit" and learn a new way to function in times of stress. I call times when clients are able to avoid going into a dissociative state a "save." To illustrate how important they are, I often have families keep track of the number of "saves" in a given day or week. Rather than focusing on the disruptive and inappropriate aspects of the child's behavior, I focus the family on noticing the positive aspects of the child's effort in countering the shutdown state. Older children and teens can learn to track these "save" moments and build in rewards for themselves for making it through the day without resorting to dissociative shutdowns. It works best to have them come up with their own set of rewards—seeing a favorite movie, time on videogames—rewards they give themselves to celebrate the pride they feel in having learned something new. Over time, of course, living a life with awareness and connection does begin to bring its own rewards, and clients are ready to dispense with the more planned reinforcements provided by themselves and others, as their new skills become second nature.

SLEEP ANOMALIES

Before concluding this chapter on "staying awake," it is important to mention that a significant minority of dissociative and traumatized children have sleep anomalies that bring them into treatment. The instability of consciousness represented by the dissociative shutdown states may be reflected in disrupted sleep habits and sleep cycles. Children may sleep too much, have reversals of day and night sleep patterns, or have extreme difficulty rousing from a state of deep sleep. Sometimes upon arousal, they are in dissociative states with distinct affects and characteristics, such as states of rage or childlike behavior.

Sleep is regulated by the reticular activating system, a primitive part of the forebrain that may be disrupted from early trauma (Perry, 2006). Sleep may have become a practiced mode of escape in order to avoid expected pain or abuse, and may have become a conditioned avoidance response. Many parents have told me that when their infants and young children were forced into visitations with the nonprimary caregiver, they went into deep-sleep states shortly before the exchanges, as if to numb the self from the stress of the disrupted attachment.

Teens with dissociative problems may purposefully reverse day and night to avoid interacting with families or to avoid school. Sleep clinics often recommend staying up one hour later over the course of several weeks until the entire sleep schedule is pushed ahead by 12 or more hours. This is easier than asking the teen to go to bed an hour earlier each night. However, as discussed earlier, the motivation for the avoidance will be the key thing to treat in these clients.

Even when the sleep pattern is not completely dysregulated, waking dissociative teens up in the morning is often a trouble zone, where deep-sleep states are often indistinguishable from dissociative shutdown, and may be accompanied by similar shifts in affect and headaches upon arousal. I have found that the most important way to address these problems is to help the teen confront what is being avoided in the morning and offer alternatives—different methods of being aroused, different school programming, or different morning routines. As with all shutdown states, the body is stating through its actions that something is intolerable. Until what is intolerable is identified and addressed, the body will use its own nonconscious method of dealing with the problem.

In analyzing sleep problems and disruptions, it is important to examine the timing of the sleep problems. A young family who had escaped from war-torn Chechnya had been awakened every morning at 5:00 a.m. by masked gunmen who raided the home and assaulted the mother. Even living in a safe environment, the three young children still woke up at 5:00 a.m., usually screaming in terror. In this case, the family was urged to create a new 5:00 a.m. ritual of a fancy celebrative breakfast to counter the memory of the timing of the trauma. The creative therapist can find opportunities in the real world to illustrate the differences between the traumatic environment of the past and the current environment where thriving is possible.

In the next chapter, we will address how regulating affect in the context of attachment helps child survivors to further erode the dissociative barriers that prevent engagement in the world around them.

11 Building Attachment Across States

Affect Regulation in the Context of Relationships

For the third time in one month, 12-year-old Timothy was in the emergency room after violently attacking his family. This time, Timothy had threatened his grandmother with a knife, knocked over the television set, and left bruises on a neighbor who had come over to help restrain him. In the emergency room, Timothy was a model of self-control. He was pleasant and cooperative with the nurses and doctors. He told them he had "learned his lesson," he was not going to do it again. He understood what upset him and he would "use words next time." His affect certainly appeared on the surface to be "regulated" at this point. Should he be discharged and sent home from the hospital? If so, how soon would the whole scenario repeat itself?

The frustrating dilemma that children like Timothy present is that their affect swings wildly between extremes. Looking at Timothy now, composed, mature, and articulate, it was difficult for the hospital emergency room staff to imagine the enraged boy that the family had been dealing with only a half hour earlier. If they were to admit him, it was unlikely the hospital would get a chance to see the kind of behavior that had triggered Timothy at home. If they were to send him home, his words did not seem like sufficient assurance that this would not happen again. In reality, Timothy's calmness did not indicate that he had learned how to calm down. He had only learned to see the emergency room as a new automatic trigger for a new conditioned state. This time, they sent Timothy home.

The most difficult affective state to work with is the arousal of anger and rage and associated aggression, as seen in Timothy. The behaviors that children enact in dissociated affective states are often dangerous to themselves and others. In fact, violent behavior is the most common reason for dissociative teens to be admitted to the Sheppard Pratt Health System's adolescent inpatient units (Ruths et al., 2002). These teens are unable to contain the extreme rage that is triggered by environmental cues, and their destructive reactions lead to revolving-door admissions in many psychiatric centers or crisis units and threaten the secure placements of many adoptive or foster children. The containment of these violent behaviors is often the main goal of admission.

To understand the wildly dysregulated affect of a child such as Timothy, let's review the importance of early attachment, which sets the stage for learning affect regulation. The attentive caregiver rocks a crying baby, laughs with a happy baby, soothes a fussy baby, and thus establishes expectancy that uncomfortable states can be soothed. The child eventually learns to self-regulate as caregivers model these regulatory processes. As observed by Carlson, Yates, and Sroufe (2009), these "interpersonal exchanges in the caregiving milieu become internalized as part of the child's repertoire of affect and behavior" (p. 43). Conversely, when early caregiving is unresponsive to overwhelming affect in the developing child, the child may be left with emotional arousal that vacillates between extremes of overarousal and underarousal.

Neurological studies lend support to the importance of early relationships to the development of healthy affect regulation (Stien & Kendall, 2004). According to Schore (2009), the underdeveloped orbito-frontal cortex, disrupted by impaired caregiving, can lead to disorganization and disinhibition of lower subcortical brain regions, which is reflected in the emotional disinhibition and overreactions of the dissociative children and teens.

The result of these deficits in the healthy integration of emotion with the higher brain centers is an affect life in disarray. Without central modulating mechanisms, the moods of the child survivor swing rapidly. These rapid swings reflect non-conscious responses to ever-present triggers without the guidance of the thinking brain to analyze and contain them. Unable to regulate emotions with learned methods of self-soothing, the child survivor looks for artificial ways to regulate mood. These can include self-injurious acts that release endorphins, or destructive acts against others, hurting the people whose attachment and love they yearn for—but fear they have lost. Children may substitute one intense feeling state for another in a furtive avoidance dance, like someone walking on hot coals, jumping from one foot to the other.

Our clients have learned in their original environments that attachment is only safe under certain circumstances. They learn to anticipate when a caregiver will be brutal or cruel and zone out at those times, developing a different state of awareness where they are disconnected from the attachment figure. This process preserves some positive attachment, while giving a certain freedom for children to express their anger and hostility about their maltreatment through aggressive or destructive acts they don't fully remember or understand. Divided awareness preserves a certain kind of pseudo-attachment, seen when Timothy mouths the words of what he plans to do when he gets back home. His attachment is not the enduring attachment that helps a child thrive and internalize self-regulation, as he cannot sustain those feelings when confronted with triggers that suggest to him that his safety is not assured.

The inescapable conclusion from the convergence of research and clinical observations is that teaching the management of affect within the context of an attachment relationship is an essential clinical strategy when working with the chronically traumatized and dissociative child survivor. It is only through developing this consistent attachment that the child's regulation of affective states can become truly under his or her own control. Ironically, true self-regulation requires attachment to someone who cares for the child, loves the child unconditionally, and expects that regulation will be achieved. Yet, attachment even to wonderful caregivers is generally compromised when a child has been severely traumatized. These deficits are both a self-regulatory and a relational problem. Thus, the clinical work involves a two-pronged approach—teaching individual strategies for managing affect in a new way, and supporting emotional communication in the context of a relationship. Both tasks are difficult undertakings, yet both are essential to treatment success.

The As in the EDUCATE model—arousal, affect, and attachment—are interrelated on theoretical, neurophysiological, and clinical levels. This chapter and the next cover affect regulation skills in individual therapy and family therapy. This chapter focuses on affect regulation skills in the traumatized child, but includes some techniques that are done conjointly with the parents, as there must be a fluid interplay between individual and family techniques when working on affect regulation in children.

REVERSING AUTOMATICITY

The Affect Avoidance Theory defines dissociation as: *The automatic activation of patterns of actions, thought, perception, identity, or relating (or "affect scripts"), which are overlearned and serve as conditioned avoidance responses to affective arousal associated with traumatic cues.* When Timothy reacts in the family environment with his combative behavior, we are seeing the initiation of an automatically activated "affect script"—a planned behavioral repertoire for rage that is inappropriate to his current context. On some level, Timothy cannot help himself. Whatever trigger in the environment he is responding to has been perceived and responded to on a nonconscious level; he is engaged in the act before he has had a chance to process what has happened or how he feels about it. While his behavior looks like the expression of intense affect, it is the expression of an overlearned affective portrayal of rage; Timothy does not experience this rage in an integrated or authentic way. This is why his affect reverses so easily when he arrives at the emergency room. This primitive "attack mode" rage is a vestige from a previous time that becomes automatically elicited when Timothy feels a survival threat. This behavioral display prevents Timothy's authentic engagement with his emotional reactions that would help him negotiate his environment more effectively.

Paradoxically, part of what we need to accomplish to help Timothy learn to calm himself down is to help him identify and consider what he really feels at the triggering moments and use that information to problem-solve in his family relationships. Like Sonya, who broke her bed when her mother tried to give away her t-shirt (see Chapter 2), Timothy is mystified about the real feelings underlying his behaviors. In Chapter 2, I introduced the idea of healthy mind: *The healthy mind effectively selects the information that will allow it to seamlessly manage transitions between states, between affects, between contexts, and between developmental challenges, in a way that is adaptive to each shifting environmental demand.*

Based on this definition, Timothy must learn to be able to shift seamlessly between contexts and to develop more appropriate responses that fit his current life. For Timothy to do this, he must learn to identify what triggered his reactions and what he felt about that, and then use his feelings adaptively as signals to correct problems in his world. Timothy will need to be able to focus on those transition moments when he automatically enters the rage-filled state. He will need to defeat the automaticity, and replace it with awareness. He will need to select what is relevant for his current world, knowing what he feels and why, and learn how to respond to his family based on that new awareness, rather than base his responses on outdated survival programs. All of this is a tall order for a boy such as Timothy, but not impossible. First, Timothy must understand his own affects and become motivated to tune into them.

AFFECT EDUCATION: IDENTIFYING
THE PURPOSE OF FEELINGS

Our effort to help the child survivor manage shifting affect states begins with psychoeducation. Tomkins's (1962, 1963) model of affects as signals provides a clear and straightforward way to help the child survivor understand the roles and benefits of the affects they have learned to shut out or turn off. To begin the discussion of affect, I ask the young client or teenager if they hope to learn to drive one day. The client responds, "Of course!" I ask the client how his mother would feel if he told her that he would love to learn to drive, but has no intention of following any of the road signs—he will drive following his own rules, ignoring stop signs, yield signs, and red lights. *"Would your mother let you learn how to drive if this is what you planned to do?"* I ask. "Of course not, but I wouldn't do that," answers the child. *"But you are doing that already with your feelings,"* I respond. *"You are trying to be in the 'driver's seat' of your own life, but you are not using the road signs and signals that tell you where to go, what to approach, what to avoid, and when to use caution. Those road signs are your feelings, which should be assisting you, not controlling you or being ignored by you."* Each feeling, I explain, has a purpose rooted in our biology that helps us keep in mind information about the environment and our experiences that we have gathered over time. Fear, I explain, tells us there is something to avoid, as it may have been a source of danger in the past. Sadness tells us we miss something or someone that we love and it helps us keep that connection. "What does anger do?" they will ask me.

Most children have been taught that anger is a "bad" emotion and that they should not feel any. I correct this notion immediately, telling them that anger is the "self-defense" emotion that tells others to back off or get out of their space. It tells us when someone is violating our personal boundary. Anger gives us the warning and incentive to do something about this invasion. Once you have the information about what or who is invading your space, it becomes your choice of how to respond. I then ask children to think back to times they were angry so that they can remember having used anger in an appropriate self-defensive way. I praise them for having listened to the emotion and responded well. I explain that when boundaries are violated when a child is too young to fight back, then their anger has learned that it has no purpose and may go underground, only to assert itself uncontrollably later on. I teach children that they need to reclaim and "own" their anger and find a way to use its message to assert their rights in an appropriate way. I compare anger to the sensory perception of pain. Pain serves an important evolutionary purpose of having an organism know when something is hurtful or toxic and must be avoided. Even though pain is unpleasant, it is necessary, and people can't survive without it. For example, patients with pain insensitivity (dysautonomia) often die from injuries that they don't have the sensitivity to prevent. Similarly, I explain that trying to turn off your anger will result in putting yourself in situations in which you might allow others to take advantage of you.

Children and teens are often very relieved to hear this information, as they have felt ashamed of their anger and its results. I explain that the negative results of their anger are because they are not more accepting of it, so they can't use it for its real purpose. I further explain that the strong anger that they currently harbor relates to a past need to be protected when their boundaries were violated. Their anger is valid. Unfortunately, in the past, they were too small and not strong enough to use their anger to fight back the way their body was telling them to. Now, all of their stored up anger has gotten stronger and stronger and is looking for a way to be released. The anger is so eager to express itself, it may do so when it is not really appropriate and may be misdirected.

These messages about anger were reassuring for Timothy. He was mortified about his rage-filled behavior and this message helped to relieve his phobic avoidance of discussing the violent reactions he had at home. Anger, he learned, was something that could be understood and handled, something that was even worthwhile and useful; rage-filled actions did not have to be the inevitable result.

Another feeling that clients have tried to dissociate from and that often expresses itself without their awareness is the feeling of sexual arousal. My psychoeducation about sexual feelings was described in Chapter 7. After explaining about the "tickly" sensations that all people share when their private parts are touched, one can add that these are feelings that are intended for older people of the same age to share, but not for adults to share with children. Again, we emphasize that these are good feelings to have, even though some people may act on the feelings in the wrong way and engage in inappropriate behavior. Like anger, it is important that sexuality not be seen as a child's private shame, but as universal feelings that all humans share. Opening the door to discussion of this confusing area can be clarifying and might allay the anxieties children may have if they have been sexually abused.

Psychoeducation about feelings covers several other important areas that may be confusing to children and their parents. The families and children must learn to make the distinction between feelings and actions. For some families, these two concepts are tied too strongly, and the families must learn that having a feeling does not mean that certain actions are inevitable. If feelings have been associated with destructive behaviors in the past, children and parents wrongly assume that the feelings are the problem. As feelings are reframed as helpful and not inevitably associated with negative reactions, children and families begin to learn to tolerate feelings in themselves and others.

Families and their children must also learn how to differentiate between their own feelings and those of others. Traumatized children easily pick up on parents' moods of anger and depression and must learn how to create barriers between their own feelings and those of others. *"Feelings,"* I explain, *"like colds, don't have to be contagious if you protect yourself. Protecting yourself from other feelings means respecting the boundaries of your family members so as not to presume they are feeling the way you are feeling."* Families and children can learn cue words for communication of feelings, such as "I'm in a bad mood but it's not because of you," or "Give me some space," so that moods are not inevitably shared.

Another key differentiation that must be taught is that feelings themselves are not the trauma. The phobic avoidance of feelings associated with trauma can lead to a sense of equivalence between the two. Once children understand that feelings are simply their body's signal system, that feelings are distinct from actions and are not necessarily contagious, they are ready to learn how to regulate them more effectively.

AFFECT AWARENESS AT TRANSITION MOMENTS

Awareness of affective states is one of the building blocks of consciousness itself. The awareness of self is built on the differentiation and memory of affect states that link a person's autobiographical memory and produces a coherent sense of self. Affects are the "psychic glue" of identity (Monsen & Monsen, 1999). By focusing on the transition moment when a child such as Timothy goes from calmly watching television to out-of-control rage, the therapist can help the child survivor develop affect management skills that will help them in future interactions. These skills involve identifying triggering events and associated feelings, tolerating the feelings, learning to moderate their intensity, and learning to make new behavioral choices during moments of intense affect. If rage is perceived as being associated with a dissociated self-state, the child must forge a bridge to that dissociated self so they can explore underlying feelings that may be masked by rage-filled behavior.

Timothy had identified that his rage-filled behavior was caused by an "angry voice" that sounded like his grandfather. He did not want to listen to it and was humiliated by the actions he had engaged in when he felt the voice "taking over."

Using the EDUCATE model discussed in Chapter 7, Timothy was encouraged to "Understand what was hidden" (U) and "Claim it as his own" (C). He appreciated the "angry voice" as a manifestation of his survival instinct and as an important part of himself that could not be ignored. Through "listening in," we were able to find out from the "angry voice" some of the incidents that led to his intense rage at home.

Triggering Moments

In some ways, just being a child is a traumatic trigger for traumatized children, as children are always in a powerless position with respect to adults. They are constantly being told what to do, being given limited options, and made to feel like their lives are not under their own control. Thus, with traumatized children triggering moments are everywhere. When your clients and parents say "nothing triggered this event," you can be certain that there was some event that reverberated in the echo chamber of traumatic memory and deprivation, and led to the problem behaviors. Rage reactions are at their core a way to protect the self from perceived dangers. The therapist must discover what dangers the angry part of the child or teen is perceiving and find ways to build in protection.

One of Timothy's triggers was having his grandmother turn off his TV shows in the middle of the program. This, of course, would irritate any child and likely causes a fair share of tantrums in homes with nontraumatized children. However, for Timothy, this sent him biting, kicking, and throwing dishes, making it increasingly unlikely that he could continue to live with the family that loved him. The following dialogue describes the process of evaluating the triggering moment before Timothy's intense explosive reaction.

Therapist:	*Sounds like you really had a hard time last week at home. Your mom is pretty worried about you.* [Therapist emphasizes worry and not anger.]
Timothy:	I know. I lost it. Only once I think. [Actually, he "lost it" multiple times. We explore the one he is "willing" to remember.]
Therapist:	*Let's look at that time you lost it. What day was it?*
Timothy:	I don't know. I guess Tuesday.
Therapist:	*What time was it? Before or after dinner.*
Timothy:	It was definitely before dinner, because I was watching my show. That's what started it.
Therapist:	*Really.*
Timothy:	Grandma always starts with me then. [He views her as a "perpetrator," even though he is the one who injured people. However, to get the story, I go with his perception at this point.]
Therapist:	*What did she do?*

Timothy:	She told me to wash up for dinner and wouldn't let me finish my show.
Therapist:	*She wouldn't let you finish your show?*
Timothy:	No.
Therapist:	*How did you feel about that?*
Timothy:	I don't know what gets into her. She does it on purpose. [Timothy avoids the feeling question. We will have to get to that later.]
Therapist:	*What do you mean "on purpose?"*
Timothy:	She knows how much I like the show.
Therapist:	*You mean it feels like she wants to hurt you on purpose by turning off your show?*
Timothy:	Yeah, on purpose, on purpose. [This phrase seems to have a much deeper meaning for Timothy, and seems to be the trigger for him. I want to find the source of that.]
Therapist:	*What a terrible feeling to know someone hurts you on purpose. That's familiar to you, isn't it?*
Timothy:	Of course, my grandfather did it all the time. He knew what he was doing. It wasn't an accident the time he burned me. He told people it was an accident, but it wasn't.
Therapist:	*So when your grandma turns the TV off, it feels like she is hurting you on purpose, like your grandfather used to do. No wonder you acted like you were fighting for your life.*
Timothy:	Yeah, I lost it.
Therapist:	*Is that when "angry voice" seemed to be there?*
Timothy:	"Angry voice" hates her for doing that.
Therapist:	*"Angry voice" thinks it's just about the same thing—turning off the TV, or burning you like your grandfather did. Do you agree with "angry voice" that it's the same thing?* [I phrase it in a way that he can see the differences.]
Timothy:	Well, not exactly. But why does she do it, then?
Therapist:	*It seems like she is just doing it to hurt you, and it makes you wonder if she really loves you when she does that. I have watched your grandma, and it looks to me like she really does love you. Maybe we should find out about why she turns off the TV. You and the angry voice inside you have a right to know and understand that.*

Purposeful actions that the person knew would cause Timothy distress triggered this powerful traumatic memory that made him feel unloved and worthless. Before this feeling is examined, the reaction to the trigger is automatic. Upon examination, however, the overwhelming feeling can be seen as relevant to his past, and not necessarily relevant to now. Helping Timothy recognize that he is actually reacting to the feeling that he is not loved can lead to a new, more adaptive behavior—communicating and finding reassurance. Family work with Timothy's grandmother became an important part of treatment at this point. I needed to build empathy between them, and help Timothy experience her direction as love and not as deprivation or "hurting him on purpose."

Survivors of early childhood abuse will find abundant signals in the actions of others that will trigger feelings of being unloved and undeserving. When triggered, these feelings are often too painful and overwhelming for the child to tolerate. They often lead to uncontrollable rages, which frequently occur in dissociated and isolated states of identity that have never experienced love.

IDENTIFYING AND EXPRESSING AFFECTS: ESTABLISHING A FEELING VOCABULARY

Traumatized children and teens often have no differentiation skills to describe their affective experiences. In our early sessions, I ask clients to identify what makes them sad, happy, scared, afraid, ashamed, disgusted, or jealous, along with any other feelings that come up in our conversation. As they describe events associated with each of these, I record them in a notebook for our use, as I am helping them organize their affective life so they have a new vocabulary of associations for describing feelings that have seemed nameless before.

Figure 11.1 shows 14-year-old Deborah's depiction of the feeling "grief," which is "how you feel if you lose your mother." The intensity of this depicted affect also became a gauge in therapy against which to judge other disappointments and losses that were not so acute as this original and profound loss when she was abandoned at an orphanage. The jagged line above the lip on the depicted imaginary character that is part of Deborah's internal fantasy world is a scar from an injury that this imaginary character experienced in her birth home before adoption. Deborah herself was unaware whether she had sustained such an injury and herself had no visible scar. However, preverbal experiences may find expression symbolically in artwork or somatic memories.

Representing feelings through role playing, doll play, or drawings helps the child or teen become more adept with emotional language and increases skills in differentiating the variety of affective states that children experience. Drawings provide a method of containing the intensity of feelings while still capturing their essence. By drawing themselves in different situations, children can learn to differentiate feelings from one another and begin to group certain kinds of feelings together. I also have a deck of feeling cards that show a variety of facial expressions that help prompt children to describe their feelings, and all clients are invited to add their own feeling cards to this ever-growing collection.

Different colors can be picked to represent different feelings, and the child can create graphs to show how high on the graph the different colors reach. The child can check in with the feelings graph at the beginning of each session, coloring a bar with the designated color to the height that represents how big the feeling is that day (see Figure 11.2). Having many different colors at different heights on

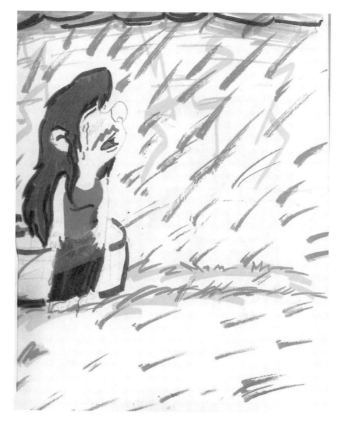

Figure 11.1 Deborah depicts feelings of grief. Used with permission.

the graph helps illustrate that one's emotional life is complex and composed of many different feelings. If each feeling is represented by a different imaginary friend, or internalized dissociative state, the graph can help to illustrate that the whole self really does have all of these feelings, even when they feel divided. The therapist might ask the child to focus inward and allow each of the different feeling states to feel a little bit of a neighboring feeling. This exercise helps the child with dissociated feeling states begin the process of blending the states as a move toward eventual integration.

Some emotions may be hard to name, but describing the somatic associations to the feelings—headaches, stomach aches, and other pains or strange sensations—can help the child and therapist develop a common affective language. The role of therapist throughout treatment is to help the child or teen know that their feelings are acceptable, understandable, normal, and an important source of information from which the child can learn. The therapist role is often to amplify feelings

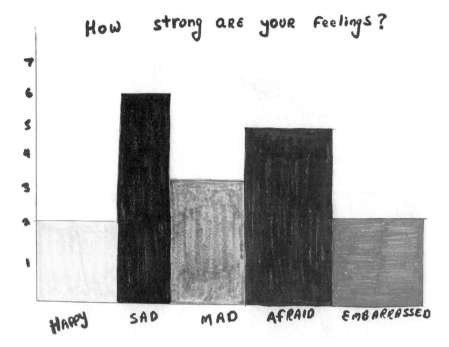

Figure 11.2 A feelings graph that helps children depict the intensity of various affects. Used with permission.

children are prone to avoid, and help lower the volume on feelings that are over-aroused by validating and providing opportunities for expression.

METAPHORS AND IMAGERY TO REINFORCE TOLERATING AFFECTS AND FLEXIBLE SHIFTING

Visual imagery can help reinforce affect regulation strategies by providing practice in noticing affects, tolerating affects, and helping children become less avoidant of their affective lives. The following are examples of some of the metaphors and imagery I use with children.

The Ocean, and the Ebb and Flow of Emotions

Most of the young people in my area have visited the Atlantic Ocean, and I ask children to picture themselves standing on the beach with the ocean in front of them and their feet resting firmly and securely on the sand. Then, I ask them to picture the waves coming one by one towards them, looking big and overwhelming as they approach but evaporating into suds along their ankles as the waves come to shore. I explain that their own feelings are similar to these ocean waves, appearing huge and overwhelming at first, but if they stay with their feet firmly planted on the ground, they can observe the "wave of feeling" as it comes. I tell them to be patient and observant as they watch the feeling "break" and get smaller. The next feeling will come and it also might look huge and overwhelming but it, too, will fade as a small splash around their feet.

Practicing this imagery of watching the ocean waves safely from the shore can serve as an exercise to condition the child toward tolerance for overwhelming feeling without overreaction. This is a form of mindfulness training used in Dialectical Behavior Therapy (DeRosa & Pelcovitz, 2008; Linehan, 1993) that helps a client stay with a feeling while observing it, rather than being overwhelmed by it.

Nine-year-old Tracy (introduced in Chapter 7) was sexually abused at the age of 7 by her grandfather while her mother was at work. When experiencing severe separation anxiety in school, Tracy was taught to name each feeling that she visualized as a wave coming toward her. During her anxiety attacks, Tracy would imagine waves and say to herself: "Here comes fear, it is smaller now. Here comes missing my mother, it is smaller now. Here comes my heart beating strongly, it is calming down. Here comes my mom's voice saying, you are all right, you are all right." The rhythmicity of the waves and her love of the ocean imagery helped Tracy to calm herself and stay in the classroom.

The Windshield Wiper and the Ongoing Processing of Emotional Information

I tell my clients that they must become accustomed to "keeping their windshield wipers on all day." Keeping the windshield wipers on means ongoing efforts at processing, understanding, and filing away events that arouse emotional reactions during the course of a day. Too often, criticisms, perceived rejections, or negative attributions stimulated by events start "clouding their windshields." By the end of the day, children may feel depressed and overwhelmed, without being able to put their finger on exactly what is bothering them. I teach children to make short comments about feelings that arise during the day so they can process and file each incoming piece of information that stimulates an affective reaction. By doing this, the sum total of their affective arousal does not overwhelm them at the end of the day.

Sometimes it helps to record these small events in a notebook to discuss with their parents at the end of the day, or with me in our next therapy session. This reinforces the young person's habit of noticing how he or she is reacting to things, so that we can develop countering strategies over time. The goal is for their "windshield wiper" to become automatic so that they can process these small affective disturbances with little effort and move on with their day.

Safety Imagery for Comfort and Relaxation

Helping children and teens learn how to find an optimal level of comfort and safety is an important component of affect tolerance. A safety zone can be developed through use of imagery or through a repetitive activity. This imagery or activity can be used as a retreat if feelings become too overwhelming at home or school. Safety imagery can involve beach scenes, or places children have seen in movies or books. Some children like to pick a favorite animal and imagine themselves as that animal in a peaceful location—under the sea, for example, or in a forest by a lake. The therapist can also suggest imagery that helps an angry part of the mind retreat to safety as well, like an imaginary soft room that can be punched without injury, or a special room with an imaginary pet tiger or snake that helps the angry self feel as powerful as the animal. This can become a place for the angry part of the self to find safety and relaxation without acting out.

As discussed in Chapter 9, some children who are motorically overaroused need some type of activity to calm themselves down. Video games on handheld devices can be used to restore a sense of calm during arousing therapy sessions, along with card games, pick-up sticks, throwing a ball back and forth, and other activities that involve focus, manipulation of materials, and behaviors that don't involve higher levels of thinking. Parents need to understand that these kinds of activities are stress relievers for many overaroused traumatized children and help children to restore their nervous system to an even keel.

Images of Power to Shift Direction

Children and teens who enter rage-filled states will no doubt express to you that they feel these switches are inevitable and uncontrollable. While they tell you they are regretful, even mortified, about what they have done in these other states, they perceive them as something that cannot be changed. Having them envision the self as powerful enough and in control enough to change becomes a first step in managing these extreme states.

I try to find an image of shifting direction that is particularly salient and appropriate to the clients I am working with, which may be based on an activity they enjoy, such as biking, skateboarding, surfboarding, or running during a sports game. I ask them to hold in their mind the image of themselves making a split-second decision to turn to the right instead of to the left. I ask them to imagine the sensations in their mind and body associated with making this quick decision and to find something to anchor them to this mental image. For girls, holding on to a wristband or bracelet could serve as a cue; for boys, it could be touching a belt buckle or clasping their hands together. The clients are taught to practice seeing themselves at a moment when they easily, seamlessly, with strength and fortitude choose to steer themselves in a different way. Imagery suggestions that connote personal power and determination helps solidify this important concept in their mind. To give them an opportunity to practice doing this, I instruct clients to hold on to this image of strength and self-direction throughout the day, even when they are not affectively aroused. Timothy used the image of his bike on a forked path to practice in his mind the idea that he could decide at any moment to shift the course he was taking, when feelings of fear and insecurity were aroused in his family. Eventually, you want the client to be able to use the image to help them choose another way to behave when extreme rage is aroused, but this may not happen immediately.

PROVIDE ALTERNATIVE ACTIVITY FOR
ANGER EXPRESSION

The client is rehearsing in his mind that he will have the strength and presence of mind to initiate a new path, and it is the therapist and family who must work out ahead of time with the client what the new path will be. It is easiest for families and children who are dealing with these extreme behaviors to have a physical place to go to that cues new behaviors—such as a "blow-off-steam area" or a "calm-down space." This space within the house, which can be the child's own room, the family room, the basement, or even the garage (if it is a warm and safe place), should include a variety of activities available to the child or teen. It is important to talk with the client to help develop ideas for supplying this special place, and using the calm-down area should be viewed as a very positive and heavily reinforced achievement. The first activity available must be one in which the client can expend physical energy to begin the process of dissipating the anger. Possible activities might be hitting a punching bag, breaking cardboard boxes, hitting a soft couch, or engaging in exercise on a treadmill. It is also important to have other kinds of activities in this space that serve to distract and to refocus the child's energy. There can be a bin of favorite puzzles or Legos and opportunities for creative expression with clay, or crayons, markers, and paper. Ideally, the client should move from the activity involving physical discharge to one involving creativity and focus. The end of the calm-down cycle might involve connecting with a beloved family pet.

Some families have even found it helpful to have "fire drills," where the child practices quickly running to the calm-down space to avoid inappropriate aggression. These drills for younger children can be staged throughout the day, initiated by an agreed upon signal. The child should be rewarded for succeeding even during the practice "fire drill." The goal, of course, is for the child or teen to be able to make the independent decision to go to the calm-down space when necessary. However, approximations toward this ultimate goal should be acknowledged and praised.

Parents and children must agree on the specific language that parents will use in encouraging utilization of the calm-down area. During confrontations, often the parent's tone of voice or escalating anger becomes an even more potent trigger, escalating the child's rage further. Simple words such as "time to take some space," or "room time" without much inflection in the voice may suffice. Some amilies use signs that the children have created ahead of time, giving helpful messages such as "You know what to do" or "Use your power to choose wisely." These calm-down spaces combined with the child's envisioning his own power to choose another response set the stage for the possibility of change.

HOW TO USE BEHAVIORAL REINFORCEMENT TO ASSIST WITH LEARNING AFFECT REGULATION

Behavior reinforcement programs are standard tools of trade in working with children and adolescents. While these can be useful, they can also backfire with dissociative children and teens who may not be able to keep the rewards in mind when intense affect states overwhelm them. Often, therapists and clients expect reward systems to accomplish more than they reasonably can with this population. However, there is a role for these programs within the total context of treatment interventions if the therapist keeps several cautions in mind. An emphasis should be placed on reward for making different choices at critical periods of affect arousal, rather than simply good behavior. A child who successfully calms down using alternative strategies or finds a nonaggressive solution to affect arousal is demonstrating key skills and should be praised and rewarded for the skill shown in making new choices. Children can be reinforced as well for getting control of their rage in only 10 minutes when it took 30 minutes yesterday, and earn tokens, points, or privileges for this achievement. It is important to make sure that what you are rewarding is not the absence of acting-out episodes, but the *actual skills* being utilized in calming down more quickly or making new choices at moments of key stress. Long-term rewards should be framed not as rewards for good behavior, but opportunities to have more privileges and age-appropriate resources because the child or teen has earned the trust of the family.

Emphasis is always placed on the critical, challenging moments when the child starts to enter an aggressive state but self-corrects, and utilizes other outlets for stress. As discussed in Chapter 10, I call these "save moments" and urge families to praise the child for the new path taken. Some families resist the idea of putting so much emphasis on things the child "should know already," but I try to help them see that their traumatized child doesn't have the automatic learning of these skills that other children have, and they may need to learn these small steps toward change and be recognized for them. I also encourage children and families to report "save moments" to me so we can evaluate together how well the child averted a potential disaster.

Finally, in establishing rewards for the child to change his behavior, it is important that the rewards have some meaning to the dissociated part of the self that may harbor the most rage. By utilizing "listening in" exercises, you can find what kinds of incentives might have meaning for this part of the self that is precipitating the misbehavior, and then make internal bargains to encourage cooperation.

For example, with Timothy we might ask if the "angry voice" would agree to avoid aggression against his grandmother in return for having Timothy earn time playing a favorite video game.

Timothy became increasingly skilled at utilizing his calm-down space that his grandmother and mother had created for him. He had Legos, mystery books, and old newspapers that he liked to crumple and jump on. Over time, he wanted to tell me about every moment a disaster was averted, and was able to identify what made him angry, what it reminded him of, and how he chose another path.

BUILDING ATTACHMENT ACROSS STATES

True healing occurs for a dissociative child survivor when attachment is consolidated across all states. Ultimately, explosive rages reflect a breakdown in the relationship between child and caregiver. Triggers for rage-filled behaviors will inevitably be interactions with their caregivers, and the child's rage-filled explosion against family members exemplifies this severe breach in attachment. That breach is generally more profound than the parents or therapist realize.

Most children and teens who have angry parts of the self that enact dissociated affect scripts in the family initially believe that the angry part of the self is *not* the child of these caregivers in a literal way. Early in my career, I discovered that many children who were adopted in the preschool or early school age years retained a sequestered part of their identity, often with a different name, the birth name, sometimes fluent in the birth language, whom they felt had never really been adopted by the new caregiver. In these early years of my therapeutic work, I used to do ritualized symbolic re-adoptions, with dolls representing the pre-adoptive self and found that the families and children experienced relief from these exercises and began to feel a sense of deeper connection. As I worked with severely dissociative children, I found that this part of the self that "does not have a mother" was often at the core of the extreme rage acted out against the parent. Then I learned that even children who were not adopted, who had lived with their biological parents from birth, if they experienced significant early interpersonal trauma, often retained a dissociative part of their identity that did not feel attached to the parent. Even children who have suffered from severe medical trauma may harbor a part of themselves who feels estranged, alienated, or unattached to their parents. When trauma has overwhelmed a child's ability to be soothed, this ruptures the parent-child bond in a fundamental way, which is often represented by a dissociative split into an attached and unattached identity state. Healing this rift in attachment does more to heal dissociation than does any other intervention that I have found. Uncovering the rift is the first step in this healing.

Often, even in the initial interview, I ask if the child perceives that there is a voice, an imaginary friend, or dissociated identity state, that does not like or feel attached to his or her primary caregiver. Almost inevitably, I find it is an angry dissociated state that has no sense of closeness to the parent. This phenomenon becomes self-reinforcing in families. As the child reacts in anger toward his parent, the parent responds by becoming rejecting, critical, and punishing. It is the dissociated part of the child that perceives the parent's rejecting critical stance, but the parent's disapproval means little to this dissociated identity state, as that part of the self feels little attachment to begin with.

Thus begins a vicious cycle in which both the child's and parent's anger and negativity reinforce one another. When the child is in a positive mood and enjoying positive attention from the parent, the parent has little awareness that these positive interactions are not being encoded, remembered, and stored across the child's whole mind, but instead are only selectively remembered by the friendly "attached" portion of the child. Meanwhile, the angry child state becomes more and more disconnected, and more and more angry as he perceives little opportunity to access the love and affection doled out when the child is calm.

Early on in the therapy, I try to have the parent communicate messages of attachment to the child's whole self. These communications, which I sometimes prepare ahead of time, or coach the parent to say in my presence with the child, may go something like this: "*You know I love the whole you. I love the funny you, the silly you, the baby you, and even the you that broke my CD player. I even love the voices in your mind that sometimes say mean things. It is all part of you, and it is you that I love. Even the angry part of you that has wrecked things in the house, I love. Come here. I want to hug all of you. Did the hug get all the way through? I want to be sure that even the little baby you that I didn't even know before you were adopted feels the hug, too.*" These speeches can be modified to address the circumstances that match the life and experience of each child. If the child has clear different names of identity states, the parent can mention loving the " 'Marcie' part of your mind just as much as I love you."

These interactions where the parent embraces and addresses love to the whole child feel profoundly relieving to the child. Although they may hesitate at first, children and teens report to me that dissociated parts of the self that feel unloved readily accept the love of the parent. This exercise may seem counterintuitive to some parents who fear they are accepting bad behavior. To encourage them to comply with this exercise, I ask them to imagine that the angry part of the self is like an angry 2-year-old screaming, "I hate you, I hate you." Would they say back to the 2-year-old, "I hate you, too?" Or would they scoop up the angry 2-year-old and try to dispel the rage with love? I explain that these dissociated parts of self are stuck in time in these early years and need the kind of love the parents might give a 2-year-old. The children report to me the parts of self that have felt unattached enjoy the parental attention directed to them in these exercises. In fact, just this exercise alone can have some effect on modulating the intensity of children's rage reactions.

Following my instructions, Timothy's mother told him that she understood about "angry voice" and loved him as a part of Timothy. When she hugged Timothy, she said, "I want to be sure you feel it all the way deep inside to every little part of you."

REASSURANCE OF SAFETY

When the angry reactions do not abate using all the techniques described above, it is often a safety issue that has been overlooked. Rage is part of the "fight or flight" reaction and signifies that the child is perceiving danger from some source in the environment. Evaluating where the child perceives this danger may be coming from becomes an important therapeutic intervention. After months of revolving-door hospital admissions for explosive anger, I asked Timothy if the "angry voice" inside of him knew that his perpetrator grandfather was gone for good. Timothy immediately began to argue with me. "He could come back anytime he wants. He could Google us and find our address. He could be waiting for me after school," Timothy insisted. Despite the reality that a protective order was in place and the grandfather had not been seen for six years, Timothy believed that his grandfather could carry out his threats of killing Timothy for telling the secrets of his abuse. The "angry voice" inside of Timothy kept him hypervigilant and ready for an attack at a moment's notice, and needed a reality check about the likelihood of the grandfather's return.

I engaged Timothy in a lengthy conversation regarding his safety and I asked him to be sure the "angry voice" was "listening in." With his mother and grandmother present, we discussed in depth what the legal protections for Timothy were, and how fast the police might get to the house if his grandfather showed up. We discussed how threats are a form of control and intimidation that are mainly used to frighten the child into silence. We discussed the risks for his grandfather of trying to follow through on the threats and how much more powerful Timothy now was compared to his grandfather, as Timothy was bigger and stronger, and had the power to get his grandfather in severe legal trouble if he showed up. These realities had not been considered to this depth before, and Timothy perceived that the "angry voice" was listening intently to the discussion. At the end of the discussion, Timothy reported to us that the "angry voice" conceded that the need to keep his attack skills so honed was no longer as necessary and that he would choose to wait "deep on the inside" for the day that his grandfather, or someone like him, might attack him. Timothy's behavior improved dramatically after this discussion, and the brutal attacks on family members lessened in severity and finally subsided.

Sometimes, simply identifying the danger that is feared can serve to comfort and reassure a rage-filled part of the self. For example, you might ask the child, "Is part of you afraid that you will be returned to the orphanage? Are you afraid you will you be punished the way you were in a previous home? Are you worried your parent will go back to using drugs? Are you worried your mom will go back to your abusive step father?" Naming the previously unnamed fear and addressing the child's concerns honestly can help to reassure parts of the self that are acting out as an expressing of their profound insecurity. (See Appendix J for a clinician checklist about aggressive behavior.)

Although I have mainly discussed working with rage reactions, clients can regulate and modulate intense feelings of sadness, sexuality, fear, or shame harbored in a dissociated part of the self using similar methods. The therapist works with the child and family to identify triggers and to modify the environment to reduce triggering. The therapist also works to promote a healthy attachment between the caregiver and child, including the part of the child represented by that dissociated feeling state. The therapist also addresses any ongoing fears or beliefs, whether realistic or unrealistic, to which the dissociated part of the self is clinging.

In the next chapter, we will explore family interventions in more depth. I will discuss how Timothy's family provided him with "empathy implosion" for his early trauma, which assisted in modulating the intensity of Timothy's anger and insecurity.

12 Child-Centered Family Therapy

Family Treatment as Adjunct to Dissociation-Focused Interventions

Plaintively, with wide eyes and a beseeching tone, Mrs. Patrick said, "I want the 'old Janie' back!" This request, more common than you might imagine, is based on the parent's desire to move back in time before the trauma, or to avoid acknowledging the multifaceted and complex person that her son or daughter has become. *"Development can only move in one direction—forward,"* I responded. *"You will never get the old Janie back, and that is not what you really want. What you really want is a new Janie, a new Janie that may get angry, show outrage, or disappointment, but will stay attached and feel loved through all her changes of state or difficulties in life."*

Traumatized children and teens cannot become fluent in affect management and regulation without family support to reinforce skills learned in therapy. Families must learn how to tolerate their children's expressions, even of anger and disappointment, while staying connected in a loving way. This is often a challenge, as families who have been traumatized, or had a child who was traumatized, often avoid speaking of the trauma, as this may arouse guilt for their role in not effectively protecting the child. When a traumatized child is adopted or placed in foster care, the new parents may want to focus only on the positive future and avoid the past, for fear of further traumatizing the child. Thus, families may engage in a collusion of mutual dissociation around the topics of trauma or other family secrets that arouse intense affect.

When working with traumatized children and their families, it is important to establish new ground rules that allow communication about previously off-limit topics. The therapist must help the families avoid defensive and self-justifying reactions to their child's hostility and blame by teaching families to provide a safe environment for the appropriate expression of feelings. Meeting with families also offers opportunity to educate them about the effects of trauma, how dissociation may express itself, and to build empathy and understanding for their child's symptoms.

Case studies of dissociative children in treatment suggest that family involvement is an essential component of the treatment of dissociative children. These traumatized and overwhelmed families need psychoeducation, support, and coaching on parenting strategies (Wieland, 2011b). As pointed out by Waters (1998), parents can serve as cotherapists in the treatment and their cooperative involvement in the therapy predicts treatment success (Silberg &Waters, 1998). Waters emphasized the importance of education about dissociation when children appear to deny even witnessed behaviors, and the importance of creating predictable routines and family rituals that serve a grounding function.

For some families, I use 15 minutes at the end or beginning of each hour-long session to touch base with the family. When working with teenagers, I try to have a family session at least once a month, where issues related to family communication and the teen's functioning in the family can be discussed. Whether or not the parent comes into any individual session, I encourage the families to leave me voice messages with updates on the child or teen's behavior, so that I am kept current about their challenges and behaviors over the past week.

THE THERAPIST STANCE

As therapist to the child, it can be tricky to try to manage the tension of alliances when parents want you to take their side during conflicts. However, I never shift my role from child therapist, even in family sessions, as the children or teens will perceive this as a betrayal, and have subsequent difficulty trusting a therapist that appeared to side with their parents against them. I warn parents in advance that family sessions may be hard on them, and that I may seem to be taking the child's side more than their own. If they have previously engaged in more conventional family therapy, they may be used to family therapists who appear to take a neutral stance toward family members or who frequently side with the parent to help the child learn to "behave." My stance is very different, as I am always representing the child's viewpoint, helping the child to find words to express what might have felt inexpressible, and helping the parents understand the child's reasons for frightening or aggressive behaviors. When my approach is explained as trying to provide as much safety as possible for the expression of emotions and the parents can see how well the child is responding, they come to appreciate this child-centered therapy approach—although they may need to brace themselves for some difficult sessions.

PSYCHOEDUCATION

Educating the parents about affect, trauma, and dissociation follows principles already covered in earlier chapters. However, there are some important points that are necessary to emphasize to parents as they prepare for the journey of treatment with their child survivor. Just as I have emphasized the adaptive value of the child or teen's symptoms to the client, this must be thoroughly explained to parents. Beleaguered, with resources stressed, and often at their wit's end, parents are quick to judge behaviors as disrespectful and provocative on purpose, and become impatient with their children. Emphasizing how aggression, for example, likely reflects the child's own feelings of lack of safety and need for self-protection gives parents a perspective that they can hold onto during challenging times. Explaining that self-harm may be the child's way of communicating feelings of low self-worth and powerlessness can be important for parents trying to understand their child's difficult behavior. By far the most important point that parents need to understand is that their children's reactions are rarely a personal attempt on the part of the child to be rude, obnoxious, or resistant to the parent. While it may feel this way on the surface, it is essential for the parent not to personalize these types of behaviors. These behaviors have meanings that extend far beyond the relationship between the child and parent and understanding their broader meaning can help decrease parents' defensive reactions and help them tune in more effectively to what the child really needs from them.

It is also important to prepare parents for what to expect from the treatment process. Parents should be warned that as their child becomes more comfortable in the realm of affective expression, the child could increase their emotional displays at home. Like a plumbing system that has been turned off for a while, when it starts to run again, there may be sudden explosive bursts and occasional drips, until the "plumbing system" of affects becomes more regulated (Silberg, 1999). As the parent comes to understand that the child's affective changes may, at first, not feel under the child's control, the families can structure the environment to help channel and direct the child's changing affective states into the most appropriate contexts. For example, regressive states are most appropriate at bedtime, when soothing and cuddle time with favorite transitional objects is most appropriate. After school is the best time for offering "wind down" time—a time when the child can be silly or playful. This may be followed with a more structured homework time. By structuring in these various time periods throughout the day, parents can help their child learn to match affective states to the appropriate context, moving the child in the direction of the healthy mind that is our ultimate goal.

Finally, a key goal of the therapist is to instill in families hope that their child can get better, along with an appreciation of their child's unique strengths and potentials. Traumatized children can be surprisingly resilient, and conveying our belief in them and an expectation of their ultimate success helps to promote this resilience.

EMPATHY IMPLOSION: COMMUNICATING HURT, PAIN, BETRAYAL, OR ANGER IN FAMILY THERAPY

The communication of feelings directly to a parent serves as an antidote to the affective dysregulation of dissociative children and teens. Creating a context in which affective communication feels safe is the single most effective way to build deeper attachments between the child and parent. Using words to express anger, hurt, pain, or disappointment, rather than acting out in angry or self-harming behaviors, connects the child's affect to the higher brain centers, helps cement the attachment relationship, and helps dissolve dissociative barriers. It is music to my ears when I hear children tell their parents how they "pissed them off," hurt their feelings, made them scared, or even caused them to feel unloved. If parents can sit and listen nondefensively, the intensity of the child's affect is modulated. The attachment breach from the time of trauma is repaired bit by bit every time one of these interactions occurs. Whether the child's expression of hurt, pain, or anger is based on a minor event, or is related to the overwhelming pain from the original trauma itself, these interactions are therapeutic building blocks of affect regulation and attachment.

Janie was 4 years old when she was adopted from a Korean orphanage. At age 16, Janie was still hypersensitive to any perceived criticism or rejection from her adoptive mother. Janie often wanted homework assistance when her mother was busy winding down from a long day and starting to prepare dinner. Her mother simply saying "Not now" would trigger Janie into feeling overwhelming abandonment, rejection, and thoughts of self-harm. She felt unloved, and that she was "stupid," as her schoolwork seemed too hard. The combination of rejection and self-doubt would propel Janie into self-loathing, despair, and abandonment anxiety and she would scream or slam the door to her room while cursing at her mother.

Janie's mother came to one of her daughter's therapy sessions, complaining of how demanding Janie was and wanted my help in explaining to Janie that there was no need to overreact to her mother cooking dinner. Janie was too old to be so demanding, her mother complained. Of course, Janie's mother was right. However, Janie needed to express to her mother exactly how being rebuffed at dinnertime made her feel, not as a way to assign blame, but in order to vent her feelings in the context of their enduring attachment. I explained to Janie's mother that Janie had never benefited from that early learning in the toddler years that relationships endure despite mild breaches or separations. Instead, Janie learned that her whole world could be turned upside down and disrupted profoundly in a moment's notice. Therefore, it is not unexpected that Janie would feel insecure when she feared her mother was angry with her or not available. This explanation provided an opportunity for Janie and her mother to recognize what they had missed out on in Janie's early years. In addition, Janie's mother dropped her defensiveness and became more open to dealing with Janie's demanding behavior. The conversation proceeded like this:

JANIE [LOUDLY]: It's like you don't care at all. I could flunk out of school for all you care. You just leave me like that. I feel so hurt.

MOTHER [ENCOURAGED TO LISTEN NONDEFENSIVELY]: When I don't help you right away, it's like I don't care at all. It's like I'm leaving you on your own when you really need me.

JANIE: Yeah! That's right! [Janie was relieved that her mother seemed to understand.]

MOTHER: I am so sorry. The last thing I ever want to do is to have you feel abandoned. I will always be here for you, no matter what. [Mother acknowledges Janie's deepest feelings and validates them, and reassures her.]

JANIE: Well, it sure feels like it.

MOTHER [AGAIN URGED TO NOT BE DEFENSIVE]: I am so sorry. That is not my intention.

THERAPIST: *How could Mom show you at the time that she does not mean to cause you feelings of abandonment? How can she show you she does want to help you, just not then?*

JANIE: She shouldn't turn her back on me.

At this point, Janie and her mother worked out a new strategy for dealing with Janie's demands at dinnertime. Janie's mother would turn to face Janie and reassure Janie of her love, before explaining that she had to cook dinner. This session helped reframe Janie's behavior for her mother. What her mother originally viewed as inappropriate and overdemanding behavior on the part of a 16-year-old was reframed as the behavior of a hurt and traumatized child who needed help to avoid being triggered during their interactions. For Janie, the opportunity to express her hurt and have it validated helped further cement the relationship between her and her mother and allay the insecurity from her past.

The same format of validation for feelings can be used for both minor and major difficulties in the parent-child relationship. At its essence, all developmental trauma is a betrayal of the promise of a safe childhood. All children view parents as representing the promise of protection against harm. Therefore, all parents must apologize when their child has been harmed, even if the events were out of the parent's control. These apologies are profoundly helpful to child survivors and help to moderate the anger of their betrayal and strengthen the child's connection to the parent.

In one emotional therapy session, I asked Timothy's mother and grandmother (see Chapter 11) to spend the whole hour trying to put themselves in Timothy's shoes and explain to him what they thought it was like for him to be trapped by his grandfather's secret abuse. Timothy was mesmerized by hearing their attempts to describe what it would feel like for a 6-year-old boy to be powerless, abused, and forced to keep this frightening secret. He was riveted as they described to him the terror, loneliness, and pain they knew he must have felt, and sometimes angrily corrected them if they expressed something inaccurately. This "empathy implosion" strengthened his attachment to them, and helped build his own empathic skills as well.

Parents may want to deflect the rawness of emotion conveyed in sessions during which early trauma is discussed by criticizing the child's use of words or tone. I urge parents to give children the freedom to express in their own way the intensity of the hurt, pain, and betrayal they have experienced. The experience is healing for children and helps them become more connected to their parents and family.

PRACTICING IDENTIFICATION OF TRIGGERS

Family therapy sessions are also useful for determining what facial expressions, words, or tones tend to set off automatic reactions in the child or teen. Research tells us that traumatized children are selectively responsive to angry expressions

(Pollack & Sinha, 2002), and this conforms to my clinical experience with clients. Traumatized children may interpret the arch of an eyebrow, a brief look in the eyes, or other momentary facial expression on a parent or sibling as anger, and an automatic behavioral reaction of fighting can be triggered. Parents are often surprised to learn how small expressions on the parent's part can serve as a reminder of a traumatic event and associated traumatic beliefs. The parent may say "No more TV" (because it is bedtime), and the child may interpret this as being punished for no reason, triggering the child's instinct to fight. Discussing phrases or looks that trigger the child, and agreeing on new expressions, can help circumvent arguments set in motion by these unintended triggers.

Sometimes, family sessions can be used to practice desensitizing family members to each other's facial expressions. As each member of the family shows their meanest face, angriest face, or most scared face, the other family members often erupt into uncontrollable laughter. This serves to desensitize everyone to the intense affects these expressions have come to provoke. These exercises can also help reinforce the idea that feelings in the family do not have to be contagious. Many traumatized children personalize their parent's mood and view them as a source of potential danger. Parents explaining their moods to their child, such as saying, "I am in a bad mood, but it is about work," can help children and teens disengage from the contagion of bad moods in the family.

BUILDING RECIPROCITY

The essence of trauma is helplessness, and no one feels more helpless in relationships than do traumatized children. Their helplessness is often deeply rooted in the belief that they are and will be perpetual victims. They believe that human relationships are characterized by the weak and the strong—a victim and an aggressor. The mutual interactive nature of relationships eludes them as they have felt "acted upon" and, thus, have come to believe that in order to get their needs met, they must "act upon" others. One of the reasons that the child survivor chooses to act out is to find a way to gain a sense of increasing control in their world. The inappropriate acting out then engages child survivors in a self-defeating cycles, as the response from the parent often increases the child's feelings of helplessness and stimulates further acting out. To overcome their view of themselves as powerless, it is important for children to learn that they do have some power in their relationships.

Ten-year-old Samantha was adopted at age four from a family in which she suffered sadistic physical and sexual abuse (see Chapter 9). Samantha taught me the metaphor of the blood pressure cuff. Once when Samantha had to go to the emergency room for treatment, the doctors used an automatic blood pressure cuff to assess her blood pressure. She disliked the sensation and fought to have the blood pressure cuff released. She noticed that the harder she fought, the tighter the cuff became. She realized that her behavior of fighting her mother when her mother was trying to help her, like the blood pressure cuff, only got more intense by her resistance. This metaphor helped her reframe her mother's interventions in a more positive way. This blood pressure cuff is similar to a Chinese finger trap puzzle that holds the fingers in a position of restraint—the harder you try to release your fingers, the tighter it becomes. Releasing the puzzle involves a counterintuitive movement of relaxation of the fingers. I use these metaphors to explain to my clients that the ways they are trying to get out of their helpless feelings are causing them to feel even more helpless—the way out of this trapped position is through open communication and discussion with their parents or caregivers. In these discussions, it must be possible for the child or teen's view to be respected and understood by the parent, and changes made when appropriate on rules or expectations.

Families must be willing to reward appropriate communication and reasoning with opportunities to be released early from grounding punishments, opportunities to negotiate later bedtimes, or handle times for chores in new ways. The goal is not to give the child the upper hand in these negotiations, but to give the child some sense of power and control. We want children to come to realize that they are more likely to get what they want when they employ communication and reasoning, and we want to illustrate that aggressive solutions will backfire and cause more restriction. We want children to learn that relationships can be reciprocal, and built on mutual trust and cooperation. Although some authoritarian families find it difficult to accept these kinds of negotiations, I explain that this is a necessary antidote to the helplessness experienced by a traumatized child, and it is important that the family be an environment that facilitates healing. The risk is that family life becomes more and more like the Chinese finger trap, with each side becoming more rigid and recalcitrant as they try to assert their authority and power.

ENCOURAGING AGE-APPROPRIATE ACTIVITIES AND RELATIONSHIPS

"She has no friends" is a refrain I often hear from the families of the child survivor. Traumatized children often find peer relationships to be a serious challenge. Struggling during their early years to maintain a hypervigilant focus on managing relationships with caregivers, these children often have little knowledge of the give-and-take of peer relationships. They may be seen as "odd" or "off" by peers from an early age, leading to bullying and scapegoating. This adds to their trauma, as they learn that even peer relationships are dangerous. Traumatized children may try to dominate peer relationships and try to establish friendships with much younger children, which make them feel safer and in control. Conversely, they may enter into peer relationships in which they are dominated, submitting to the dominant child's whims for the benefit of a friendship. Teens who have been sexually abused may come to believe that the only basis for a relationship is their value as a sexual object; they may become promiscuous, seeking contact in the way that feels familiar. Other teens may have friendships ruined by their erratic and changeable behavior or by their apparent amnesia for planned excursions. Often, however, the children I see stay isolated from peer relationships and view them with caution, if not fear.

Yet, we know that success in peer interactions is a very important predictor of future success for children and teens. Close friendships teach children the values of trust, intimacy, and shared affection. Friendships also help children learn appropriate self-disclosure, and help build empathy through learning to understand other people's perspectives (Gifford-Smith & Brownell, 2002). Research shows that the ability to acquire friends requires both affect regulation and mentalization (appreciating the contents of other people's minds)—skills that are often difficult for traumatized children (Fonagy & Target, 1997).

For children and teens with dissociative symptoms, friendships are even more significant. Nothing motivates children or teens to end dissociative behaviors more than do peer relationships. There are a variety of reasons why peer relationships are such a key training ground for achieving the seamless state shifts, appropriate to context, that are the hallmarks of the healthy mind. Most importantly, these relationships promote the child's motivation to appear normal, act normal, and be like everyone else. Traumatized children do not want the embarrassment of being identified as "weird" or "different." Children may have wildly fluctuating states at home, but seem to somehow make it through the day without incident at school. Children have explained to me that they expend significant effort to keep themselves focused on staying present and grounded when they are with their peers. This degree of effort and intentionality to stay grounded is relaxed when they are back at home, where the embarrassment of being different is not such a big concern. A child or teen who regresses in the home environment to a younger state may expect some indulgence, change in voice, or reciprocal accommodation from parents. However, in a peer environment, such a shift may result in mocking behavior on the part of the peer observer, or a quick. "Knock it off." The peer environment often has little tolerance for dramatic and unexplained shifts in behavior, which trains the children and teens to present a more coherent and consistent self. Finally, successfully engaging with peers is intrinsically so potentially rewarding and fun that the dissociative child and teen is at an optimal level of arousal where traumatic intrusions are less likely to interrupt the child or teen's consciousness.

For all of these reasons, helping isolated children and teens achieve even one friendship can be very beneficial. Because the children are so often hesitant to create these opportunities themselves, I encourage the parents to find a likely friend through asking the teacher who an appropriate choice might be. At first, activities that do not demand too much reciprocity can be encouraged—like movie outings or ice-skating. As the child becomes more comfortable, short afternoons with structured activities where the parent is supervising is recommended. While this may seem second nature in the lives of most families, the parents of the severely traumatized child often forget to make time for these important normalizing childhood experiences, and thus therapist encouragement is often necessary. In preparing families and children for these outings, it is important to help the children maintain a sense of privacy about their traumatic histories and the working of their internal worlds.

Some teenagers newly diagnosed with a dissociative disorder may want to share this information widely, as a new ticket to popularity. This always backfires, and often ends in inappropriate or exploitative relationships. One teenage girl in my practice became involved with a young man who figured out how to get her to switch to a sexualized self-state, and used that information to repeatedly exploit her. Families and teens must be cautioned to keep information about dissociation private to prevent ostracism or exploitation.

TRAUMATIZED FAMILY BELIEFS

The task of parenting traumatized children is extraordinarily difficult, and parents need to be sensitive to their own issues and recognize impediments they may have to responding appropriately to their children. For example, some parents may themselves be coping with a history of trauma or may be traumatized by what happened to their child. Traumatized parents and parents with unresolved losses often have difficulty consistently and appropriately responding to their children. This can promote disorganized attachment in their children and predispose children to dissociative reactions (Hesse, Main, Abrams, & Rifkin, 2003). As James (1994) has sagely pointed out, parenting a traumatized child requires self-awareness, an ability to handle exploration of the child's trauma and one's own trauma, the ability to accept direction and work as a team, and the willingness to get help for oneself as needed. The work required in family therapy requires psychological stamina, and perceptiveness, capacity for insight, and self-awareness. Many parents with trauma histories will need to be in their own therapy in order to successfully handle the demands of adjunctive family therapy. Yet, I have found in my practice that most parents I have met have the love, commitment, stamina, and psychological-mindedness to engage in this difficult work.

Some parents will hold on to beliefs stemming from their own families of origin, which interfere with the healthy messages we teach children in therapy. These beliefs will need to be identified and corrected for their children to heal. Some of the traumatic beliefs of families are identified in Table 12.1.

Parents who have come from families where there has been multigenerational trauma may come to overly identify with the child's trauma. They may believe that it is impossible for the child to truly heal, as they themselves have been unable to heal (see 1 and 4 in Table 12.1). If they themselves have not successfully processed their own feelings of self-blame for trauma they suffered, they may project some of that blame on their children (see 2 in Table 12.1). Some of the parents may identify with the child's traumatic belief that whoever hurt the child is more powerful than they are, and seem as frightened as the child by the prospect

Table 12.1 Traumatic Beliefs of Families of Traumatized Children

1. You are damaged just like me.
2. I deserved it—you deserved it. This is my punishment.
3. I am helpless to parent you. The abuser is more powerful than I.
4. You can never be normal.
5. I'll always be there because you can't protect yourself.
6. I am better than the ones that hurt you.
7. You'll be just like them. I won't let you do to me what they did.
8. It's me and you against the world.

of retraumatization (see 3 in Table 12.1). Parents may also become entrenched in a paranoid belief system that danger lurks everywhere. As a result, they may become overprotective and mistrusting of the child's friends, their child's friend's parents, or even health professionals. As these parents react to their suspicions with retreat, their paranoia is reinforced and they come to believe that no one can understand the depth of suffering that their child has gone through (see 8 in Table 12.1), and may give a message to the child that she can never be safe (see 5 in Table 12.1).

Some parents may perceive the child as a victimizer and be caught in a cycle with the child, where they each alternate between victimizer, victim, bystander, and rescuer (Silberg, 2004). In these cases, family therapy is needed to help identify these counter-therapeutic roles and find ways to free parents from these collusive binds with their children. Families who have passed down cycles of abuse from one generation to another are particularly vulnerable to giving mixed messages to the child, in which they alternate between wanting to protect the child, feeling helpless in the way they themselves were helpless in stopping their own abuse, and fearing the child is "just like grandpa" or other family members who abused them (see 2 and 7 in Table 12.1).

Some adoptive parents avoid all responsibility for their behavior toward the child by attributing all the child's symptoms to what occurred prior to adoption. This can enrage the child, who feels discounted by the parents constantly bringing up the past as an avoidance strategy for dealing with the current everyday problems in the household. The assistance of other professionals to provide therapy to the parents may be necessary when the traumatic beliefs of the families serve to interfere with the child's treatment (see 6 in Table 12.1).

DISSOCIOGENIC FAMILY PATTERNS

As I have come to know the families of my clients, I have noticed some characteristics that can inadvertently promote dissociative coping styles in children and teens. Sometimes families covertly collude with dissociative strategies by subtly disallowing the expression of certain feelings in the context of the family. At other times, parents selectively reinforce certain dissociative states of functioning with their own reciprocal change of state, thus reinforcing the child's own dissociative strategy. For example, when a child regresses, the parents may treat the child in infantilizing ways, or become hostile and defensive themselves when the child enters an angry state. When these patterns exist, it is important to educate the families about their behaviors, and try to encourage new parenting behaviors during the family sessions. The following are some family patterns that are particularly challenging for the child survivor.

Authoritarian Families and Over-Controlling Families

In authoritarian families, parents have strict rules about rudeness, manners, and appropriate ways to talk to adults. These households can run perfectly well when they are raising children without the developmental disruptions of early trauma. Normal children can learn to adjust to these requirements and adjust their behaviors accordingly. However, children with traumatic backgrounds, who are prone to dissociative responding, will adapt in a surface way to these rigid household expectations, and then develop an "angry Suzie" dissociative state or imaginary friend that will express the child's rebellion. The family will be harshly rejecting to the "angry Suzie" presentation, thus further disrupting the potential for attachment. These families must come to understand that "angry Suzie" can be progressively shaped into more appropriate behavior, but they will have to be more lax in their strict behavioral rules in order to embrace the "angry Suzie" part of the child and allow expression of the feelings of hurt and rejection that the rigid rules provoke in the child.

India was a 7-year-old girl adopted from Russia at the age of 3. She lived in a family with these kinds of rigid expectations. Because of how well she performed some of the time in following their strict rules of table manners and decorum, the family found it impossible to accept her "Wild Indie" behavior, which included throwing food at the table, slamming doors, and talking back. I had to help India's family understand that the "real India" was not the way she behaved in her "perfect" moments, but that the "real India" was likely a combination of all of the different feelings and states she expressed. While the blended "India" would not be perfect, she would be real.

Parents Who Are Closely Enmeshed With Their Child

On the opposite end of the spectrum are the overly indulgent parents who accommodate the regressive behaviors of their children and are threatened by their child's increased independence and self-reliance. These parents may be eager to accept the regressed presentations of the child, and fail to help the child appropriately handle traumatic losses and move on. These families need support in appropriately pushing the child toward age-appropriate functioning.

Lisa was an 18-year-old college freshman who was abused by a neighborhood boy between the ages of 6 and 10, and suffered multiple losses. Lisa spoke to her mother three times a day, and got advice for everything, including what to wear to social events or what topics to pick for her papers. Lisa also had an angry and bitter dissociative state that blamed her mother for not having known about the abuse. As this antagonistic dissociative state expressed herself more in treatment, Lisa would avoid talking to her mother for weeks at a time, and often engaged in reckless behavior during these times. This led her mother to reprimand Lisa about her poor decision making and warn Lisa that she could only thrive in college with her mother's daily support. Lisa and her mother needed to learn to disengage from this regressive dependency to achieve a more healthy balance between support and independence. Otherwise, Lisa would continue to alternate between these extremes and not learn the self-regulation necessary for functioning independently at college. If parents evidencing patterns such as these have difficulty examining their own contribution to the child's behavior, supportive therapy for the parent may be required, as well as intermittent family sessions. As Lisa moved forward in her integration, she adjusted to calling her mother weekly, and made independent decisions about clothes and paper topics.

Divorced Households With One Abusive Parent

An increasingly common phenomenon of our society is that children, even very young children, may be required to split their time between two households. Family courts are guided toward a presumption of joint custody and expect both parents to get along for the sake of the child. Courts are not always equipped to understand that a child whose parents are divorced might also be a victim of abuse in one of those households. As a result, too frequently, children from divorced families are ordered into the unsupervised care of a parent who abuses them (Hannah & Goldstein, 2010; Neustein & Lesher, 2005). This is an extraordinarily difficult problem for the protective parent and for the child. One common coping mechanism for a child forced into this kind of arrangement is dissociation (Baita, 2011; Silberg & Dallam, 2009). To manage the differing treatment they get in each household, children may adapt by a separate persona, or dissociated state, to cope with the abusive household, and often will show amnesia for the abuse while living at the other household. While protecting the child from awareness of the dilemma of the situation, this amnesia also makes it difficult to get a disclosure of abuse. This kind of court-ordered dilemma is one of the most dissociogenic situations a child can encounter, as all of the necessary features for promoting dissociation are present: contrasting environments and expectations, abuse from which there is no apparent escape, and no opportunity to be soothed from the abuse (Kluft, 1985). I have referred in previous chapters to Adina, a child of 8 caught in this exact situation and evidencing dissociation in her clinical presentation. Adina described to me clearly that her brain was split in to two "inner people," which helped her function, depending on whose house she was in. She explained she could not remember what happened in each house, as a different half of her brain took over.

Therapy served a powerful role as the only place where both "halves" of her brain were allowed to coexist and learn about each other. This set the stage for her ability to disclose the abuse that was occurring at her father's home, although it took six months of therapy before she was willing to speak openly about the abuse. Clinicians should be particularly alert for signs of dissociation when children have alleged abuse but remain court-ordered to visit the household in which abuse was alleged. (See more about this in Chapter 14.)

SWITCHING DURING FAMILY THERAPY

The intensity of affect in family meetings can lead children to switch from state to state as they seek to avoid the intensity of affect arousal through engaging in their automatic behavioral programs. They may become angry, fearful, or regressed, curling in a ball or talking like a baby. These are wonderful learning opportunities for the families and the children. In these cases, you can witness the kinds of transition moments that might evoke state change in the home in living color right before your eyes. Both the family and child can learn from you how to handle these moments and you can teach the family and child about alternatives to the automatic behaviors. You can illustrate through your reactions that affects can be tolerated, and that communication with loving family members is the antidote to their avoidance and fear. The key strategy for the family and child is to identify the feared affect that led to the behavioral avoidance represented in the switch and find ways to accept it, talk about it, and act on it in new ways.

The case of Jennifer (introduced in Chapter 10), a survivor of sexual assault and family violence, provides an excellent illustration of intervening during switching in a family session. Jennifer and her mother were processing the sadness they both felt about the illness and decline of Jennifer's ailing maternal grandmother. Jennifer had written a poem about her love for her grandmother, and when she read the poem, her mother started to cry. Her mother's tears evoked fear in Jennifer, who remembered early years of family violence. Jennifer suddenly regressed into a 4-year-old state, and ripped up the poem, stating, "Bad poem made mommy cry."

Gently, I explained to Jennifer the difference between tears of tenderness and tears of fear, and asked her if she would help me tape the poem back together. Jennifer's mother had an opportunity to observe my encouragement of a more mature approach and followed my lead, instead of indulging the regressive behavior, as she usually did. As Jennifer taped the poem back together, she switched back to her 14-year-old self and continued the discussion. By keeping focused on the task, I illustrated to Jennifer that the task could be handled despite her fears, and that the environment did not have to switch because she did. I modeled the acceptance of her mother's sadness and encouraged sharing the moment of sadness together, rather than avoiding the intensity of the affective arousal.

Some children may switch into angry states in the course of family therapy. As long as the child is not acting destructively, I encourage the family to accept the intensity of the expressed feelings, even if they consider the expression rude. As long as there is no name-calling and no threats, I don't mind if colorful language is used if it helps the children express the depth of their feelings. Inevitably, the intensity is modulated just by the tolerance of its expression in the session. This allows the family to engage in emotional communication outside of the therapy that is more authentic, which continues to modulate the intensity of angry states. If children's authentic expression of anger can be respected and tolerated, they will no longer need to enact their rage in another state. The opportunity to express angry feelings contained in another state directly to the parents serves to erode dissociative barriers in a powerful way.

Appendix K provides a checklist for clinicians to guide family therapy with the child survivor and her family.

The role of family is key as well in the next central task of therapy, which is the "T" in the EDUCATE model, processing traumatic memories, which will be explored further in the next chapter.

13 Rewriting the Script
Processing Traumatic Memories and Resolving Flashbacks

What is the most natural thing for a child to do when she has fallen off her bike and hurt herself? Well, of course, tell her parents. It is usually upon the telling of the event that the emotional expression begins, the crying, maybe even sobbing. This sobbing serves both as a physiological release of the pain and trauma, and as an opportunity for soothing through bonding with the loving other who comforts, listens, validates, and understands. After such an experience, the traumatic event will be remembered, but not with avoidance or the development of enduring symptoms. When traumatic events that do not overwhelm the child's resources are processed with a loving caregiver shortly after their occurrence, the child's equilibrium is restored, and there are generally no enduring effects.

Like the loving caregiver, the trauma therapist has the power to provide the soothing relationships that can counter trauma. Listening to the child or teen and serving as a witness to what he or she has suffered is a key and powerful healing component. Our therapeutic attempts to process traumatic events with children should try to approximate the normalcy of telling a story in a soothing and validating relationship, as described above. The validation should be in the context of a caring relationship, allow for the expression of emotion and recounting of the events, and be as soon after the trauma occurred as possible.

Yet, children who have survived developmental trauma have many impediments that may have blocked previous attempts to be soothed after trauma, and these impediments interfere with their receptiveness to our interventions. In many cases, caregivers have been the ones inflicting the trauma, setting up an impossible bind and leading the traumatized children to believe that what they need the most following trauma is impossible to attain. Even when children find someone to soothe them, reassurance itself can become a new trigger, since they have learned that their environment does not stay safe for very long. Soon emotions associated with the trauma become a trigger as well, as they are no longer signals for useful escape or self-protection. Instead, emotions associated with the trauma signify to the child survivors that they will have little control over their environment or the promise of future safety. Self-protective memory processes help clients avoid thinking of painful events, and soon the child survivors may no longer remember what happened to them.

Rather than simply run in to your office to tell you the painful events endured and receive validation and support, like the crying child after the bike accident, your young client may present anywhere along a continuum of being flooded with overwhelming memory or denying that anything ever occurred. As therapists, we are the counterbalance to the polarity of the posttraumatic stress reaction. When memories are too intrusive, we are there to help clients evaluate what has triggered their flashback and to help them differentiate the present from the past. When clients avoid acknowledgement of traumatic events, we are there with gentle reminders that tie behaviors to known events from their past. As we struggle with our reactions, we may ourselves vacillate between feeling a pressure to hear the traumatic events, and seeking to avoid exposing ourselves to them. In addition, we may want to protect the young child survivor from the pain that comes with remembering past trauma. In these cases, therapists must navigate through the resistances of the clients as well as their own in determining how and when to delve into their clients' traumatic past. This processing of the traumatic past is the "T" in the EDUCATE model, and is the focus of this chapter.

WHEN IS THE RIGHT TIME TO PROCESS TRAUMA WITH CHILDREN AND ADOLESCENTS?

When working with adult survivors of complex trauma, it is advised that trauma processing occur in the mid-phase of treatment after a course of stabilization (Brand et al., 2012; Chu, 1998; Herman, 1992; Loewenstein, 2006; Turkus & Kahler, 2006; van der Hart et al., 2006). Processing too soon may destabilize fragile adult survivors, leading to hospitalization, self-injury, and regression. However, with children and adolescents, this blanket recommendation needs to be reevaluated as relevant to each child's unique situation. It is important to recognize that children and teens have not had as much opportunity to develop the avoidance defenses and phobia to the traumatic content that gives it so much power with adult survivors.

Over time, the overuse of avoidance defenses convinces the self that the feelings associated with the trauma are as dangerous as the trauma. This perception becomes increasingly reinforced over time, as a feedback loop of traumatic trigger, avoidance, and then relief is initiated over and over again. By the time the traumatized individual has reached adulthood, this feedback loop of avoidance and relief has been reinforced so many times that it can be very difficult to break. At this point, reminders of the trauma and the feelings associated with the trauma have become almost indistinguishable from the trauma itself.

However, with children we have the opportunity to talk to them closer to the events and more closely model the healing effect of direct support and soothing. They have not had as much time to practice the avoidance and relief cycle. Thus, children and adolescents do not require as much preparation as adults before trauma work begins. In fact, with children and adolescents, there are times when it is particularly appropriate to discuss the traumatic events sooner rather than later. For example, a child who comes to your office may actually be still in the process of enduring that trauma on a daily basis, as was my client Adina during the first six months of treatment. The longer it takes for the child to disclose on-going abuse, the longer the child may have to endure living in that environment. Sometimes, the child may no longer be living in that environment, but there may be other children who are being traumatized on a regular basis. Waiting to hear the child's experience may result in other children remaining in danger of being abused as well. Another time when it is important to discuss traumatic events is when children are being referred for therapy after abuse is discovered and there are pending legal charges. Allowing the child to share his story closer to the time of the events may insure that the details are more accurate. As therapy records could be subpoenaed, these events may need to be discussed and recorded care-fully. Another time that dealing with traumatic content earlier in treatment may be necessary is when dangerous symptoms such as aggression, sexual acting out, or flashbacks have escalated, impairing functioning. Often, this escalation of symp-toms is a form of communication that the environment has become unsafe and some important information must be revealed.

So the answer to when is the right time to tell about the trauma is—it depends. Typically, processing traumatic memories occurs in the mid-phase of therapy, after skills in affect modulation have been taught and the child has begun the process of making connections with the whole self. While you are likely at this stage during the mid-phases of treatment, there are many circumstances in which you will need to deal with traumatic material early in the treatment as discussed above—such as when disabling symptoms overwhelm the child, when legal proceedings require it, when other children may be in danger, or when the child has been waiting to tell someone of a recently experienced event. The farther away in time the disclosure is from the time of the traumatic incident, the more in-depth the processing of this event may need to be. For events close to the time of trauma where avoidance de-fenses have not developed, telling about the events, their meaning to the child, and the child's feelings and reactions can occur quickly and earlier in the treatment. However, for repeated events endured during the developmental period, for which soothing was never provided, traumatic processing may be a lengthier process, continuing through many months of therapy.

Sometimes, hospitalization can even be avoided if traumatic intrusions that reveal unprocessed trauma are dealt with in outpatient therapy at the time the in-tense symptoms appear. Marks (2011) described an intensive outpatient treatment model for a dissociative child in which the child is seen every day for two weeks to intensively process trauma when symptoms are severe and the therapy seems stuck. I use a similar methodology for traumatic processing, treating clients for several weeks intensively during their summer vacations from school, scheduling 1.5–2-hour sessions daily. These intense sessions can be cathartic and allow chil-dren to finally express anger against a former parent who hurt them severely, or reveal details of abuse that have never before been shared.

According to Blaustein and Kinniburgh (2010), "To safely explore memory, a child must have some capacity to modulate affect and physiology, must have developed some sense of safety in the therapeutic relationship and must have a sufficiently stable context outside of the clinical space" (p. 224). With children, discussing traumatic events rapidly creates a therapeutic relationship with the therapist that in itself provides an antidote to the traumatic event. Children are less demoralized about relationships than are traumatized adults and, therefore, develop the trust needed to discuss traumatic content more readily. It is also important to note that the modulation of affect and physiology required to prepare a child to tell a trauma story can be very modest with children. Sometimes simply having a soft couch to sit on and a stuffed animal or pillow to hold may provide enough soothing and modulation so that children feel comfortable telling their story. Knowing that a loving caregiver is available during or after the session also provides an important form of modulation that is typically unavailable to the adult survivor.

THE COMPONENTS OF PROCESSING TRAUMATIC MEMORY

Imagine a mirror reflecting an image from a mirror across the room, creating an infinite reflection of the same image, smaller, but reaching far back, seemingly forever. Events and emotions experienced at the time of trauma similarly leave their echoes and reflections on current-day behavior like the images in the hall of mirrors. For the traumatized child, emotional experiences rarely occur in isolation, but have long histories of associations to a long series of similar events from the past. When children's behavior appears inexplicable to themselves or to others, it is often necessary to go back through that "hall of mirrors" to find other similar events, and eventually an index event may be discovered that contains raw emotional power that is driving some current behavior. The affects and memories associated with this index event or events are often sequestered from everyday functioning, with an avoidance loop of rehearsed forgetting and dissociation. But reminders of the event are everywhere, and these reminders stimulate nonconscious trauma-based reactions.

Processing those events involves encoding the experiences is a new way, so that the information contained in the traumatic memory is consolidated and integrated and connections are developed between the limbic areas of the brain and the higher brain centers. Successful processing involves activating multiple brain functions originally associated with the traumatic event under new calmer circumstances, and providing desensitization to this originally overwhelming material.

I have found that the following components are important to include in the processing of traumatic material with the child survivor: **content of the traumatic event** (focus on memory of the events themselves), **sensorimotor experiences associated with the event**, exploring **the event's meaning** to the child, **affects** (such as anger, shame, fear, sadness, abandonment, and loneliness), and

mastery experiences that counter feelings of powerlessness. This processing must take place in the context of a **validating relationship** either with the therapist, or conjointly with a loving caregiver. The attention to the original traumatic events targeting each of these domains of experience provides ultimate resolution to the child survivor by countering the dissociative avoidance that has given rise to multiple symptoms.

Setting the Stage

The therapist sets the stage that the office is a safe place in which traumatic events can be acknowledged by referring in a matter-of-fact way to the traumatic events throughout early conversations. This is done by connecting the trauma to behaviors that are being addressed in the therapy. For example, if a child has had difficulties with sexual acting out, the therapist might casually say, "*When children come from families where parents have been too free with their bodies and not respected the privacy of children's bodies, children may get confused over what's okay to do and what isn't. I can understand how that happened to you.*"

If a child with a trauma history comes into the office after having overreacted to a peer conflict, this becomes a perfect time to tie present reactions to past experiences. For example, the therapist might say, "*I can see why you are feeling upset. That might have reminded you of the very scary thing that happened to you when you were little, when you felt really helpless—being hit like that might not feel the same to you as it does to other kids, since you had so much hitting in your life when you were younger.*" Similarly, the therapist may tie in the feelings of being targeted by classmates with past experiences: "*When someone does something to you on purpose, like that kid at school who took your pencil, it might make you angrier than other children, because you remember that your dad, used to do things to hurt you on purpose, and that was terrible for you.*" These kinds of comments throughout early sessions establish the therapist as someone who knows about the past, is not afraid to talk about it, and understands how the current environment is filled with reminders of past traumatic events. Hopefully, your young clients will soon be able to make similar associations between their own behavior and past experiences. You can help them make these connections sooner through your open acknowledgement of the connections between the past and the present.

Telling About Traumatic Events

When your client begins to tell you about a traumatic event, it is important to provide calming and safe sensory or sensorimotor stimulation, such as soft toys to hold or blankets to wrap up in. Ideally, clients have already practiced with you finding safe and healing images, and they know how to use breathing exercises to combat stress (see Chapter 9). When telling about trauma, children can be given frequent breaks and offered alternative activities to help calm them. With Timothy, victim of sadistic abuse at the hands of his grandfather, the calming needed to engage in traumatic processing only happened after he had played a few rounds of "Angry Birds." We alternated ten minutes of this video game with ten minutes of talking about traumatic events. Video games also provide instant feelings of mastery in defeating an enemy, provide bilateral brain stimulation, and provide a good motivator to intersperse with the difficulty of traumatic processing.

It may also be helpful to provide children with symbolic means of communicating their trauma story, as this can provide a safe distance from material that they can't bring themselves to disclose. They may prefer depicting the event through drawing pictures, writing about it, or acting it out with puppets or toys.

Fifteen-year-old Deborah, adopted from a Romanian orphanage at age 3, drew the picture shown in Figure 13.1, which is a cartoon-like representation of an imaginary character that was abandoned. While she did not have the actual memory of her own abandonment, she had internalized feelings of being unloved due to her stormy early history that needed to be processed. In the picture, Deborah depicted a birth mother prior to giving her child up for adoption, saying, "Everything" was wrong with her. Deborah's picture allowed us to talk about her feelings of abandonment, and I helped her appreciate her true special qualities that her birth

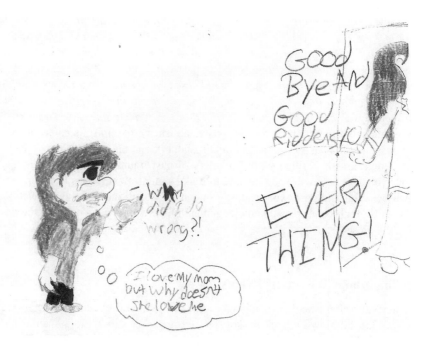

Figure 13.1 Deborah depicts feelings of abandonment. Used with permission.

mother could never have really known about. Her adoptive mother participated in the session to reinforce this message.

For older children who are not interested in play or art, writing the memories in a special memory journal may be the best approach. Some children will develop a memory book in which each page contains a picture, poem, or description of an event from their past. When children write about or depict traumatic events, I ask them to add an empowering message to the page or drawing—something that remarks on something that is different between that time and now, describing how they are different, or describing what they might have done right in the situation.

Figure 13.2 shows 11-year-old Shantay's picture of herself as a neglected infant before her adoption. She was instructed to tell something empowering to the crying baby and she wrote, "She will get better sooner than you think."

Some children will type things on e-mail or instant message, and send information to me with this electronic media, which sometimes gives them distance to say things they might not have had the courage to tell me directly. Other young children may find it safer to tell their stories to a puppet in my office rather than to me.

When children have inner voices, imaginary friends, or dissociative states that have been identified, I invite them to include that part of their mind in the

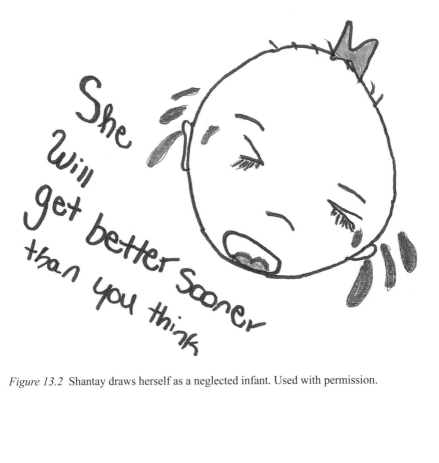

Figure 13.2 Shantay draws herself as a neglected infant. Used with permission.

activities. Checking repeatedly whether the "Sad Jane," "angry voice," or "Other Angela" is feeling okay about what is being discussed helps the child know you are connecting to their whole self during this difficult exploration.

Connecting to Sensorimotor Experiences

When the child is drawing, playing, or recounting traumatic events, and anchored with safe and calm imagery or sensory stimulation, it is useful to inquire about sensory experiences during the time of trauma—How did your tummy feel? Where in your body did you feel it? What did the pain feel like? You might ask them to draw or create other representations of the pain or other sensations. If the activity becomes too overwhelming, allow the client an opportunity to retreat to the pleasant sensory experiences that you have provided.

Connecting to the Meaning of the Events

The most painful aspect of the traumatic events is often the meaning these events hold for how the child and teen survivor views himself. I ask children questions such as, "What did you think this meant about you when this happened? Do you ever wonder why this happened to you? What do you answer to yourself?" These kinds of questions often get to the heart of the stuck thoughts that trap the child in a stranglehold. These stuck thoughts about the self are generally "shame-based" ideas, which tend to be the most painful of all affective experiences (Kluft, 2007). Shame has its roots in the early experience of ruptures in relationship with important attachment figures that leave children feeling exposed and blameworthy (Lewis, 1987). The feeling of shame may serve as an adaptive strategy of self-punishment to remind the developing child of the consequences of disrupting pleasurable experiences, such as connection to attachment figures (Nathanson, 1992). This cycle of self-punishment becomes acute for children whose early attachments are fraught with painful experiences and repeated disruptions. These lead to beliefs that they are to blame for the trauma they suffered because of some shameful characteristic of the self. Child survivors learn to avoid thinking about forbidden, shame-based thoughts, which become more powerful over time. These forbidden thoughts contain beliefs about their identity and circumstances that lead them to feel even more trapped and hopeless.

Examples of shame-based thoughts that may emerge from these discussions include: "There is something terrible about me that will always make me a victim"; "I caused this abuse because of something terrible about me"; "When people get to know me they will find out terrible things that will make them hate me."

Once we have identified these shame-based thoughts, I use a subjective units of distress scale as utilized in Eye Movement Desensitization Reprocessing (EMDR) (Adler-Tapia & Settle, 2008) and ask children to rate how much they

Table 13.1 Examples of Traumatic Thoughts With Opposite Thoughts

Traumatic Thoughts	"Opposite" Thoughts
People who know me hate me and will harm me.	People who have harmed me don't know me at all. When people get to know the real me, they will love me and not harm me.
I was weak and stupid.	I protected myself as best as I could; I now have the tools to protect myself better.
I blame myself for being there.	What happened to me was caused by other people's bad choices. I can make a good life for me with my own good choices.

believe this thought on a scale of 1 to 10. As we begin to talk about the thoughts that are evoked from the worst traumatic memories, the clients usually rate these as somewhere between 8 and 10. Even 7- or 8-year-old children can understand a rating scale. However, they might use markers or crayons to color a graph or "feeling thermometer" to show how high the feeling feels to them.

The next challenge is to come up with an "opposite thought" that promotes a counter-view to the traumatic belief. This is a very difficult thing for the child survivors to think of independently. Often, I must create and write it down for them, as the ideas contained in the opposite thought seem so foreign and unfamiliar. I ask the client to rate these opposite thoughts, as well. At the beginning, the client's belief in these is low; they will often be rated as a 2 or 3. This rating system serves as a useful measure of the client's progress in countering their trauma-based negative cognitions. Children are often proud and surprised when they see a record of these changes. Examples of traumatic thoughts alongside their opposite thoughts are included in Table 13.1.

Connecting to Affective Experiences at the Time of Trauma

Connecting to the affective experiences at the time of trauma is key for defeating dissociative barriers and resolving trauma. Once the child has connected to the negative affect, empathy and compassion from the therapist as well as from the child toward himself can mitigate the intensity and help the integration of the affective experiences.

The primary method for getting the young person to make these connections is to resonate with the emotion of the child and amplify it, expressing the feelings that the child may have dissociated, and asking the client when the earliest recollection of that emotion might be. An example of this was described in Chapter 2, with the case of Sonya, who was adopted at 9 years old from one of the worst orphanages in Siberia. In Sonya's case, amplifying the feelings of frustration and deprivation she experienced when her mother wanted to donate one of her old t-shirts to Goodwill harkened back to a cold night in the orphanage when her nightshirt was taken away from her. Highlighting how that same feeling affected

Sonya's behavior in the present and led her to break her bed helped to release her from the power of that automatic program of response.

This technique was also helpful with Sally, adopted from a Romanian orphanage at age 7, who felt compelled to engage in an odd behavior that she didn't understand. She had a habit, even at age 18, of putting her hand in the Coffeemate or other powdered creamer at coffee shops and licking her hands. While she knew this was inappropriate behavior, the compulsion to do this was very strong. I decided to enter the trauma "hall of mirrors" and attempt to find the feelings associated with this behavior and amplify them. I asked Sally to tell me what came to mind when she thought of the powder and putting her hands in. She stated she felt a gnawing feeling in the bottom of her stomach of a "hunger so big no food could ever be enough." I asked her to think about a time she remembers being that hungry. I play-acted the voice of a hungry child in an exaggerated tone, "Won't anyone give me food?"

Sally began the journey back through the hall of reflected mirrors. She remembered a time in first grade when she started to cry right before lunch. Newly adopted, Sally did not know the school routine, and didn't know that she would get lunch. This memory catapulted Sally back to the neglect of her early years. As she continued on the backwards journey, Sally remembered what appeared to be the index event. She described being hungry at the orphanage and getting up in the middle of the night with the other children and searching the cabinets for food. They would find bags of evaporated powdered milk, and they would put their hands in the bags and lick their hands. Sally was able to describe the feeling of triumph she had in discovering this milk, and acknowledged that she feels that same triumph when she dips her hands in powder at coffee shops. We discussed other things Sally could do to get the same feeling of triumph. Overcoming the pain of this traumatic memory required Sally to extend feelings of compassion to her hurt child-self from the past, and reassure her now that food is ample and available. Extending compassion to the hurt, hungry, neglected, or abused child that was once their reality is an important way to counter the child survivors' negative affect associated with a traumatic memory. "*Let's imagine you hugging that small Sally, and letting all the love flow out from your arms into her. Make sure she feels your love and knows she will find safety, warmth, and food one day and you will be with her,*" I instructed Sally.

Once the affective experience has been accessed, allowing the expression of the emotion to unfold in its own time is important. The emotionality of the moment is accepted and validated by the therapist, and this validation helps moderate the intensity of the emotion. The more the child talks about the affective experience, and gives voice to the painful affective memory, the more the experience is dissipated and integrated. Just like the child who fell off of her bike and cries uncontrollably in her mother's arms is relieved after the expression, so, too, the child survivor finds similar relief upon expression of the emotional experience related to her trauma. When the child is calmer, she can benefit from some psychoeducation about why her reaction was a natural consequence of the experienced events.

This technique of accessing emotions from the past may re-create experiences of intense anger, fear, sadness, or shame. Usually, multiple affects are associated with a traumatic event. Fourteen-year-old Eve, who had an early history of exposure to domestic violence and multiple foster placements, hid in the bathroom at school when a policeman came to talk to her Civics class. I assumed that her early exposure to police responding to her family's domestic disturbances had led to this traumatic reaction. As Eve began to describe her reaction to the policeman visiting her class, she revealed an incident from her childhood she had never before reported. Eve remembered a time she had picked up a bar of candy from a store at age 5. Her foster mother had told a policeman, who had bent her hands behind her back as a warning and told her about prison. The affective experiences associated with that incident were shame, anger, and fear, all of which she was able to express as I gave her the time and opportunity to talk about this experience. While this event seemed so minor compared to the other horrifying events of her childhood, the pain, humiliation, and fear she felt from how the policeman treated her amplified her own shame-filled belief that there was something essentially wrong with her. Eve cried, banged her hands on the table, and used colorful language to express anger and outrage toward the policeman of her memory. She challenged him, "How dare you treat me like that!" Her mother and I let these feelings progress without stopping them.

This expression in the context of validation and safety will finally metabolize the unprocessed experience. Her mother and I extended compassion for what that 5-year-old endured, and helped her reevaluate her judgment against herself for having taken the candy bar. Finally, she could extend compassion to the 5-year-old inner self as her mother and therapist, her validating witnesses, extended compassion to her. Some children doing these exercises feel that a younger version of themselves had remained as a dissociated self-state, but after these exercises, these young people often experience the younger versions of themselves integrating into the whole self.

Turning Helplessness Into Mastery

The final component of processing involves reversing the sense of traumatic helplessness by giving the child opportunities for mastery. One powerful way to accomplish this mastery over trauma is through art. As Sobol and Schneider (1998, p. 192) stated, "An image developed and changed through art-making may alter or amend internal imagery." Creating artwork creates pathways for integration of the mind. It engages the amygdala, where conditioned responses are primed, the right occipital where visual memory is stored, and the prefrontal cortex where planned action is formulated.

When children draw pictures of traumatic events, I will often ask them to change the pictures showing escape routes for trapped moments, magical interventions that relieve pain, cutting out people they do not want in the picture, or pasting things onto pictures.

Adina saw a brochure in my office for the Leadership Council on Child Abuse & Interpersonal Violence, an organization I helped found that works for justice for survivors of interpersonal violence (www.leadershipcouncil.org, reproduced in Figure 13.3). "How terrible," 8-year-old Adina exclaimed, "that the figure does not have her mouth! Can I put it back on?" Adina had been sexually abused by her father and every time she opened her mouth to explain to me what happened, she had become terrified and silent. I suggested we make multiple copies of the picture, and I encouraged Adina to cut out the puzzle piece mouths and paste them over the missing mouth of the little girl and say, "Now the little girl can tell what is happening to her! No one can keep her silent." Soon, Adina involved her mother and brother, asking them to cut out as many of the puzzle mouths as they could, pasting them over and over again on the little girl without a mouth.

Sometimes, mastery over the helplessness of trauma can occur through transformational rituals. Nine-year-old Nate had painful memories of an abusive youth pastor in his church and created a cardboard sculpture depicting the pastor as a devil. Nate wanted a way to symbolically destroy this image in order to help free himself from the hold the pastor had over him. Nate suggested we burn the sculpture, and together we created a prayer to be recited at this burning ritual, "May the burning of this object release your pain, your despair, all of your built up anger, and let it float with these ashes and this smoke back into the universe. May the universe fill you with gratefulness for the safety and blessings you now have. May

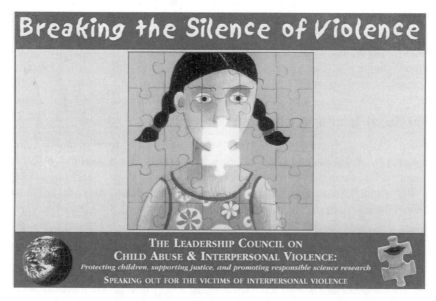

Figure 13.3 Brochure: Adina pastes puzzle mouth on picture to master feelings of being silenced. Used with permission.

the energy released in the burning of this object be transferred into energy for healing, growth, and change."

Mastery in Play

Sometimes traumatic events may have occurred before the narrative encoding of memory has developed. Recent experimental evidence suggests that some children can verbally recall unique events from as young an age as 2, even 6 years later (Jack, Simock, & Hayne, 2012). In some cases, these events surface in indirect ways—such as enactments in play or drawings (Terr, 1988). The therapist observing these scenarios should actively intervene to change the story and empower the child to become a survivor and not a victim. For example, if the child places a doll in danger, the therapist might say, *"Let's not let those bad people hurt the baby. Where could we put her that is safe?"* If the child continues to resist rescue efforts in the play, comment on those: *"You don't believe it is possible to really keep that little baby safe, but I am going to keep helping you find a way to do that, because that should not happen to any little babies."* Over time, the child will eventually model your efforts to save the characters in play from the disaster scenarios.

Eye Movement Desensitization Reprocessing

EMDR techniques provide another way that traumatic memories may be processed and mastered (Adler-Tapia & Settle, 2008). These techniques have been adapted flexibly for children so that any kind of cross-modal stimulation involving tapping, coloring, or even moving car figurines back and forth while the trauma story is told can create the bilateral stimulation that is an important component of this treatment approach. My clients express that alternating rhythmical tapping of their knees is particularly calming, and these calming behaviors can be accompanied with empowering and safety statements crafted specifically for the children and their unique issues. Examples of such statements include, "I am safe now because I have my mother with me"; "I am powerful and can make choices about my life"; "I am strong enough now to get out of situations like that one." (To utilize these techniques effectively, practitioners should enroll in established EMDR training programs.)

TELLING THE STORY TO ATTACHMENT FIGURES

My model of normal trauma processing in young children is the child running to tell her mother that she has just fallen. The witnessing of the experienced traumatic event by the child's or teen's attachment figures is where true healing can take place. Often, children have not been able to tell their parents what happened to them due to embarrassment, fear of being blamed, or fear of their parent's overly emotional reaction. When helping children talk to their attachment figure about the trauma, it is important to first assess if the individual will be able to handle hearing the information and help prepare the parent or caregiver to listen nondefensively. Then, after helping the child prepare what she wants to say, you can help the child tell her story. With proper preparation, sessions in which children talk about traumatic events with their parents present can produce powerful healing.

Children and teens need to know that their parents are strong enough to handle the intense affect and grief that accompanies the trauma. They also need to know that it is safe for them to tell these things to their parents, even though it could evoke guilt from parents who have not been able to protect their children from a trauma. Angela, a 14-year-old girl introduced in Chapter 7, came to therapy following 2 years of undiagnosed abdominal pain. She had a dissociative self-state she called the "Other Angela" that helped her cope with the pain. The "Other Angela" harbored intense rage against her mother for not solving the medical issue and leaving her in agony and bedridden for almost 2 years of her life. Angela's pain was finally diagnosed as severe gall bladder disease and surgery corrected the problem. It became apparent that processing the pain of her illness in the presence of her mother was extremely important, as she viewed her mother as a failure for not getting her proper medical help quickly enough. This view of her mother fueled the pain and rage harbored in this dissociated state. Because Angela was a taciturn young lady and hard to engage in conversation, I asked her to describe the pain with the help of the thesaurus on my computer. Using the thesaurus, Angela with the help of the "Other Angela" laboriously copied down words from the computer list, such as "excruciating, hell, terrifying." I asked her to arrange them on a paper and then to color the paper with colors that helped convey the intensity of the feeling. Although she tried to cover the words with red and black scribbles, the words capturing her pain could still be discerned through the coloring (see Figure 13.4).

When this activity was done, I told Angela that she needed to express to her mother what the pain had been like for her. Angela was timid at first and avoided eye contact. Then, she slowly read her list of words while her mother listened with tears streaming down her face. When Angela finished reading, her mother looked at her empathically and told her how very sorry she was that she had been unable to get her properly diagnosed sooner. Angela's mother promised her that if the pain returned, she would go to the tertiary medical center in their area and get an emergency appointment, and asked Angela to forgive her for letting her down. Angela's mother had been a kind and attentive mother, who had taken her daughter to multiple specialists and accepted their opinions. However, her acceptance of Angela's anger and disappointment was an important step in healing the dissociative rift within Angela, who could not make sense of both a mother who was loving and attentive, and a mother who could not help relieve her pain.

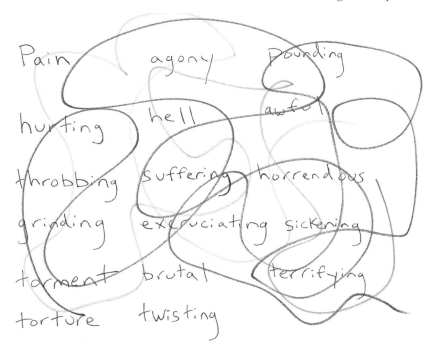

Figure 13.4 Angela's words for pain. Used with permission.

In the session following this family meeting, Angela had a bounce in her step and a new brightness in her eyes. When I asked her how the "Other Angela" had accepted her mother's acknowledgment of responsibility and willingness to listen to her feelings, Angela said, "A wall fell down." The opportunity for a young person to process traumatic information directly to a primary attachment figure can heal traumatic stress and repair the divisions within the self more rapidly than any other technique.

RESOLUTION WITH ABUSERS

As evident from many of my clients' stories, the trauma endured by many child survivors was inflicted by an attachment figure—a mother, father, grandparent, or even a sibling. This becomes a problematic area for intervention, as varying agendas based on loyalty to the offenders may lead to contrasting approaches about how these situations should be handled. With a sibling perpetrator, families may be eager for the family to get back to normal and have the child resume living with the older sibling. For abusive fathers who continue to be married to the mother, the family may urge reconciliation and forgiveness, or avoid the matter entirely.

The ideal resolution for children with parents who have perpetrated against them has been outlined by the Center for Sex Offender Management (2005). While developed for the case of sex offenses specifically, the principles in this approach can apply to any situation in which abuse or neglect has been inflicted on a child by a caregiver. Center for Sex Offender Management guidelines, based on expert consensus, recommends reunification with an abuser only after the abuser has received appropriate treatment, is aware of the risks of reoffending and how to mitigate them, and is able to apologize to the child in a sincere way at a point in time when the child is ready for this to happen. Careful monitoring by both the child's therapist and the offender's therapist should guide the reunification process. The reunification moves from letter writing to supervised therapy sessions, to public visits, and only to unsupervised private visits after extensive monitoring and therapy by the therapists of each party.

Unfortunately, this blueprint for ideal reunification rarely occurs. Often, the family courts order reunification before either party has completed therapy, and before any acknowledgement of wrongdoing. These premature reunifications can be disastrous to the child survivor, who may be overwhelmed by exposure to the feared perpetrator, and caught in feelings of extreme ambivalence between wanting to please the abusive parent and feeling anger and hatred. Placing children in these situations magnifies their dissociation and prevents its resolution. For example, for a time after disclosure of abuse by her father, Adina was required to visit with her father in a supervised setting. When asked how that felt she replied, "My face is smiling but my brain is crying." Through this colorful language she captured the feelings of dissociation inherent in her predicament. She wanted to please her father and the supervisory center and smiled appropriately, but simultaneously experienced rage and confusion—her "brain crying."

The ambivalence of attachment to the abuser can be understood as a cycle that I term the Cycle of Traumatic Attachment. Recognizing that her abuser harmed and betrayed her, the child is plunged into feelings of worthlessness and thoughts that she deserved what happened to her. This leads her to feel unlovable, and one way out of these feelings is to hold on to the belief that, in fact, her abuser did love her. Then, she realizes again that the person who supposedly loved her harmed her, again plunging her into feelings of worthlessness. In other words, in order to maintain their attachment and to feel that they are in fact lovable, these children must accept that they deserved what happened to them and deserve to be harmed. This cycle is depicted in Figure 13.5.

This paradox binds abused children to a relationship that is demeaning and destructive. In my experience, children cannot handle the complexities of negotiating this paradox while in direct contact with an abusive parent or caregiver, especially before that parent has authentically apologized and taken responsibility for the offense. If forced into premature contact, these children will continue to utilize dissociation to cope with the inherent contradictions of the situation. Children may alternate between identification with the abusive treatment they received and engage in self-destructive acts, or lash out in unproductive anger at

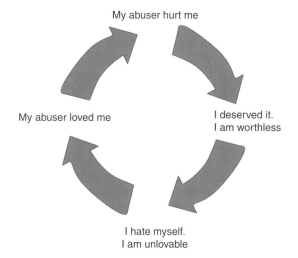

My abuser hurt me

My abuser loved me

I deserved it.
I am worthless

I hate myself.
I am unlovable

Figure 13.5 The Cycle of Traumatic Attachment.

others for the ways they were treated. Survivors of child sexual abuse may have even more difficulty extricating themselves from this cycle, as the abuser has often groomed the child and presented the abuse as an expression of love. The intimacy of the relationship and the betrayal involved leaves sexual abuse survivors particularly confused about what love is and whether their personal value is based on their role as sexual objects.

If not forced into reunification prematurely, children and teens can make significant progress working on these conflicting feelings toward their perpetrators in therapy. One technique I utilize is asking the child to talk directly to dolls that represent the perpetrators. I encourage children to verbalize their feelings to the dolls, explaining what felt unfair to them, and how it has affected their view of themselves. The purpose of this exercise is to provide an opportunity for the abused children to voice the feelings that they have had no opportunity to express, and to restore a sense of personal power. This process empowers children and enables them to view themselves as stronger, better, and morally superior to the offender, thus reducing the offender's psychological power over them. As the offender's power diminishes, the strength of dissociated feelings that identify strongly with these offenders also diminishes. Sometimes I ask teens to express their feelings in letters to the abuser or for children not yet as fluid with writing to dictate the letter to me. Children have dictated amazing, strong, and powerful letters that encapsulate their rage, indignation, and new learning about relationships that provided an empowering antidote to the helplessness. Most of these letters never get sent, but occasionally, if the offender has been ordered into therapy and the child agrees, these letters can be sent to the therapists of the offenders and used in their work.

Ten-year-old Marcie wrote a letter to her father who abused her before her parents separated when she was 5. This letter, which was never sent, is reproduced here. The letter helped Marcie work through her feelings of outrage, and helped her view herself as survivor and not victim.

Dear Dad,

It hurt me so bad when you abused me.
You have no right to do that.
Because of you my life was not normal.
Real love is compassion, kindness, caring, lovingness—
Supporting me not hurting me, never harming me.
Real love is making sure someone is safe and making me feel good about myself and helping with feelings.
Love means never forcing me to do things..
Despite what you did my life can be extraordinary
I don't have to be like you—I can be a singer
I can be anything I want just not you because you did horrible things to me—
you need to know you made me feel terrible, it's uncalled for, selfish, mean, cruel
I can be a singer, actress, I can write songs and poetry
You need to learn to keep hands to yourself
Be respectful, be kind, not hurtful, don't be so selfish, think of how others feel.
I make it through a lot of hard things and I can make it through this too.

Marcie

Many abused children who enter therapy need to find some internal resolution with offending parents who are no longer in their life because parental rights have been terminated, the parents have been sent to jail, or have fled. In these cases, some treatment settings encourage the children to forgive their abusive parent or caregiver, telling children they "have to forgive" because the person "will always be their parent." This type of forced forgiveness is counterproductive and leads the child to reenter the Cycle of Traumatic Attachment. Noll (2005) studied forgiveness in adult survivors of sexual abuse and found that forgiveness can be helpful if it is limited to feelings of letting go, dispensing with revenge, and moving on with one's life. However, when forgiveness is associated with a conciliatory attitude toward the offending parent, and letting the parent back into their life, the clients showed more symptomatology.

Many children move through stages in their understanding of how to reconcile the fact that their own parent has harmed them. These stages might include believing they can change or heal the parent, extreme anger and rejection, indifference, and finally acceptance of the parent for who he or she is without blaming themselves. Therapists cannot rush this process but rather should provide ample opportunities for children to explore what love means, why they deserve love and care, and why their parent may have been unable to provide the love they deserve.

At age 10, as Adina reached the end of a 2-year therapy following her disclosure of sexual abuse, she told me she was ready to give up her feelings of anger and revenge fantasies toward her father. She created the picture shown in Figure 13.6 of the "Gooderator." Adina stated that she could take the awful feelings about her

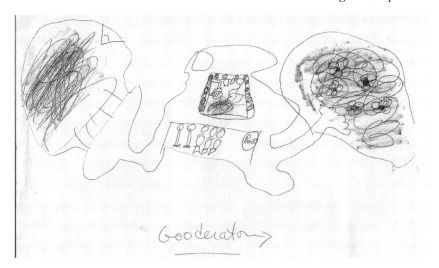

Figure 13.6 Adina's picture of a "Gooderator" that transforms bad feelings about her father. Used with permission.

father that were like "dirt," put them in the Gooderator, and have them come out the other end as a "flower." Her picture symbolizes Adina's desire to leave behind her angry feelings about her father and transform these feelings so that she could move on with her life.

FLASHBACKS

It can be frightening and disorienting for the therapist to witness a flashback in the office. Like the dissociative shutdown states described previously, these flashback events appear to be involuntary and even seizure-like, outside of the apparent control of the child or teen, and may be accompanied by physiological markers of arousal, including sweating, rapid breathing, or involuntary movements. I have watched many teenagers relive an apparent rape with jerking movements of the hips, and screams of "no." Witnessing such an event can frighten even experienced therapists.

Flashbacks appear to reflect the neurological effects of trauma on the brain. According to Martin Teicher (personal communication, November, 2010), the flashback may be a subclinical seizure experience located primarily in the right side of the brain. During these seizures, the nerves cells fire in repetitive patterns of closed feedback loops, without correction and stabilization from the prefrontal cortex, which could analyze the differences between past and present. During flashbacks, the past is experienced as now, and the physiological sensation of fear is acute. As disruptive as flashbacks can be, they may have a purpose. From an evolutionary point of view, it is adaptive for an organism living in a traumatic environment to have a rapid and hypervigilant warning system for potential dangers. I explain to clients that one reason that the flashback keeps coming back is because the brain is giving the child a warning—something you experienced in the past could come back and harm you again. Until their brain is completely convinced that the events in the flashback are not going to reoccur, the flashbacks will continue as a warning. I ask the child to work with me to figure out what in the environment the child is being warned about.

The transition moment is key, as it is the instant when a current experience feels so overwhelming that the body goes into this warning mode. Often, the reason the flashback is occurring is because the traumatic trigger in the environment is a situation or person that is closely reminiscent of the original traumatic event, and they have not yet identified how to respond to this trigger in a safe way. This conception explains flashbacks as an adaptive warning mechanism that helps the mind get away from trauma. The wisdom of the flashback is recognized as a way to help them know when unsafe things are occurring so that they can "get away quick." Often, I tell the young person that until all of the possible warning information is extracted from the flashback, like juice from an orange, the flashback will continue to occur. The information is extracted by utilizing the prefrontal cortex—thinking, planning, and matching functions—to create a new pathway to intercept the automaticity of the flashback experience.

Thus, when a child or teen presents with sudden onset of flashbacks, it is important to explore whether something unsafe is occurring in his or her current world. The exploration of what is unsafe can lead to uncovering traumatic reminders associated with past traumatic events. For example, 15-year-old Belinda was hospitalized for flashbacks of a rape she had experienced a year earlier. Exploration finally revealed that a current boyfriend was acting in threatening ways. The flashback served as her warning system of the possibility of future danger with the new boyfriend. Resolution of her acute symptom required dealing with the previous trauma as well as her current relationship with her boyfriend.

Time Machine Technique

The Time Machine Technique is a procedure for reducing intense flashbacks, which incorporates many of the components of processing traumatic memories. This technique allows children or teens to imagine going back in the past to undo a traumatic event, substitute mastery for powerlessness, and change his view of himself in relation to the perpetrator. This exercise is most appropriate for children and teens with flashbacks that have persisted for six months or more. It should never be used with recently experienced traumatic events, and should never be used for children who are preparing to go to court to testify about the traumatic events experienced. It is also inappropriate for children or teens victimized by having been coerced to pose for online pornography, because for these children the crime has not literally stopped.

In preparation for the exercise, I tell children and teens that, although we can never change the past events that have happened to them, we can change the way they are experiencing it. I tell them that currently, their mind is convinced that the traumatic event is still relevant and real, and as a result their mind is "practicing" experiencing this event over and over again. It is as if their mind is caught in a feedback loop going over the same event time and time again, like a broken CD player. I explain that I have a way for them to get out of it, so their mind can rehearse something more pleasant and empowering. While some may argue we must honor what is really true, I counter that the child's mind thinks it is really true that the past trauma is happening over and over again. We will substitute really true ideas—that they are safe, that they can be powerful, and we will use the children's amazing imagination to accomplish this. Most children or teens who are tormented by their flashbacks are willing to try the technique.

I begin the time machine exercise by asking children to tell me the flashback they experience, emphasizing primarily what happens *right before* the most terrifying or traumatizing aspect of it. I ask them to include a lot of sensory details and help me see the environment, what they are thinking, and lead me up to the traumatizing moment. They are often very relieved that they do not have to tell me the worst part of the event. Then, I ask them to give themselves any superpowers that they would like to have. Most teenagers and children describe themselves as becoming invisible to the perpetrator at the key moment, and then having the power to fly away from the trauma. Generally, they do not pick violent endings, but if they do, I encourage them to think of something that saves themselves but does not involve further violence. When they do give themselves superhuman strength, they often simply toss the perpetrator away and then get out of the way.

I then ask children to say something to the perpetrator as they are leaving. Finding these sentences is a very important part of the exercise. If this part of the exercise is too difficult for them, I will help them craft a statement such as, "You thought you hurt me, but I am stronger than you." "You will remember this forever, but I will move on with my life." "I could forgive you if I choose, but will you ever forgive yourself?" "How can you live with yourself when you hurt someone so much smaller? You are a coward." These statements generally describe the power and moral superiority of the child or teen, in contrast to the weakness, cowardice, and moral depravity of the perpetrator. Finally, I ask them to end the story in the arms of a safe person, feeling soothed and comforted.

Once we have the elements of the story, I ask clients to close their eyes, assume a relaxed posture, and I tell the whole story back to them, including the sensory details the child provided prior to the worst part of the trauma. As I tell the story, I add new vivid sensory details describing their use of their superpowers as the end of the story is changed. The process of telling the story back takes 15 to 20 minutes, and clients usually react with feelings of peace and relief. The client is then asked to continue to rehearse this new ending by imagining it right before they go to sleep, or when they feel that the flashback experience may be imminent. Some clients like to make a picture or a collage of the moment when they reverse the helplessness they felt during the trauma and their new superpowers take over. These pictures can then be hung on the wall above their bed, or affixed in some other prominent place in their home to remind them of mastery rather than helplessness.

When rehearsed frequently over time, this exercise may allow new brain pathways to be developed so that the over practiced circuitry of the traumatic memory is replaced by new connections that are accompanied by feelings of safety and empowerment.

There are several cautions to the use of this exercise that need to be kept in mind. If you try to do this exercise too soon following the trauma, or before some of the basic foundations of treatment have been achieved, the clients can react with increasing guilt or self-blame. They may interpret the superpowers part of the exercise to mean that they should have done something different and, thus, are to blame for what occurred. In addition, if this exercise is done at the wrong time, the clients may feel that you are not respecting their experience or are denying the validity of their suffering. Thus, before doing this exercise, it is important to talk honestly with the young person about what it can do and what it cannot do, and gauge the reaction. If the child is offended or deeply reluctant, it is best not to pursue this treatment technique.

Gina was an ambitious, athletic 15-year-old who had never told anyone the details of her traumatic experiences, which occurred when she had visitation with her father between the ages of 8 to 10. When she was 11, her father remarried and moved out of the state, and he never pursued ongoing visitation and they lost touch. Eventually, multiple traumatic symptoms appeared—eating disorder symptoms, self-harm, a voice in her mind that she said showed her scary pictures, and conflicts with her mother, some of which she forgot about immediately after they occurred.

On the surface, Gina was compliant and cooperative in therapy. However, she would never really discuss the voice in her mind or the scary pictures, which she said she preferred not to think about. Gina insisted that the scary pictures were not that relevant; she just pushed them out of her mind. On further inquiry, Gina revealed that she had never really told anyone about the traumatic events that occurred during the visitations with her father. She had told all previous therapists that it was too painful to go into, and they had accepted this, and allowed her to talk about other things. I explained to Gina that her mind was telling her that it was not yet safe to forget the bad things that happened to her. Those scary pictures in her mind were her mind's way of giving her a perpetual warning about the dangers that are out there. These dangers may seem real and terrifying to her younger self, who still remembers the trauma and does not have the skills to discern what is safe to leave in the past and what needs to be kept in the forefront of her mind to remind her to be careful. Thus, the scary pictures function as a perpetual reminder. I suggested to Gina that perhaps a better way to handle this perpetual memorial in her mind was to tell someone about the past trauma she experienced and sort through how to understand it. I asked her to check with the voice in her mind whether telling about this would be okay. She told me the voice in her mind agreed that this might help, and for the first time revealed that the "scary pictures" were of things that happened to her when she visited her father. She agreed to tell me some of the story about the trauma.

Haltingly, but with determination, Gina described her father taking her on a long ride through the rolling hills of West Virginia to an abandoned shack at the foot a mountain. There, she recalled that her father would go into a room where people were using drugs, smoking, and sniffing powder. She recalled waiting in a small room on a cot, and she recalled that the men in the house would visit her in the room and abuse her. Gina did not want to go into more detail about the abuse. I described the time machine technique and Gina wanted to try it. I asked her to identify the moment before the most terrible thing happened, and she stated that it was the moment she entered the little room and lay down on the cot. I asked her to send compassion, love, and understanding to the younger self who had to endure that pain, sadness, fear, and feeling of abandonment, and tell her, "I know how you feel." Gina chose the superpowers of being able to fly and creating force fields around people. I asked her to describe to me how she would handle the situation with her new superpowers. She stated she would watch the first person to enter the room, which was usually her father, and would then create an invisible force field around him so that he could not move. He would look at her in confusion as he would try to extricate himself from his new invisible prison. She would then create these invisible force fields around all of the people in the other room, and they would not have access to their drugs while imprisoned in the confines of the force field. I asked her what she would say to her father, and she stated she would tell him, "You are weak, and I am strong. You are not my father and never can be again." Then she stated she would fly out of the house and back to her mother's arms in her new home where she currently lived.

After telling this story, Gina smiled and stated that it was the first time that she had realized that she could choose to take away her father's position as her father. Thinking through what she wanted to say to him allowed her to engage her higher-thinking centers and formulate thoughts about disconnecting from his power over her. Gina realized that her father's power had prevented her from telling anyone about what happened to her, as he had always told her not to tell, "or else." She did not know what the "or else" was, but knew that it was the power of that threat and her father's authority that had kept her silent all of these years.

As Gina lay back comfortably in a chair, I had her countdown from 10 to 1 while she imagined entering a magic elevator that could take her back in time and change events in a special time warp space that changes psychological reality. I repeated her story to her, making the details of the winding West Virginia road very vivid, and including a sense of anxiety but anticipation that this time could be different. When I described the details to her of her father trapped in the force field, I evoked sensory details of his facial expressions in shock and defeat, and recognition of her new powers. When I described her flying through the air, I created vivid images of the wind in her hair and the scenery below. Finally, I described the emotional and physical comfort of being in her mother's arms and the safety of her future.

When the exercise was over, I asked Gina about her feelings, and the voice and the scary pictures. Gina described feeling a sense of safety and relief and said she was now thinking about the experience with her father in a new way. Although Gina had not yet disclosed the details of the most horrifying parts of the story, this imagery exercise allowed her to gain a new level of insight and strength in dealing with her traumatic history. She told me the inner voice "also enjoyed the experience" and was going to "sort through the picture file" and take away ones she did not need anymore.

Over time, Gina reported that the voice became less and less prominent and the scary pictures were replaced with "reminder pictures" that conveyed messages about tasks, obligations, and worries, but no longer horrifying images. Gina also reported that as her mind became more fluid, the reminder pictures faded, and she only experienced the normal nagging thoughts and fears that serve as minor warnings or adjustments that help guide behavior. As therapy progressed, Gina became more forthright about the abuse experiences, but the power of those experiences was much diffused by this exercise. Gina reported that she practiced imaging this scene frequently and engaged in imaginary dialogues with her father, where he faced what he did to her and even apologized. She accepted completely that this was in a different time warp, and she knew that her real father had never apologized and probably never would.

The most interesting superpower that one client reported was the power to burn words indelibly onto someone's forehead with her eyes. She burned the words "I am a rapist" into her rapist's forehead, stating that his shame would follow him wherever he went. It is inspiring to see the creativity and resilience of young people as they allow their imagination to focus on their internal strengths and inner drive for recovery.

Cautions in Assessing Flashbacks

Flashbacks have become a household word, and even young children may use this word to describe internal experiences, some of which may not actually be flashbacks. Thus, it is important when a family or client come to you complaining about "flashbacks" that you assess what they mean by the term. Some children describe hyperventilation episodes, aggressive acting out, or panic attacks as flashbacks. Some children or teens may use this handy label, which produces immediate sympathy from their family or therapist, but not in reality be experiencing a flashback at all.

Most behaviors related to trauma have both an operant and classically conditioned component—they are both affected by the current environment and stimulated by a past environment. So even legitimate flashbacks and intrusive traumatic reminders that appear to be the random firing of unintegrated neural firing patterns from past experience, can be shaped by the current environment to become relatively stronger or weaker. It is important to look at how the child's environment—family, school, and other people the child spends time with—reacts to the child's flashback experiences, as those environmental contingencies can play an important role in determining how enduring these patterns become. In special schools for emotionally disturbed children, it is important to have a balanced approach when children or teens present with flashbacks triggered by school events. Having a crisis room where the child can go to process and receive one-on-one assistance is important. It is also important that if the child goes to the crisis room that there are built-in rewards for returning to the classroom quickly, so that avoidance of class does not become an end in itself and, thus, a reinforcer of the flashback experience. This caution applies to all settings where children and adolescents can develop secondary gains for holding on to symptoms that provide opportunities for the avoidance of responsibilities.

An Exception to Every Rule

As with all rules, there is always an exception. The traumas experienced by some children remain inaccessible to awareness, despite a safe and supportive family, a skilled therapist, and a stable environment. I have found this pattern in some children who have been severely and chronically traumatized and then been adopted into safe homes. A minority of these children seem to put the past trauma behind them completely and totally. It almost appears as if they feel that their survival now depends on adapting to the new home by erasing the traumatic events from consciousness. When a child or teen has no recall for the past, it can become burdensome and irritating for the therapist to continually bring up trauma. In these cases, it is best to focus on current problem-solving, with an emphasis on building trust, to stay alert for how the past may be affecting their current life, and to let them know that if and when their mind is ready, information may come forward, but they can be perfectly fine even if this never occurs.

FORENSIC CONSIDERATIONS

When discussing traumatic events with a child or teen, clinicians must be mindful of any current criminal investigations. If there is an ongoing criminal investigation, discussion of traumatic events should only be done in coordination with the forensic team that is investigating or prosecuting the case. The clinician should refrain from any techniques involving imagery, or relaxation techniques involving suggestion. These may be easily misconstrued as hypnosis and thus negatively affect the credibility of the child if he or she is called as a witness. When a therapist is working with a child who may be testifying in court, therapy should avoid traumatic processing. Instead, therapy should focus on providing reassurances of safety, supporting the child's bond with the safe parent, and encouraging mastery statements that empower the child.

If the traumatic events are not accessible to memory consistently, but only accessible when children switch into a dissociated state of mind or different identity state, it is probably not advisable to have them testify, as the court will be suspicious of memories that are not consistent. The clinician should have open communication with the investigator and decide on a methodology for rapid transmission of any new details that emerge in therapy. Sometimes with young children, details of severe maltreatment may emerge over time, and key pieces of evidence may be told to the therapist that were not included in earlier forensic interviews. This is frequently the case with younger children. For example, 5-year-old Charlotte disclosed sexual abuse by her father on weekend visitation only after her mother asked about dried blood she found in Charlotte's underwear. Charlotte gave sufficient information in the forensic interview for prosecution, but later in therapy revealed that father's friends had participated in the abuse with other neighborhood children. This information was key to the ongoing investigation and the search warrant on one of the newly named offenders led to evidence against the original suspect. When new details arise during therapy, the clinician must keep verbatim notes on the child's disclosures, not interrupt, be careful not to ask leading questions, and preserve the record for the ongoing legal proceedings.

The next chapter will expand further on forensic considerations as we examine how child therapists interface with a variety of systems in supporting the growth of the child survivor.

14 Interfacing With Systems

The Therapist as Activist

As a therapist, you hold on to a vision of the world as it should be, rather than accommodating to the way things are. Our work often feels like an uphill battle as we seek to improve our clients' lives while systems with which we interface often seem oblivious to the needs of our clients. We know continuity of care is important, yet changing insurance companies, foster care companies, or school placements can result in the child being forced to change therapists. We know that many of our clients require ongoing services, yet managed care companies increasingly require short-term solutions. We teach our clients that their brains are adaptive and not sick, yet families are often told that their children will likely have lifelong disabilities due to biological psychiatric illness. We work to protect our clients from unsafe environments, yet courts often return children to unsafe caregivers.

Despite these obstacles to helping our clients heal, there are ways to navigate each of these barriers. Communicating with various systems that exert control over the life of the child survivor is a key principle of trauma treatment, as the interventions of the clinician need to be supported and reinforced throughout the many milieus in which a child lives, learns, and plays (Perry, 2009; Saxe, Ellis, & Kaplow, 2006). No matter what treatment model one uses, system dilemmas will arise that require a thoughtful, child-focused, and trauma-sensitive response.

CONTINUITY OF CARE: CHALLENGE RULES AND POLICIES THAT MAKE NO SENSE

There are many situations that can result in children being switched to a new therapist, usually based on the convenience of the bureaucracies that are responsible for the children's care. A therapist is switched to another division in the same agency that serves a different population; her entire caseload is transferred to someone new. A child is switched to a new foster care agency that doesn't have a contract with the child's current provider. A school has a policy that the child may not see outside therapists despite the fact that she has just begun to make progress with a new therapist. I have encountered all of these situations and my answer is always the same—continuity of care if a child is doing well with a therapist is more important than an agency rule or regulation.

Sometimes, simply pointing out that you want an exception is enough to convince the system to allow you to continue seeing the child. At other times, you may need to ask to talk to a higher-level administrator. In one setting in which I consult, I was told that if I accepted a referral from a psychiatrist who worked in a different program site, the child would have to switch psychiatrists because the insurance company required that the child have a therapist and psychiatrist in the same out-patient site. If I agreed to accept this new policy, I would no longer be able to collaborate on cases with this psychiatrist, and every time he referred a child for treatment for dissociation, he would be forced to abandon his own client. After several phone calls up the hierarchy, I found the administrator whose job it was to enforce this rule. The administrator agreed that this policy would interfere with my client's care and made an exception. Sometimes, agency "rules" are simply lore that one administrator tells another without question, and then clinicians assume that because an administrator said it, it is immutable. By repeatedly challenging rules and asking for exceptions, I managed to stay the therapist for Balina, described in the Preface, who had nine foster placements in 9 years. In order to maintain our therapeutic relationship, I had to get on the panels of her changing foster care agencies, sign up to be a therapist at her special school, and accept a sliding-scale fee structure. I have found that when policies that hurt our clients are challenged, these rules can often change.

SUFFICIENT TREATMENT LENGTH: EXPLORE PAYMENT OUTSIDE OF PRIVATE INSURERS OR MAKE SPECIAL CONTRACTS

Many traumatized and dissociative children require treatment for several years or more, which is often not available within private insurance mandates. In a preliminary study of treatment outcome on dissociative children using pooled data from two clinicians, we found an average treatment length of 12 to 24 months was associated with the best outcome (Silberg & Waters, 1998); but some clients required treatment for more than 5 years. Myrick et al. (in press) examined treatment outcomes with severely dissociative young adults engaged in multiphased trauma treatment. When they assessed the clients participating in their treatment study at the 30-month follow-up, there was significant reduction in destructive symptoms and increase in adaptive functioning, and many of these clients had already been in treatment for a considerable length of time even before participating in the study. Even 30 months is a significant treatment length that may be outside the benefits structure of many managed-care companies. After survivors of early trauma have achieved symptom reduction, the availability of the therapist when the child faces new developmental challenges is often important.

Despite managed care requirements dictating short treatment lengths, there are options for longer-term care available. In 1984, the Victims of Crime Act (VOCA) established a compensation program to reimburse crime victims, and every state in the United States now has a fund that will pay for treatment services for victims of crime (http://crime.about.com/od/victimassistanceprograms/Victim_Assistance_and_Compensation_Programs_By_State.htmVictims Assistance programs). I have found these funds to be very generous, often covering years of therapy for child victims of abuse and neglect, and occasionally even covering hospitalizations. In most states in which I have accessed these funds, their availability does not depend on the successful prosecution of the perpetrators of the alleged crime.

Sometimes insurance programs provided by state governments are more generous with length of treatment than private insurers. When treatment length is an important consideration and a private insurance company is refusing to cover additional treatment, many of my clients have successfully switched to the public insurance option. Rules and regulations for these programs are continually being modified, so it is important to explore the current status of mental health coverage in your state program and determine if it may be a better option for your client.

It is also possible to negotiate with the private insurance companies to approve longer treatment coverage for children and teens with complex traumatic histories. In my experience, talking with a clinician from the managed care company about the significant adverse experiences your client has experienced, along with the success you have had in keeping your client out of the hospital and able to attend school, can be very helpful in getting these treatment plans renewed. Many private insurers are pleased to have clinicians on their panels who are experts in trauma, and they may be willing to develop special rates or special protocols for handling traumatized children. Don't be reluctant to appeal decisions about continued care. When you succeed in talking to a clinician higher up on the hierarchy, it is possible you can convince her of the ongoing need by being specific about the interventions your client needs and the risks to the client who does not receive appropriate care.

If the client doesn't have insurance, or the insurance company refuses to cover the client's treatment, there may be other options. Some states have free clinics funded by public funds or private grants, where clients can receive specialized trauma services. Also available in many jurisdictions are state-funded special education programs that provide therapy on site. A number of my clients have attended a state-funded special education program administered by the Sheppard Pratt Health System. In these programs, therapy can continue for many years while the children attend this special school.

WORK COLLABORATIVELY WITH OTHER TREATMENT PROVIDERS

While knowledge of the effects of trauma is becoming more widespread, many clinicians have received no training on providing trauma treatment and tend to view the symptoms displayed by trauma survivors through a different diagnostic lens. I have found that the most important thing to stress in your consultations and collaboration with colleagues who have no specialized knowledge or training in childhood trauma are pragmatic considerations—what is working and why, and whether it may be useful to try a different approach. It is hard to argue with success, and easier to argue for an alternative way to approach things when the previous method utilized didn't work. Diagnostic battles over whether the disorder is best characterized as dissociative disorder, posttraumatic stress, or bipolar disorder are less important than arguing for specific interventions that might be helpful, no matter what label is used. Affect regulation exercises and imagery work can be effective even for bipolar disorder, so it is important not to get caught up in these controversies when we are trying to intervene to stabilize the client.

Because it is descriptive of specific behaviors, I have found that introducing the concept of Developmental Trauma Disorder (van der Kolk, 2005) can resolve a lot of treatment team debates over what is wrong with clients with a history of severe trauma. However, I have successfully treated traumatized children and adolescents, even in settings where the clinical directors completely disagreed with my diagnostic formulation. There could be no disagreement with the observed improvement of the client based on the interventions I used. Sometimes the varying perspectives expressed by different members of a treatment team can reflect the contrasting internal conflicts of a dissociative client struggling with competing impulses. The process of resolving the team's opposing views can often propel the clients to resolution of their own internal conflict.

When working with members of the team with differing viewpoints, it is best to keep discussions focused on pragmatic considerations rather than theory. If your client feels caught between differing viewpoints of team members, empower your client to think for herself and judge what is right, based on what works for her. If you use your knowledge about trauma to educate others, without preaching or judging others' points of view, you may make a wider impact.

Many of your clients may be working with psychiatrists or other medical professionals who are prescribing medications. These may be for symptoms of attentional problems, depression, anxiety, mood dysregulation, hyperarousal, or disturbed thinking. While there is controversy regarding the overuse of psychiatric medications among children and adolescents (Parry & Levin, 2012; Sroufe, 2012; Whitaker, 2010), it is important to evaluate each situation on a case-by-case basis and maintain a close working relationship with providers who are prescribing medications. As the therapist, sometimes you are in the best position to report your client's reactions to new medications, and whether the medication appears to be assisting or interfering with the therapeutic process.

It is important to maintain ongoing positive relationships with your clients' schools, as well. Therapists can help teachers and administrators understand why children are having traumatic reactions to noise in the classroom, to teacher feedback, or to limit-setting. The therapist can brainstorm with the school about mitigating the effects of situations that cause the child to decompensate and about developing ways to assist the child in navigating a school day. Providing the school counselor or nurse with an agreed-upon list of strategies for managing anxiety or flashbacks is often much appreciated. In my experience, the traumatized children I work with require someone at the school who is perceived as a safe person to go to during crisis moments, and may need to be provided a special pass to leave class as needed. Returning the child to the classroom quickly after utilizing planned strategies should be an ongoing goal.

When children cannot manage in the classroom, the therapist may need to meet with administrators at the school to determine what kind of specialized placements are available. The therapist's presence at these meetings can be very useful in helping to determine the specific resources that will best assist the child in functioning in a school setting. Access to special placements is often a difficult thing to achieve and a therapist presence advocating for the resources needed by the child may make the difference. Rather than relying on diagnoses, it is important when meeting with school officials to be practical and descriptive of what the child can and cannot do, and what resources would be of most assistance. The therapist can also advocate for availability of a resource room or resource specialist, opportunities for the child to leave the classroom when overwhelmed, a smaller class setting, and contact with school professionals who are knowledgeable about triggering, flashbacks, and other elements of the child's trauma-based responding.

INTERFACING WITH THE LEGAL SYSTEM: KEEP YOUR INTEGRITY

Many clinicians feel intimidated by the legal system and are unfamiliar with the ground rules of the legal environment. Many lawyers use bullying tactics in approaching mental health professionals, acting as if the legal interests of their clients for whom they are zealously advocating have precedence over the mental health interests of the client for whom you are advocating. Many clinicians dread the time-consuming nature of getting involved in the courtroom and are uncomfortable with the adversarial nature of the legal system. I understand these hesitations, but have found that it is necessary to have some familiarity with the legal system and how it operates in order to help my vulnerable clients. If therapists stick to what they know and to the ethical principles that guide their work, they should be able to successfully navigate the legal system.

Often, mental health professionals assume they have no power to defeat court orders that harm children. Mental health experts do have the power to be clear, data-based, and ethical. You can play a role in helping to educate the legal system in your testimony about trauma and its impact on children. Judges are often hungry to hear this kind of information and grateful to mental health experts who share their expertise. My main admonishment is to not let the power of the legal system bully you into compliance with things that harm children. Maintain your integrity while educating the court about what your client really needs.

Do Not Accept Court Appointments That Violate
Your Ethical and Legal Obligations

At the outset of getting involved in a case, examine any court order that names you and be certain that you are willing to accept the terms of involvement as spelled out in the order. If you do not accept these, make it clear to the court immediately that you cannot ethically do what they are asking and tell them why.

When I got the initial court order for my client Adina (Chapters 2, 6, 12, 13), the order stated that the therapist was not allowed to report allegations of abuse to state agencies. Instead, the court order stated that the therapist could only report these allegations to a "parent coordinator," who would then determine whether these reports would be reported to Child Protective Services. Because the court had wrongly determined that previous allegations were unfounded, this order, in-geniously crafted by the attorney for the abusive father, had restricted the therapist from making more abuse reports. This order directed me to violate both my code of ethics and the legal mandate from the state in which I practice. If I followed the court order, I would jeopardize my license by failing to comply with my state's legal requirement that mental health professionals report suspicions of abuse. I ex-plained this immediately to the parent coordinator and agreed to inform the parent-ing coordinator of any abuse allegations that arose in treatment, but I did not agree to let her decide whether the abuse disclosure would be reported to Child Protective Services. In fact, when Adina did disclose the sexual assaults from her father that were occurring on weekend visits, I informed the parenting coordinator, but only after I had faxed a graphic picture drawn by Adina to the supervisor of Child Pro-tective Services. I would not let those who wanted to squelch further disclosures by Adina conscript me into supporting their efforts to suppress the truth. Once the case was heard in court, it became clear that the "parent coordinator," although appear-ing neutral, was, in fact, a paid witness for the father, and was eager to testify that she did not believe the disclosures. Had I relied on her court-sanctioned power to screen out my abuse suspicions, Adina would never have been protected.

Other court orders that I ask to be amended are orders that ask me to do psychological testing on parents to determine whether allegations of abuse are founded, or where a child should reside. I explain to the courts that in order to assess whether abuse has occurred or to determine the mental health needs of a child, it is *the child* who needs to be assessed primarily, and not the parents. When I am court-appointed to write a "custody evaluation" in situations in which there are allegations of abuse, I request that the court rewrite the order as a "mental health evaluation to determine issues of child safety and protection."

Many custody evaluators use psychological testing on parents to determine child custody. I explain to the court that psychological testing of parents cannot tell you if a parent is an abuser. In addition, results of psychological testing are frequently misinterpreted to conclude that women who have been victims of domestic violence and have symptoms of posttraumatic stress have personality disorders, resulting in them being considered unfit to retain custody of their children (Erickson, 2005).

Parental Alienation or Parental Alienation Syndrome, a construct often used in family court, is based on a simplistic theory that children who accuse a parent of abuse or feel angry at a parent were brainwashed into that point of view by the other parent. Although the theory has received wide dissemination in the family law community, it has neither a logical nor a scientific basis. There is a relative absence of any empirical or research support for the reliable identification of the syndrome of Parental Alienation, or the validity of its theoretical underpinnings. The National Council of Juvenile and Family Court Judges rejected the use of parental alienation syndrome Parental Alienation Syndrome (Dalton, Drozd, & Wong, 2006), and legal and psychological research has concluded that it has no scientific merit or legal utility (Bruch, 2001; Hoult, 2006; Meier, 2009). Despite this, children's allegations of intrafamilial abuse are increasingly being attributed to alienation. In these cases, the courts often respond by punishing the parent believed to be alienating the child (i.e., the parent seeking to protect the child from abuse) by giving custody to the other parent— the alleged abuser (Neustein & Lesher, 2005). This happened to Adina and Billy (Chapter 8), along with several other children whose treatment is described in this book.

The popularity of parental alienation in family courts appears to be due to the widespread myth that most allegations of abuse that arise in custody disputes are false. Research, on the other hand, has found that it is surprisingly rare for false allegations of sexual abuse to arise during a custody dispute (Faller, 2007; Thoennes & Tjaden, 1990). The myth that allegations in the context of divorce are likely due to parental alienation provides a simplistic approach of shifting the blame when complex questions of how to protect children from abuse arise in court.

The problems created for vulnerable children whose protective parent (usually their mother) has been accused of "parental alienation," or "coaching," has come to the attention of the federal government's Department of Justice, Office of Violence Against Women. Along with George Washington University's Domestic Violence and Legal Empowerment Program (www.DVLEAP.org) run by Joan Meier, I am part of a cooperative agreement to conduct research to help determine the factors that lead to children being placed in the custody of abusers. To determine these factors, I am examining "turned-around cases"—cases in which a child is placed in the custody of an abusive parent, and a later judicial finding corrects the error and protects the child. The cooperative agreement supports the development of a curriculum based on this research to help improve judicial decision-making in custody cases. The results of this research thus far indicate that accusations of "parental alienation" leveled by the alleged abuser against the protective parent is one of the chief reasons for these disastrous outcomes where children are forced by the court to spend time in the control of abusers.

As a therapist trying to maintain allegiance to children and integrity in your work, be suspicious of all court orders that ask you to treat children or parents for "alienation." In providing treatment to children or guidance to parents, you should rely on observable evidence of behavior. Lack of specificity and clear definitions result in diagnoses based on vague impression or attribution of unconscious processes that no one has witnessed. If required by the court to document "alienating behaviors," write down a specific list of behaviors you will consider to be "alienating," and which behaviors you will not consider "alienating," and document why. In a recent court case, a mother was accused of "alienation" because her 4-year-old child used the word "Daddy" for the stepfather who raised her. When the child was 3, her biological father suddenly appeared on the scene. Because the child did not switch over to calling her biological father "Daddy" immediately, the mother was considered to be guilty of alienation. Courts must understand why conclusions such as this ignore children's developmental realities, and practitioners must educate courts rather than buying into the court's flawed reasoning.

If a child does not want to see a parent, carefully examine the child's relationship with the parent. A relationship between two people is best understood as between those two people, and research suggests that a child's estrangement from a parent is most likely due to how that parent treats the child (Johnston, 2005). It's profoundly disrespectful to children to ignore their perceptions about the reasons for difficulties in a relationship and to assume it is the fault of a third party, the basic premise of parental alienation theory.

You should reject or ask to have rewritten any court orders that would compromise your scientific objectivity or that require a clinical approach to your clients that is not based on sound evidence. For example, a court order might require you to "not report," or interpret in another way, a future disclosure of abuse, as did the court order I had received before treating Adina. You cannot make decisions about a possible situation in the future that you have had no opportunity to assess. Similarly, dismissing allegations because a previous interviewer failed to substantiate abuse is not a valid reason to disbelieve a child. Disclosures of abuse follow known patterns and are dependent on age of the child and relation to abuser, and sometimes several interviews are required before disclosure (Olafson & Lederman, 2006). As a mental health practitioner, your work must be rooted in empirical data rather than misguided notions based on legal advocacy.

Similarly, if you are ordered to work with a family in which your job is to reunify children with someone who is actively causing harm to your client, you should reject that job as unethical. Sometimes, even court-ordered supervised visits can be harmful to a client, as a child may be reacting with traumatic re-experiencing to the sight of an abusive parent or the sound of their voice (see case of Estie, Chapter 9). Nine-year-old Billy described his traumatic triggering during supervised visits in this way, "Every time I see him it reminds me of what happened, like watching a movie growing worse and worse every minute and every second." When children have posttraumatic reactions to contact with an abuser, this needs to be conveyed to the court, so that the court has the best information by which to judge the impact of its decisions.

Abuse-Proofing

There are many instances in which it is unclear if a young child has been abused or not, and you may be asked to help with reunification. In these cases, I have developed a protocol that I term "abuse-proofing." I conduct a series of prescribed sessions with the parents and the children in which I rehearse with the children appropriate boundaries, safety rules, and rehearse with them that they may not keep secrets. Both parents are required to reinforce the injunction of no secrets and agree to specific guidelines of what is safe and appropriate behavior. Rules are developed that specifically address the allegations that have been made and parents apologize if the children believe that any of those rules were broken. Sandra Hewitt (2008) has developed a similar protocol for the reunification of young children following abuse allegations that cannot be proven. She similarly advocates the development of clear rules and monitoring the children's safety over time. My protocol includes more sessions in which there is specific training around never keeping secrets. This "abuse-proofing" procedure has led children to reveal abuse promptly following reunification, and provides a methodology to reassure families that reunification, even after abuse allegations, may be possible, if required by the court.

Calinda was 4 years old when she first disclosed that her father had touched her "tata" during weekend visits. The medical evidence was ambiguous and Calinda's language was undeveloped at age 4. As a result, the forensic interview did not yield a definitive result. The judge ordered the family to participate in my abuse-proofing protocol. I held six sessions with both parents, Calinda, and her 7-year-old older brother. At my prompting, both parents encouraged the children to always tell the truth and never to keep secrets. The father went over specifically rules for safe touching with Calinda and her brother, and made a "solemn promise" that none of those rules would ever be broken. The court increased their time with their father over the course of six months until the children visited every other weekend. Calinda continued in therapy with me and I reinforced the principles of the abuse-proofing protocol regularly. Two years after the initiation of the abuse-proofing program, Calinda told her mother, "Daddy broke his promise." She described an incident of digital vaginal penetration to her mother, her pediatrician, a doctor in the emergency room, and her therapist. Further paternal visits were suspended following the substantiation of this new report by the medical personnel. The father agreed again to supervised visits rather than have a judge hear the new testimony from the multiple professionals who had documented the new allegation. The children did not mind these supervised visits, and continued to see their father for several years until he moved out of the area and lost contact with his children.

Do Not Be Hesitant to Go to Court If You Can Help Your Client

There are many reasons that a clinician may be subpoenaed to testify on issues related to child clients—child protection issues, criminal issues, foster placement issues, or custody or visitation issues relating to divorce. These are often very important moments in the lives of children in which the course of their future will be determined. Your input could literally save your client's life. If you have information that may help a court understand what your client has dealt with and what the sources of harm in their environment have been, it is important not to avoid these opportunities. To safeguard your ethical obligations to your clients, you must discuss with them what you might say and find out what your clients want you to say, along with what things they prefer you not discuss. While you cannot guarantee that you can always avoid confidential material on the stand, having these discussions can help guide your testimony. It is unethical to give an opinion to the court that is in direct conflict with your client's expressed wishes. You cannot ethically treat your client if you have knowingly violated your client's expressed wishes to you. If you feel that you cannot in good faith represent what your client has told you as being in his or her best interest, you need to avoid court at all costs, to preserve the therapeutic relationship. Keep in mind that it is profoundly disrespectful to your client not to respect the client's opinions and you might consider referring out if you consistently feel you must disregard your client's wishes and self-described viewpoints. For example, if a child does not want to see a parent, and you believe it is in the child's best interest to see that parent, you should not advocate on the stand for your own point of view rather than the child's. If a child does not want to see a parent, examine carefully that child's relationship with the parent. Ignoring the child's perception about the reasons for difficulties in that relationship sacrifices your alliance with your client, and is also inconsistent with the literature about why children refuse visitation (Johnston, 2005).

Some therapists have the misconception that it is always unethical to testify in court. It is only unethical to do this if you testify to recommend something that your client expressly opposes, or if you testify to things that are beyond the scope of your expertise or knowledge. As a therapist, you can testify to your patient's diagnosis, the impact of his diagnosis on his behavior and emotions, prognosis, and treatment recommendations (Kleinman, 2011). You cannot testify about people you have not met, but you can testify about your client's fears and perceptions about people, whether or not you have met the person in question. State mental health associations provide review courses on legal and ethical guidelines that can help you in navigating the unique legal and ethical requirements of your own jurisdiction.

Some children have observed the faulty systems they have been caught in, and yearn to make changes. They are often more acute observers than we realize. At the end of Billy's treatment for sexual abuse, he told me he wanted to be a judge, and I responded, "Is that so you can believe children when they tell you they are abused?" He corrected me immediately. "No," he stated, "so I can believe the *evidence*."

STRIVE TO BE AN EXAMPLE OF THE HUMANE WORLD YOU ARE TRYING TO CREATE FOR YOUR CLIENTS

Our clients will often reenact in their environments the traumatic binds that have characterized their chaotic lives (Chu, 1998; Courtois, 2010; Loewenstein, 2006). As they enter systems of care, they may provoke staff into reactions that create familiar patterns. Although physical restraint may trigger flashbacks, out-of-control behavior may lead professionals to use these very interventions that traumatized children fear the most. Viewing themselves as unworthy and unlovable, these children may be so provocative or enraging that systems of care impose restrictions or consequences that make them feel even more unworthy.

Sandra Bloom (1997) created the Sanctuary Model, a model for affecting change in institutions, such as residential centers for traumatized youth, that helps the environments model a humane, client-focused approach. The model encourages an atmosphere of respect, open communication, flexibility, safe conflict resolution, and self-care throughout all levels of the system. Treatment provided in this kind of environment is more likely to resist the traumatic reenactments child survivors may attempt to provoke. There is less need for use of restraints, less staff turnover, and a greater feeling of well-being among staff and clients alike (www.sanctuaryweb.com/sanctuary-model.php).

Whether or not your treatment setting has been trained in the Sanctuary Model, you can try to embody the values described by Sandra Bloom in your interactions with mental health professional colleagues, schools, medical providers, direct staff who care for your clients in residential placements, families, and the clients you treat. As each individual within a system tries to be the best example of health and openness to change that they can be, the system as a whole will be influenced in that direction. A healthy society requires an individual commitment from each participant within that society. Each of us can begin that process in the systems in which we live and work with traumatized young people.

15 Integration of Self
Toward a Healing Future

We chatted casually about her new school friends and her Christmas wish list as Tanya drew a picture using the crayons and large drawing pad in my office. Children often entertain themselves when we talk, using the art supplies, puzzles, and clay that fill my child-friendly office. Suddenly, she put down her crayons and looked up at me expectantly. "Aren't you going to ask me about my picture?" 10-year-old Tanya said teasingly. "*Well, of course,*" I answered, "*tell me about your picture.*"

"It is me staying together over day and over night," she proclaimed triumphantly. She had encapsulated her newfound integration in the remarkable picture shown in Figure 15.1. Tanya's drawing of herself clearly overlays the changing contexts of day and night, and she stays undivided, despite the line that bifurcates the day and the night. Through this picture, Tanya demonstrated that she had met the challenge confronting the dissociative child survivor—to stay connected while contexts change, to seamlessly manage the transitions of states, appropriate to changing environmental contexts. She demonstrated the healthy mind we are seeking for our clients.

Nine months earlier, Tanya had presented as a classically dissociative child. Warring voices in her mind told her to act out against her parents, act out sexually at school, and refuse to do homework. Sexually abused by a babysitter and exposed to domestic violence during her preschool years, Tanya had developed a dissociative coping style to deal with her conflicted feelings. "I just make up a person for each new feeling. I don't know how I do it," she told me. "It just happens." Therapy had progressed rapidly from education about trauma and dissociation, to practice in blending her feelings by having each imaginary character explain to one another their own fragmented feeling states in letters and pictures. The fragmented feeling states made bargains and cooperative agreements that allowed Tanya to stay more focused at school and in control of her behavior. As her behavior improved, she made some new friends. The trauma of her sexual abuse was processed through drawing and processing pictures depicting the events. Family sessions took place in which the parents described the actions they took against the teen offender and apologized for not knowing and understanding sooner. Family sessions also helped identify triggering events in

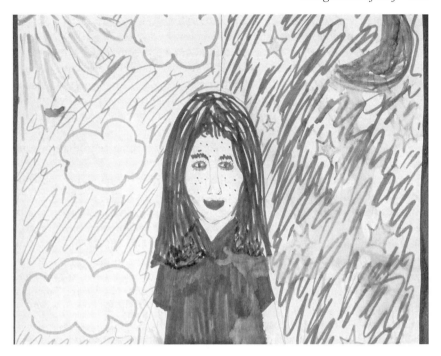

Figure 15.1 Tanya's picture of "staying together over day and night." Used with permission.

the environment—particularly fights between her parents that reminded her of past traumas. Her father attended therapy as an adjunct to our treatment, which increased the sense of safety and security in the family. Tanya was highly motivated for treatment at the time she came in, and the family was committed to the therapy. Tanya's self-portrait provides evidence of the effectiveness of the therapeutic interventions and her rapid growth.

The last E of the EDUCATE model is the "Ending Stage of Therapy." This is the hard work of the end stage of therapy, as parts of the self that were segregated blend back into the whole complex self. The road toward integration will not always follow the smooth course of Tanya's therapy. Temporary surges forward and then several steps backwards is the more characteristic pattern. The complexity of life transitions—grade changes, school changes, divorcing parents, and marrying parents—can serve as bumps on the road to healing or sometimes surprising gifts that spur treatment ahead. A foster child finds an adoptive family that truly knows how to meet her needs. A struggling student has a fourth grade teacher that understands his needs, and suddenly he has more confidence in himself. A survivor of incest experiences a date rape and feelings of betrayal and powerlessness are reactivated. Hopefully, the skills that the child survivors have learned in therapy—to honor their whole self, to tune in to their body states, to regulate their feelings, and to seamlessly manage transitions—will serve them well with whatever opportunities or hardships come their way.

During this last stage of therapy, the child or teen becomes ready to move on with the challenges of growing up—making friends, achieving academically, and developing interests and hobbies. Staying connected to a therapist during this period of time can be helpful, as clients leave behind a self-conception tied to their traumatic history and learn to see themselves based on an identity of achievement and success. Having a therapist to "coach" them forward, help them navigate the inevitable setbacks, and recognize how far they have come can be a powerful motivator for continuing to progress in therapy.

However, the realities of life mean that therapy may not be part of the child survivor's life throughout their childhood. Some may have the benefit of a treatment lasting several years, while others only receive help for several months. Because of my affiliation with a long-term residential program and special school where children can attend for years, I have had the opportunity to work with many children for the span of several years. Some I have followed from school age years through college and beyond, able to see how the insights gleaned and skills learned when they were younger served them in their later years. Financial realities have made longer-term treatments less feasible in many settings. Yet, therapists who only have an opportunity to work with a child or teen for a short time can still help their clients achieve important steps on the road to health.

DEALING WITH SETBACKS AND CHALLENGES

Reinforcing the Differences Between Now and Then

Inevitably, new situations will arise in the life of your young clients in which scenes from their past will seem to be replayed. Although there will be new characters and new situations, the same central driving themes and emotional color will be present. While these can be retraumatizing to the child survivor, these situations provide important learning opportunities. These situations can either thrust the young person back to a time of trauma, or catapult your client into a new future by helping illustrate the differences between the past and the present. Helping clients recognize that their abuse is in the past, and that they now have new capabilities to deal with stressful events, is one of the most important therapeutic challenges during the ending stage of therapy.

Miranda (see Chapter 10) had been abused in a preschool setting by a teacher and had been threatened that her family would be harmed if she told anyone about what happened. The weight of keeping this secret left her passive and lacking in personal confidence. At 14, Miranda finally revealed her secret to her family, and when she entered treatment, she went into dissociative shutdown states and had flashbacks and impulses to self-harm. Over time, she learned to manage these and was moving forward in her treatment. Yet, she still displayed a bland affect and seemed to have little zest for life. A surprising event helped illustrate for Miranda that "now" was different than "then." A new boyfriend who was showing some preliminary signs of being abusive surprised her in the cafeteria and stole her iPod in front of the teacher and other witnesses. He was suspended, and this public event garnered her a huge amount of support among the students and faculty. The principal of the school even checked in with her regularly to see how she was doing. The emotional tenor of this event was similar to what Miranda had experienced before—being exploited and hurt in a school setting by someone with power over her. However, the public nature of the witnessing of the events and the public support following the event were clearly different. Rather than allowing this experience to reinforce her victimization and further deplete her sense of self, Miranda accepted the experience as a "redo" of the past events, illustrating to her that people cared about her and would stand up for her in times of need. In the end, the event helped jumpstart Miranda's sense of confidence.

When clients experience a situation they find difficult, the therapist can help them focus on aspects of the situation that are different from what they experienced in the past. In this way, these experiences become valuable lessons in the client's strengths and support systems, rather than opportunities to feel revictimized.

The Cycle of Traumatic Demoralization

When the progress of therapy in the last stages of treatment seems stuck, I find the clients are often trapped in a cycle that I term the Cycle of Traumatic Demoralization. This cycle is depicted in Figure 15.2.

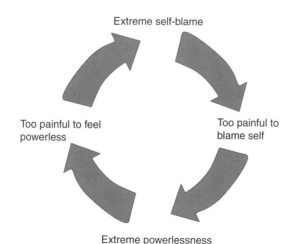

Figure 15.2 Cycle of Traumatic Demoralization.

Self-blame and powerlessness are two competing poles of a cycle of demoralization that traps some survivors of severe trauma. Both feelings are painful, and the child survivor may flee from one to the other, trying to escape the painful feelings each evokes. Survivors blame themselves for the trauma and view the self as causing, and thus deserving, what happened to them. To escape the trap of self-blame, survivors move toward recognizing that what happened to them was not their fault and that they did not cause their own suffering. The feeling brings some relief at first, but quickly evokes a sense of powerlessness, as they must accept that the events just happened to them for no reason. To escape an overwhelming sense of powerlessness, survivors move back to the position of self-blame, as there is at least some sense of power in realizing that they had some control over what happened to them. They move back into thinking that they did have control, they could have changed things, and it is their fault that they didn't. However, accepting power means accepting blame and survivors are again thrown into feelings of intense self-blame. Thus, they move round and round in the cycle without ever moving forward.

There are many places to intervene in these cycles. Contemplating the powerlessness people might feel in a natural disaster, and the clear conception that a natural disaster cannot be someone's fault, has been a useful metaphor for some survivors who were abused by caregivers. They can see themselves as having to pick up the pieces after a "tsunami" and more easily accept that maybe what happened to them was an inexplicable "act of God." They can consider that people are always learning about new kinds of earthquake and tsunami warning signs, but people cannot stop the events from happening, only develop better methods of prediction and coping. Similarly, survivors can learn from the past without feeling responsible for the past, and use past information to plan for new problems they may face in the future.

For children and teens who struggle with a lot of feelings of self-blame, I help them engage in a self-forgiveness ritual. Often, there is one aspect of their behavior before or during the trauma that they ruminate about and for which they can't forgive themselves. For example, Lila, in treatment at age 16, was abused during visits to her uncle on holidays and summer vacations. Her parents flew her across the country to visit an uncle and at age 9 Lila had imagined telling a particular flight attendant and being rescued from the abuse. She blamed herself for never telling this flight attendant, and of course, for never telling anyone during the years of her painful ordeal.

Self-forgiveness involves three steps. In the first step, the child or teen is asked to identify clearly and then completely accept the action for which they would like to forgive themselves. In Lila's case, it was the action of not telling the flight attendant about the impending abuse she would be suffering. This stage involves increased awareness of that moment in time where there might have been a choice to act differently. The second step involves understanding all of the reasons behind one's previous choice. Lila was able to identify the consequences she feared in the family for telling, her mistrust of what the flight attendant would actually do, and her fear that the abuse might get worse if she told. I tried to help Lila re-create her own mindset at age 9 when she thought of telling. To help her do this, I asked her to think about any 9-year-olds that she knows and to try to imagine how they think. During this step, it is also useful to help clients understand what power they did use to cope with traumatic circumstances. For example, Lila realized that she had used her power to play subtle tricks on her uncle.

The third step in the self-forgiveness paradigm involves a "recommitment." In this step, clients identify a new action or behavior they are committing to as a lesson learned from the traumatic experience. In Lila's case, her recommitment was to tell her story at a local fundraising event for abuse survivors in order to convince other 9-year-olds that they should tell. Another recommitment some children make is to speak up immediately if anyone is taking advantage of them or someone else. Once the client has decided on her recommitment she is asked to focus healing, gratitude, and forgiveness inward to the part of herself she blames. I instruct clients to grant complete forgiveness to the self. This ritual of self-forgiveness is also helpful to clients who have lingering feelings of self-blame for acting-out behaviors that harmed other people prior to getting treatment. In this case, attempting to seek forgiveness from the person they have harmed and making amends is also an essential part of the process.

ANSWERING THE EXISTENTIAL QUESTIONS: THE CHILD AS PHILOSOPHER

Many children use the last stages of therapy to contemplate deep philosophical questions such as: "Why does God allow evil in the world?" "What is love?" "Can I love and hate someone at the same time?" No longer splitting their awareness between conflicting ideas, these paradoxes and existential riddles seem to take on more salience to child survivors. I tackle these types of questions with humility and a belief that faith in something larger than what our eyes can perceive can be a positive force for change. At times, I will involve the religious leaders of the child or teen's faith, asking them to meet with us and explore together some of the powerful questions that I myself cannot answer, such as—Why did God let this happen to me? Will my uncle go to hell? Will I go to hell for what he did to me?

A Catholic priest, Father Ray Chase at St. Vincent's Children's Center, has been a wonderful cotherapist to help resolve religious struggles of my Catholic clients struggling with the aftermath of trauma. I urge clinicians to partner with religious leaders in their community to address the unique spiritual needs of abused children and teens so that they can find answers to their questions within their own religious traditions.

Children or teens must ultimately find their own answers to these questions, but they can be guided and facilitated by therapists who are themselves well grounded. Treating traumatized children and teens can be debilitating and demoralizing, and engaging in one's faith community or other resources that restore a sense of grounding, perspective, hope, and connection to something bigger is also important in the life of therapist. A good reference on the importance of therapist self-care and how therapists can restore a sense of balance to their lives is Ferentz (2012).

Some of these children have looked at the face of evil in their lives in a way more real than any of us can imagine. When children ask me about good and evil, I tell them I imagine the world as a giant seesaw, with good on one side and evil on the other, and it is everyone's responsibility to drop as many little drops of goodness as possible on the positive side of the seesaw.

Another question children struggle with at the end of treatment is the meaning of love. Many abused children have been told that they must love a parent just because it is their parent—even if that parent harmed them. Others have told them that it is wrong to love a parent that hurt them. I tell my clients that no one can tell them what love is or who they should love, as love is an individual feeling and we all resolve this issue in different ways. In my experience, once healthy, child survivors psychologically disconnect from an abusive parent and do not extend love to the person that harmed them. However, some child survivors feel that they are able to love the parent without feeling obligated to them or justifying the behavior of the abuser. In the end, it is most important to allow questions of forgiveness and future relationships with abusive caregivers to be solved individually on a case-by-case basis (Courtois, 2010).

GROUPS AS AN ADJUNCT TO TREATMENT

Group therapy can provide a powerful adjunct to individual treatment as children and teens progress on their healing journey. I find these programs most helpful at the end stages of treatment when clients have resolved many of their symptoms and have positive energy to share with one another. Groups can provide a number of important benefits. They can reinforce mindfulness and affect regulation skills in a supportive atmosphere (Miller, Rathus, & Linehan, 2007), help children focus on positive role models such as in the Real Life Heroes Program (Kagan, 2008), and provide psychoeducation where cognitive-behavioral and affect regulation skills are reinforced, such as the Structured Psychotherapy for Adolescents Responding to Chronic Stress (SPARCS; DeRosa & Pelcovitz, 2008).

I have used groups for building peer support, enhancing motivation, and developing skills among dissociative adolescents whose dissociation was an impediment to their social, academic, and life functioning. One group exercise was to identify all of the skills necessary for driving a car, and list how the clients' dissociation could interfere with successful driving. The group then developed some operational goals that could help convince their parents that they were ready for a license—such as three months without evidence of switching behaviors and no episodes of uncontrolled rage. Other topics included handling school bullies without dissociating, and skills for managing arguments with parents. Sometimes, the wisdom and insight of young people can be remarkable. As a final project in one of my groups for dissociative girls, group members prepared a list of insights

Table 15.1 Insights From a Group for Dissociative Girls

Your body is a temple. Respect it.

Honor all parts of yourself. You have wisdom you may not yet know.

You have a right to your feelings. If someone does not accept your feelings it is their problem not yours.

If something is getting you panicky, it may remind you of something from the past. Notice the differences.

People are constantly expecting you to behave in certain ways. You don't have to do it.

Don't necessarily believe what people tell you about yourself. Trust yourself.

Dissociation has helped you cope. You will know when you won't need it anymore.

Never use dissociation as an excuse. Accept responsibility for all of your behavior even if it is embarrassing.

As you solve problems in the real world, your dissociative world will become less important.

they wanted to share with other teens entering the group for the first time. Their insights are listed in Table 15.1.

USING LETTERS TO COMMENT ON GROWTH IN TREATMENT

It is important for families and children to memorialize how far they have come, and to take pride in the efforts made to deal with their traumatic past. I often compose letters from me to the child, and encourage the child and family members to write letters to themselves and each other to comment on progress and to mark the end of therapy. These letters give family members the chance to express their pride and relief, reiterate apologies, or convey a sense of hope for the future. My own letters to the clients acknowledge my belief in the clients' potential to fulfill their own life goals. The last therapy session often involves this letter-writing exercise, and leaves client and therapist with a meaningful keepsake of the therapy experience. Following is a reproduction of a letter that Timothy's mother wrote at the end of a two-year treatment. In her letter, she expressed pride in Timothy and hope in his future.

Dear Timothy,

It's been six years now since this hard journey appeared before us. It began when you said, "Don't let me go to my granddad's, I'm afraid he's going to hurt me again!" And for a few seconds, I went deaf and the world stopped turning. Something then clicked inside me and I went into Mama-Tiger mode; I would never let him near you again.

It's been a hard road we've traveled, with sad times, scary times, and broken hearted times. But I have to tell you Timothy, that you are the strongest person I know. You've helped me to be strong, even when I was sure I couldn't be for one more minute.

These have been proud and blessed moments I've had, watching as you've chosen this new path, the one where you're taking charge of your own actions and reactions, and really your future. And it's all by using your strength and courage as fuel; instead of having fear and anger push you where you don't want to go.

It goes beyond words how grateful I feel when I see your confident smile, hope in your eyes, and peace in your heart. I still want to wrap you up and hold you safe, but I'm fine with just holding your hand now-and-then as we hike along this path a while.

I love you Timmy, always!

Your Mom

INTEGRATION

Daniel Siegel (2010) describes integration as the ongoing goal of all psychotherapy and defines integration as the "linkage of differentiated elements of a system" toward increasingly higher levels of complexity (p. 64). At the end stages of treatment, child survivors will have linked and integrated many differentiated elements of the self and no longer rely on dissociation to compartmentalize their experiences. They will have integrated their warring self-conceptions so that they can embrace the many facets of their identity without conflict. They will have integrated their affective life so that they will be able to use them as a guide for their behaviors and future choices. They also will have integrated their understanding of their traumatic past with their beliefs about who they are and will have new aspirations about who they want to be and could be.

Waters and Silberg (1998a) identified physical and psychological changes that are observable as children reach the end of treatment—a renewed curiosity, spontaneity, and a look of health. In my experience with dissociative children, integration is usually a gradual process, marked by sudden revelations of newfound abilities. Often without dramatic rituals or symbolic metaphors, children simply report feeling more whole, connected, and integrated. They may report that inner voices or imaginary friends are gone with little or no fanfare, and begin to show improvements in their everyday functioning.

While the process of integration is gradual, there may be occasional moments of triumph when the therapist and client both realize that a corner has been turned. Lisa came into my office with a lightness in her step and said, "My boyfriend breaking up with me hurts. But I know I'm going to be okay, and somehow I don't feel the need to cut myself over it." Similarly, Timothy had a fight with his mother and noticed that instead of yelling back, he retreated to his room. The voice in his mind that would prompt him to fight back was silent, and he was able to choose a different strategy for dealing with conflict. These clients realized that they had a new level of integration when they no longer felt compelled to follow their old scripts. They recognized that old patterns had been broken and thus new possibilities were available to them.

Table 15.2 provides a list of healthy cognitions for child survivors. The ability to believe and act upon many of these cognitions is a sign that child survivors have successfully broken the hold of their traumatic pasts. These cognitions

Table 15.2 Healthy Cognitions for Child Survivors

My brain is adaptive, not sick.

I am grateful to myself for my survival strengths.

I can forgive myself for any failings and move on.

I can risk attachment and trust.

I can be in charge of my behavior and choose my future.

Love is more powerful than hate. I can break the cycle.

Abuse is not my fault. Responsibility for it lies out of my control.

I am powerful and able to determine my own future.

Suffering is not inevitable for me.

I am intrinsically lovable.

I will gain autonomy and increasing self-determination.

My caregivers are strong enough to protect me and prevent future suffering.

include: the ability to love themselves, belief in their ability to master their future, and belief in relationships as a source of love and safety. This list is aspirational, as it may be a lifelong struggle to completely embrace all of these concepts. Yet in drawings or surprising revelations, clients may articulate these new beliefs or show evidence of these beliefs in their behaviors. These cognitions reinforce the viewpoint that the behaviors and symptoms of the child survivor were inevitable results of the trauma they suffered, and not the result of personal failings, psychiatric disorders, or brain dysfunction.

Metaphors of Integration

For children and teens who have seen their divided self-concept as central to their identity, therapists can use metaphors of "close hugging," "ingredients in a recipe coming together," or other images to symbolize and fortify the integration of the mind as the child imagines the parts of themselves blending together (Waters & Silberg, 1998a). Children and teens often find their own metaphors to describe the psychological changes they experience during integration. Lisa used milk as a metaphorL, "When I think of my old self, I think I was like skim milk—not all of me was really there. I think I am whole milk now." Angela stated, "It feels like a wall fell down in my mind." Six-year-old Stephanie described the imaginary parts of her mindL, "Sliding down a rainbow into a pot of golden cookies."

Flow and the Transcendent Self

At the opposite end of the continuum from the blocked, disconnected mind of the dissociative child is the mind during the experience of flow. Csikszentmihalyi

(1993) introduced the concept of "flow" to describe a unique state of consciousness involving total absorption where the intentions, skills, and challenges presented to the self are all at an optimum level. A person could be playing music, climbing a mountain, or engaged in his customary work activity, but if he is "in flow" the experience is similar. Csikszentmihalyi describes the pleasure that people feel when able to achieve this state of extreme integration. They feel limitless energy, minimal anxiety, and a sense of control over their actions.

The connection between flow and dissociation first became apparent to me when I was working with a severely dissociative teenager who was coping with the aftereffects of sexual abuse from an older brother. She told me that her only experience of feeling "real" was when she was on her high school crew team, rowing in synchrony with the rest of her team, each teammate putting their oars in the water at the exact right moment. At these times, she felt totally absorbed and fully present. During therapy, we used her feeling while rowing with her crew team as an index of how close she was able to approximate that state of being "real" in other aspects of her life. While both dissociative states and flow involve a narrowing of focus, in the dissociative state, mental energy is being used to push some mental contents out of awareness. The effort used in maintaining a dissociative state depletes energy, while being in flow is described as energizing and effortless.

Clients who have achieved integration of the self are certainly not in a state of flow all the time, but the capacity for more frequent moments of flow is there, as the full potential of the self is now accessible. This full potential includes a level of development of the self even beyond flow. Csikszentmihalyi (1993) described some individuals that achieve a level of evolution that he calls the "transcendent self." These individuals incorporate into their sense of self the desire to improve the lives of others and obtain a sense of meaning and satisfaction from viewing themselves as part of a bigger picture.

This level of integration is also observable in many of the young people that I have had the privilege of treating. One of the most rewarding characteristics you might notice in child survivors toward the end of treatment is the desire to find a way to use their own misfortune to help others. Clients may tell you they want to be therapists who work with children, or they want to be lawyers, senators, or judges to help change in some way the plight of children who have experienced trauma as they did.

Adina exemplifies the characteristics found in children who thrive following treatment, able to use their experiences to spur what is sometimes called "post-traumatic growth" (Tedeschi & Calhoun, 2004). She was a survivor of child sexual abuse and the trauma of erroneous family court decisions that had sent her to live with her abuser, despite her disclosures to multiple professionals. Finally safe from the abuse at age 8, she received therapy for two years. At the end of treatment, Adina, now 10, told me, "I feel like I got better from some weird sickness. My life is picture perfect. I can feel now. My brain is connected." Several years later, Adina surpassed the physical and emotional integration represented by this statement and seemed to achieve the higher levels described by Csikszentmihalyi.

Poised and confident at the age of 15, Adina was asked to participate in a hearing organized by the Office on Violence Against Women to help educate professionals about the needs for legal reforms to protect women and children in custody cases. Adina told her story tearfully and pleaded with the audience to listen to "the voices of children." Adina was asked by a participant whether she feels angry and resentful that she had to struggle so hard to finally get free of the abuse she suffered. Adina took a moment to think and then answered slowly, "No. There will always be bad people in the world but I must have been put here for a reason. Not all kids could be as brave and strong as I was in being able to tell what happened. And not all kids could stand up here and educate others. In a way, I am lucky that I can use my experiences to help others." The audience was speechless at her candor, wisdom, and high level of personal integration that such a statement revealed.

Both Lisa and Jennifer are now practicing medical professionals, married with young children of their own. Sonya is a physical education instructor. Angela is studying neuroscience in a demanding college program. Timothy is able to attend regular high school and has been moved out of special education classes. His mother and grandmother no longer consider sending him away to residential treatment. Sometimes children have gone on to repeat the mistakes of their parents. But most of my clients who completed treatment and whose families were involved with their therapy are now thriving. They made an energetic return to the trajectory of normal life with its ups and downs—touched by trauma, but not frozen in the traumatic past. The resilience, creativity, and hope they display continues to amaze me, inspire me, and make the hard work of therapy with the child survivor worthwhile.

The true measure of treatment success is when recovery from trauma extends to the next generation. Balina, whom you met in the Preface, a former foster child and veteran of nine foster homes in 9 years, made an appointment to see me at the age of 24 to discuss her 3-year-old son. Recently employed as a case manager for the Department of Social Services, Balina told me about the struggles she endured when her son was born premature at 24 weeks gestation. Born with severe digestive problems, he had endured multiple separations from his mother during hospitalizations. "His medical problems are affecting him psychologically," she told me. "I want him to grow up healthy, and not cope like I did, with dissociation and aggression. Will you help me learn to manage his tantrums and fears? I want to be the best mother possible to him." When I saw them together, I saw his secure attachment to her, and Balina's ability to be playful and set age-appropriate limits, and I knew this little boy had a promising future in her care. Balina had decided that the cycle of abandonment and maltreatment was ending with her. This remarkable little boy, cheerfully molding play dough in my office, and looking up expectantly for his mother's generous smiles and encouragement, was living proof of the end of the cycle of developmental trauma.

References

Adler-Tapia, R., & Settle, C. (2008). *EMDR and the art of psychotherapy with children.* New York: Springer.

Ainsworth, M. D. (1964). Patterns of attachment behavior shown by the infant in interaction with his mother. *Merrill Palmer Quarterly, 10,* 51–58.

Albini, T. K., & Pease, T. E. (1989). Normal and pathological dissociations of early childhood. *Dissociation, 2,* 144–150.

Altman, H., Collins, M., & Mundy, P. (1997). Subclinical hallucinations and delusions in nonpsychotic adolescents. *Journal of Child Psychology and Psychiatry, 38,* 413–420.

American Psychiatric Association. (2000). *Diagnostic and statistical manual of mental disorders* (4th ed., text rev.). Washington, DC: Author.

Amy. (2009, October 25). Victim impact statement of girl in Misty Series. *The Virginian-Pilot.* Retrieved from http://hamptonroads.com/2009/10/document-victim-impact-statement-girl-misty-series

Anderson, M. C., & Huddleston, E. (2012). Towards a cognitive and neurobiological model of motivated forgetting. In R. F. Belli (Ed.), *True and false recovered memories: Toward a reconciliation of the debate* (Vol. 58, pp. 53–120). Nebraska Symposium on Motivation. New York: Springer.

Armstrong, J., Putnam, F. W., Carlson, E., Libero, D., & Smith, S. (1997). Development and validation of a measure of adolescent dissociation: The Adolescent Dissociative Experience Scale. *Journal of Nervous and Mental Disease, 185,* 491–497.

Arseneault, L., Cannon, M., Fisher, H. L., Polanczyk, G., Moffitt, T. E., & Caspi, A. (2011). Childhood trauma and children's emerging psychotic symptoms: A genetically sensitive longitudinal cohort study. *American Journal of Psychiatry, 168,* 65–72.

Arvidson, J., Kinniburgh, K., Howard, K., Spinazzola, J., Strothers, H., Evans, M., … Blaustein, M. E. (2011). Treatment of complex trauma in young children: Developmental and cultural considerations in application of the ARC Intervention Model. *Journal of Child & Adolescent Trauma, 4*(1), 34–51.

Baita, S. (2011). Dalma (4 to 7 years old)—"I've got all my sisters with me": Treatment of Dissociative Identity Disorder in a sexually abused young child. In S. Wieland (Ed.), *Dissociation in traumatized children and adolescents: Theory and clinical interventions* (pp. 29–74). New York: Routledge.

Barnier, A. J., Cox, R. E., & Savage, G. (2008, October 7). Memory, hypnosis and the brain. *Scientific American.* Retrieved from http://www.scientificamerican.com/article.cfm?id=hypnosis-memory-brain

Becker-Blease, K.A., Freyd, J.J., & Pears, K.C. (2004). Preschoolers' memory for threatening information depends on trauma history and attentional contexts: Implications for the development of dissociation. *Journal of Trauma & Dissociation, 5*(1), 113–131.

Bell, V., Oakley, D.A., Halligan, P.W., & Deeley, Q. (2011). Dissociation in hysteria and hypnosis: Evidence from cognitive neuroscience. *Journal of Neurology, Neurosurgery and Psychiatry, 82*, 332–339.

Benbadis, S.R., O'Neill, E., Tatum, W.O., & Heriaud, L. (2004). Outcome of prolonged video-EEG monitoring at a typical referral epilepsy center. *Epilepsia, 45*, 1150–1153.

Blaustein, M.E., & Kinniburg, K.M. (2010). *Treating traumatic stress in children and adolescents: How to foster resilience through attachment, self-regulation, and competency.* New York: Guilford.

Bloom, S. (1997). *Creating sanctuary: Toward the evolution of sane societies.* New York: Routledge.

Bonanno, G.A., Noll, J.G., Putnam, F.W., O'Neill, M., & Trickett, P.K. (2003). Predicting the willingness to disclose childhood sexual abuse from measures of repressive coping and dissociative tendencies. *Child Maltreatment, 8*, 302–318.

Bowlby, J. (1988). *A secure base: Clinical applications of attachment theory.* London: Routledge.

Bowman, E.S. (2006). Why conversion seizures should be classified as a dissociative disorder. *Psychiatric Clinics of North America, 29*, 185–211.

Bowman, E.S., Blix, S.F., & Coons, P.M. (1985). Multiple personality in adolescence: Relationship to incestual experience. *Journal of the American Academy of Child and Adolescent Psychiatry, 24*, 109–114.

Boysen, G.A. (2011). The scientific status of childhood Dissociative Identity Disorder: A review of published research. *Psychotherapy & Psychosomatics, 80*, 329–334.

Brand, B.L. (2001). Establishing safety with patients with Dissociative Identity Disorder. *Journal of Trauma & Dissociation, 2*(4), 133–155.

Brand, B.L., Armstrong, J.G., & Loewenstein, R.J. (2006). Psychological assessment of patients with Dissociative Identity Disorder. *Psychiatric Clinics of North America, 29*, 145–168.

Brand, B.L., Classen, C.C., Lanius, R., Loewenstein, R., McNary, S., Pain, C., & Putnam, F.W. (2009). A naturalistic study of Dissociative Identity Disorder and Dissociative Disorder Not Otherwise Specified patients treated by community clinicians. *Psychological Trauma: Theory, Research, Practice, & Policy, 1*(2), 153–171.

Brand, B.L., Lanius, R., Vermetten, E., Loewenstein, R., & Spiegel, D. (2012). Where are we going? An update on assessment, treatment, and neurobiological research in dissociative disorders as we move toward the DSM-5. *Journal of Trauma & Dissociation, 13*(1), 9–31.

Brand, B.L., McNary, S.W., Myrick, A.C., Loewenstein, R.J., Classen, C.C., Lanius, R.A., … Putnam, F.W. (2012). A longitudinal, naturalistic study of dissociative disorder patients treated by community clinicians. *Psychological Trauma: Theory, Research, Practice, & Policy.* Advance on-line publication. doi: 10.1037/a0027654

Briere, J. (1996). *Trauma symptom checklist for children.* Lutz, FL: Psychological Assessment Resources.

Briere, J. (2005). *Trauma symptom checklist for young children.* Lutz, FL: Psychological Assessment Resources.

Brown, D., Scheflin, A., & Whitfield, C.L. (1999, Spring). Recovered memories: The current weight of the evidence in science and in the courts. *The Journal of Psychiatry and Law, 26*, 5–156.

Brown, R., Cardeña, E., Nijenhuis, E., Sar, V., & Van der Hart, O. (2007). Should conversion disorder be reclassified as a dissociative disorder in DSM-V? *Psychosomatics, 48*, 369–378.

Bruch, C.S. (2001). Parental Alienation Syndrome and parental alienation: Getting it wrong in child custody cases. *Family Law Quarterly, 35*, 527–552.

Burkman, K., Kisiel, C., & McClelland, G. (2008, November). *Dissociation and complex trauma among children and adolescents in the child welfare system in Illinois.* Presentation at the 24th annual fall conferences of the International Society for the Study of Trauma and Dissociation, Philadelphia, PA.

Busch, A.L., & Lieberman, A.F. (2007). Attachment and trauma: An integrated approach to treating young children exposed to family violence. In D.O. Oppenheim & D.F. Goldsmith (Eds.), *Attachment theory in clinical work with children* (pp. 139–171). New York: Guilford Press.

Cagiada, S., L. Camaido, & A. Pennan. (1997). Successful integrated hypnotic and psychopharmacological treatment of a war-related post-traumatic psychological and somatoform dissociative disorder of two years duration (psychogenic coma). *Dissociation, 10,* 182–189.

Carlson, E., Yates, T., & Sroufe, L.A. (2009). Development of dissociation and development of the self. In P. Dell & J. O'Neil (Eds.), *Dissociation and dissociative disorders* (pp. 39–52). New York: Routledge.

Carrion, V.G., & Steiner, H. (2000). Trauma and dissociation in delinquent adolescents. *Journal of the American Academy of Child & Adolescent Psychiatry, 39*, 353–359.

Carrion, V.G., Weems, C.F., Eliez, S., Patwardhan, A., Brown, W., Ray, R.D., & Reiss, A.L. (2001). Attenuation of frontal asymmetry in pediatric posttraumatic stress disorder. *Biological Psychiatry, 50*, 943–951.

Center for Sex Offender Management (CSOM). (2005, December). *Key considerations for reunifying adult sex offenders and their families.* Retrieved from http://www.csom.org/pubs/FamilyReunificationDec05.pdf

Chu, J.A. (1998). *Rebuilding shattered lives: The responsible treatment of complex posttraumatic and dissociative disorders.* New York: Wiley.

Cloitre, M., Stolbach, B.C., Herman, J.L., van der Kolk, B., Pynoos, R., Wang, J., & Petkova, E. (2009). A developmental approach to complex PTSD: Childhood and adult cumulative trauma as predictors of symptom complexity. *Journal of Traumatic Stress, 22*, 399–408.

Cohen, J.A., Mannarino, A.P., & Deblinger, E. (2006). *Treating trauma and traumatic grief in children and adolescents.* New York: Guilford Press.

Collin-Vézina, D., & Hébert, M. (2005). Comparing dissociation and PTSD in sexually abused school-aged girls. *Journal of Nervous & Mental Disease, 93*, 47–52.

Coons, P.M. (1996). Clinical phenomenology of 25 children and adolescents with dissociative disorders. *Child and Adolescent Psychiatric Clinics of North America, 5*, 361–374.

Corwin, D., & Olafson, E. (1997). Videotaped discovery of a reportedly unrecallable memory of child abuse: Comparison with a childhood interview taped 11 years before. *Child Maltreatment, 2*, 91–112.

Courtois, C.A. (2010). *Healing the incest wound: Adult survivors in therapy* (2nd ed.). New York: Norton.

Csikszentmihalyi, M. (1993). *The evolving self: A psychology for the third millennium.* New York: HarperCollins.

Dalenberg, C. (2000). *Countertransference and the treatment of trauma.* Washington, DC: American Psychological Association.

Dallam, S.J. (2002). Science or propaganda? An examination of Rind, Tromovitch and Bauserman (1998). In C. Whitfield, J. Silberg, & P. Fink (Eds.), *Misinformation concerning child sexual abuse and adult survivors* (pp. 109–134). New York: Haworth Publications.

Dallam, S.J., Gleaves, D., Cepeda-Benito, A., Silberg, J.L., Kraemer, H.C., & Spiegel, D. (2001). The effects of child sexual abuse: Comment on Rind, Tromovitch, and Bauserman (1998). *Psychological Bulletin, 127*, 715–733.

Dalton, C., Drozd, L., & Wong, F. (2006). *Navigating custody and visitation evaluations in cases with domestic violence: A judge's guide* (2nd ed.). Reno, NV: National Council of Juvenile and Family Court Judges.

Damasio, A.R. (1999). *The feeling of what happens: Body and emotion in the making of consciousness*. New York: Harcourt.

De Bellis, M.D., Keshavan, M.S., Clark, D.B., Casey, B.J., Giedd, J.N., Boring, A.M., ... Ryan, N.D. (1999). Developmental traumatology. Part II: brain development. *Biological Psychiatry, 45*, 1271–1284.

De Bellis, M.D., Keshavan, M.S., Spencer, S., & Hall, J. (2000). N-Acetylaspartate concentration in the anterior cingulate of maltreated children and adolescents with PTSD. *American Journal of Psychiatry, 157*, 1175–1177.

Dell, P.F. (2006). A new model of Dissociative Identity Disorder. *Psychiatric Clinics of North America, 29*, 1–26.

Dell, P.F. (2009). Understanding dissociation. In P. Dell & J. O'Neil (Eds.), *Dissociation and the dissociative disorders: DSM V and beyond* (pp. 709–825). New York: Routledge.

Dell, P.F., & Eisenhower, J.W. (1990). Adolescent Multiple Personality Disorder: A preliminary study of eleven cases. *Journal of the American Academy of Child & Adolescent Psychiatry, 29*, 359–366.

DeRosa, R., & Pelcovitz, D. (2008). Group treatment for chronically traumatized adolescents: Igniting SPARCS of change. In D. Brom, R. Pat-Horenczyk, & J.D. Ford (Eds.), *Treating traumatized children: Risk, resilience and recovery* (pp. 225–239). London: Routledge.

Diamond, S.G., Davis, O.C., & Howe, R.D. (2008). Heart rate variability as a quantitative measure of hypnotic depth. *International Journal of Clinical and Experimental Hypnosis, 56*(1), 1–18.

Diseth, T. (2006). Dissociation following traumatic medical procedures in childhood: A longitudinal follow-up. *Development and Psychopathology, 18*, 233–251.

Dodd, J. (2009, September 4). Shawn Hornbeck: Jaycee Dugard brainwashed, in shock. *People Magazine*. Retrieved from http://www.people.com/people/article/0,,20302413,00. html

Duggal, S., & Sroufe, L.A. (1998). Recovered memory of childhood sexual trauma: A documented case from a longitudinal study. *Journal of Traumatic Stress, 11*, 301–322.

Dutra, L., Bureau, J., Holmes, B., Lyubchik, A., & Lyons-Ruth, K. (2009). Quality of early care and childhood trauma: A prospective study of developmental pathways to dissociation. *Journal of Nervous and Mental Disease, 197*(6), 383–390.

Edwards, V.J., Fivush, R., Anda, R.F., Felitti,V.J., & Nordenberg, D.F. (2001). Autobiographical memory disturbances in childhood abuse survivors. *Journal of Aggression, Maltreatment & Trauma, 4*(2), 247–263.

Eisen, M.L., Goodman, G.S., Qin, J., Davis, S., & Crayton, J. (2007). Maltreated children's memory: Accuracy, suggestibility and psychopathology. *Developmental Psychology, 43*, 1275–1294.

Ellement, J. R. (2010, January 16). Former Catholic priest's bid for new trial rejected: Use of recovered memories upheld. *Boston Globe.* Retrieved from http://www.boston.com/news/local/massachusetts/articles/2010/01/16/former_catholic_priests_bid_for_new_trial_rejected/?page=full

Erickson, M. F., & Egeland, B. (2002). Child neglect. In J. Myers, L. Berliner, J. Briere, C. Hendrix, C. Jenny, & T. Reid (Eds.), *The APSAC handbook on child maltreatment* (2nd ed., pp. 3–20). Thousand Oaks, CA: Sage.

Erickson, N. S. (2005). Use of the MMPI-2 in child custody evaluations involving battered women: What does psychological research tell us? *Family Law Quarterly, 39*(1), 87–108.

Fagan, J., & McMahon, P. P. (1984). Incipient multiple personality in children. *Journal of Nervous and Mental Disease, 172*, 26–36.

Faller, K. C. (2007). Coaching children about sexual abuse: A pilot study of professionals' perceptions. *Child Abuse & Neglect, 31*, 947–959.

Felitti, V. J., Anda, R. F., Nordenberg, D., Williamson, D. F., Spitz, A. M., Edwards, V., … Marks, J. S. (1998). Relationship of childhood abuse and household dysfunction to many of the leading causes of death in adults. The Adverse Childhood Experiences (ACE) Study. *American Journal of Preventive Medicine, 14*(4), 245–258.

Ferentz, L. (2012). *Treating self-destructive behaviors in trauma survivors.* New York: Routledge.

Fergusson, D. M., Boden, J. M., & Horwood, L. J. (2008). Exposure to childhood sexual and physical abuse and adjustment in early adulthood. *Child Abuse & Neglect, 32*, 607–619.

Finkelhor, D., & Browne, A. (1985). The traumatic impact of child sexual abuse: A conceptualization. *American Journal of Orthopsychiatry, 55*, 530–541.

Fonagy, P., & Target, M. (1997). Attachment and reflective function: Their role in self-organization. *Development and Psychopathology, 9*, 679–700.

Ford, J. D. (2009). Neurobiological and developmental research: Clinical implications. In C. A. Courtois, J. D. Ford, & J. L. Herman (Eds.), *Treating complex traumatic stress disorders: An evidence based guide* (pp. 31–54). New York: Guilford Press.

Ford, J. D., & Cloitre, M. (2009). Best practices in psychotherapy for children and adolescents. In C. A. Courtois, J. D. Ford, & J. L. Herman (Eds.), *Treating complex traumatic stress disorders: An evidence based guide* (pp. 59–81). New York: Guilford Press.

Ford, J., & The Developmental Trauma Working Group. (2011a). *Development Trauma Disorder Structured Interview for Children (DTDSI-C 10.3).* Farmington, CT: University of Connecticut. Available from the author, jford@uchc.edu.

Ford, J., & The Developmental Trauma Working Group. (2011b). *Developmental Trauma Disorder Structured Interview for Parent/Caregivers (DTDSI-P/C 10.3).*

Ford, J., van der Kolk, B., Spinazzola, J., & Stolbach, B. (2011, November). *The Developmental Trauma Disorder field study and the DSM-5: Overview, clinicians' survey results, and structured interview methodology.* Panel presented at 27th international conference, International Society for the Study of Trauma and Dissociation, Baltimore, MD.

Freyd, J. (1996). *Betrayal trauma: The logic of forgetting childhood sexual abuse.* Cambridge, MA: Harvard University Press.

Freyd, J. J., DePrince, A. P., & Gleaves, D. (2007). The state of betrayal trauma theory: Reply to McNally (2007)—Conceptual issues and future directions. *Memory, 15*, 295–311.

Friedrich, W. N. (1997). *The Child Sexual Behavior Inventory (CSBI).* Odessa, FL: Psychological Assessment Resources.

Friedrich, W. N., Gerber, P. N., Koplin, B., Davis, M., Giese, J., Mykelbust, C., & Franckowiak, D. (2001). Multimodal assessment of dissociation in adolescents: Inpatients and juvenile sex offenders. *Sexual Abuse, 13*, 167–177.

Frost, J., Silberg, J. L., & McIntee, J. (1996, November). *Imaginary friends in normal and traumatized children.* Paper presented at the 13th international conference, International Society for the Study of Dissociation, San Francisco, CA.

Galliano, G., Noble, I. M., Travis, L. A., & Puechl, C. (1993). Victim reactions during rape/sexual assault: A preliminary study of the immobility response and its correlates. *Journal of Interpersonal Violence, 8,* 109–114.

Gates, J. R., Ramani, V., Whalen, S., & Loewenson, R. (1985). Ictal characteristics of pseudoseizures. *Archives of Neurology, 42,* 1183–1187.

Gifford-Smith, M. E., & Brownell, C. A. (2002). Childhood peer relationships: Social acceptance, friendships, and peer network. *Journal of School Psychology, 41,* 235–284.

Gold, S. (2000). *Not trauma alone: Therapy for child abuse survivors in family and social context.* Philadelphia, PA: Brunner/Routledge.

Goodman, G. S., Ghetti, S., Quas, J. A., Edelstein, R. S., Alexander, K. W., Redlich, A. D., … Jones, D. P. (2003). A prospective study of memory for child sexual abuse: New findings relevant to the repressed memory controversy. *Psychological Science, 14*(2), 113–118.

Goodman, G. S., Quas, J., & Ogle, C. M. (2010). Child maltreatment and memory. *Annual Review of Psychology, 61,* 325–351.

Grabe, H. J., Spitzer, C., & Freyberger, J. H. (1999). Relationship of dissociation to temperament and character in men and women. *American Journal of Psychiatry, 156,* 1811–1813.

Greenhoot, A. F., Brunell, S. L., Curtis, J. S., & Beyer, A. M. (2008). Trauma and autobiographical memory functioning. In M. L. Howe, G. S. Goodman, & D. Cichetti (Eds.), *Stress, trauma and children's memory development* (pp. 139–170). New York: Oxford University Press.

Grimminck, E. (2011). Emma (6 to 9 years old)—From kid actress to healthy child: Treatment of the early sexual abuse led to integration. In S. Wieland (Ed.), *Dissociation in traumatized children and adolescents: Theory and clinical interventions* (pp. 75–96). New York: Routledge.

Hannah, M. T., & Goldstein, B. (2010). *Domestic violence, abuse, and child custody: Legal strategies and policy issues.* Kingston, NJ: Civic Research Institute.

Herman, J. L. (1992). Complex PTSD: A syndrome in survivors of prolonged and repeated trauma. *Journal of Traumatic Stress, 5,* 377–391.

Hesse, E., Main, M., Abrams, K. Y., & Rifkin, A. (2003). Unresolved states regarding loss or abuse can have "second-generation" effects: Disorganized, role-inversion and frightening ideation in the offspring of traumatized non-maltreating parents. In D. J. Siegel & M. F. Solomon (Eds.), *Healing trauma: Attachment, mind body and brain* (pp. 57–106). New York: Norton.

Hewitt, S. K. (2008). Therapeutically managing reunification after abuse allegations. *Journal of Child Sexual Abuse, 17*(1), 17–19.

Hildyard, K. L., & Wolfe, D. A. (2002). Child neglect: Developmental issues and outcomes. *Child Abuse & Neglect, 26,* 679–695.

Hoffman, K., Marvin, R., Cooper, G., & Powell, B. (2006). Changing toddlers' and preschoolers' attachment classifications: The circle of security intervention. *Journal of Consulting and Clinical Psychology, 74,* 1017–1026.

Hornstein, N. L., & Tyson, S. (1991). Inpatient treatment of children with multiple personality/dissociation and their families. *Psychiatric Clinics of North America, 4,* 631–648.

Hoult, J. (2006). The evidentiary admissibility of Parental Alienation Syndrome: Science, law and policy. *Children's Legal Rights Journal, 26,* 1–61.

Hughes, D.A. (2006). *Building the bonds of attachment: Awakening love in deeply troubled children*. Northvale, NJ: Jason Aronson.

Hulette, A.C., Fisher, P.A., Kim, H.K., Ganger, W., & Landsverk, J.L. (2008). Dissociation in foster preschoolers: A replication and assessment study. *Journal of Trauma & Dissociation, 9*, 173–190.

Hulette, A.C., Freyd, J.J., & Fisher, P.A. (2011). Dissociation in middle childhood among foster children with early Maltreatment experiences. *Child Abuse & Neglect, 35*, 123–126.

International Society for the Study of Dissociation. (2003). Guidelines for the evaluation and treatment of dissociative symptoms in children and adolescents. *Journal of Trauma and Dissociation, 5*(3), 119–149.

Jack, F., Simcock, G., & Hayne, H. (2012). Magic memories: Young children's verbal recall after a 6-year delay. *Child Development, 83*, 159–172.

Jacobsen, T. (1995). Case study: Is selective mutism a manifestation of Dissociative Identity Disorder? *Journal of American Academy of Child & Adolescent Psychiatry, 31*, 1077–1085.

James, B. (1994). *Handbook for treatment of attachment-trauma problems in children*. New York: Simon & Schuster.

Jang, K.L., Paris, J., Zweig-Frank, H., & Livelsey, W.J. (1998). Twin study of dissociative experience. *Journal of Nervous and Mental Disease, 186*, 345–351.

Johnston, J.R. (2005). Children of divorce who reject a parent and refuse visitation: Recent research and social policy implications for the alienated child. *Family Law Quarterly, 38*, 757–775.

Johnson, T.C. (2003). Some considerations about sexual abuse and children with sexual behavior problems. *Journal of Trauma & Dissociation, 3*(4), 83–105.

Kagan, R. (2004). *Rebuilding attachments with traumatized children; Healing from losses, violence, abuse and neglect*. New York: Routledge.

Kagan, R. (2008). Transforming troubled children into tomorrow's heroes. In C. Brom, R. Pat-Horenczyk, & J.D. Ford (Eds.), *Treating traumatized children: Risk, resilience and recovery* (pp. 255–268). London: Routledge.

Keen, J. (2008, September 24). Mo. teen recounts '02 kidnapping. *USA Today.* Retrieved from http://www.usatoday.com/news/nation/2008-09-24-hornbeck_N.htm

Kenardy, J., Smith, A., Spence, S.H., Lilley, P.R., Newcombe, P., Dob, R., & Robinson, S. (2007). Dissociation in children's trauma narratives: An exploratory investigation. *Journal of Anxiety Disorders, 21*, 456–466.

Kim, K., Trickett, P.K., & Putnam, F.W. (2010). Childhood experiences of sexual abuse and later parenting practices among non-offending mothers of sexually abused and comparison girls. *Child Abuse & Neglect, 34*, 610–622.

Kisiel, C., Liang, L., Stolbach, B., Maj, N., Spinazzola, J., & Belin, T. (2011, November). *The complexity of clinical profiles among children and adolescents exposed to caregiver related traumas.* Paper presented at the 27th international conference, International Society for the Study of Traumatic Stress, Baltimore, MD.

Kisiel, C., & Lyons, J.S. (2001). Dissociation as a mediator of psychopathology among sexually abused children and adolescents. *American Journal of Psychiatry, 158*, 1034–1039.

Kitzmann, K.M., Gaylord, N.K., Holt, A.R., & Kenny, E.D. (2003). Child witnesses to domestic violence: A meta-analytic review. *Journal of Consulting & Clinical Psychology, 71*, 339–352.

Klein, B.R. (1985). A child's imaginary companion: A transitional self. *Clinical Social Work, 13*, 272–282.

Klein, H., Mann, D.R., & Goodwin, J.M. (1994). Obstacles to the recognition of sexual abuse and dissociative disorders in child and adolescent males. *Dissociation, 7*, 138–144.

Kleinman, T. (2011). Targeting and child protection: Should psychologists stop doing evaluations of children? *Trauma Psychology Newsletter, 6*(3), 6–7.

Kluft, R.P. (1984). MPD in childhood. *Psychiatric Clinics of North America, 7*, 9–29.

Kluft, R.P. (1985). Childhood Multiple Personality Disorder: Predictors, clinical findings and treatment results. In R.P. Kluft (Ed.), *Childhood antecedents of Multiple Personality Disorder* (pp. 168–196). Washington, DC: American Psychiatric Press.

Kluft, R.P. (1991). Hypnosis in childhood trauma. In W.C. Westar, II, & D.J. O'Grady (Eds.), *Clinical hypnosis with children* (pp. 53–68). New York: Brunner/Mazel.

Kluft, R.P. (2007). Applications of innate affect theory to the understanding and treatment of Dissociative Identity Disorder. In E. Vermetten, M.J. Dorahy, & D. Spiegel (Eds.), *Traumatic dissociation: Neurobiology and treatment* (pp. 301–316). Washington, DC: American Psychiatric Publishing.

Kolko, D. (2002). Child physical abuse. In J. Myers, L. Berliner, J. Briere, C. Hendrix, C. Jenny, & T. Reid (Eds.), *The APSAC handbook on child maltreatment* (2nd ed., pp. 21–54). Thousand Oaks, CA: Sage.

Konigsburg, E.L. (1970). *(George)*. Forge Village, MA: Atheneum.

Kunzelman, M. (2012, January 30). Court to weigh restitution for child porn victim living in Pa. *The Mercury*. Retrieved from http://www.pottsmerc.com/article/20120130/NEWS03/120139949/court-to-weigh-restitution-for-child-porn-victim-living-in-pa-

Lanius, R.A., Williamson, P.C., Boksman, K., Densmore, M., Gupta, M., Neufeld, R.W., … Menon, R.S. (2002). Brain activation during script-driven imagery induced dissociative responses in PTSD: A functional magnetic resonance imaging investigation. *Biological Psychiatry, 52*(4), 305–311.

Laporta, L.D. (1992). Childhood trauma and multiple personality disorder: The case of a 9-year-old girl. *Child Abuse & Neglect, 16*, 615–620.

LeDoux, J. (1996). *The emotional brain*. New York: Touchstone.

Leibowitz, G.S., Laser, J.A., & Burton, D.L. (2011). Exploring the relationships between dissociation, victimization, and juvenile sexual offending. *Journal of Trauma and Dissociation, 12*(1), 38–52.

Leonard, M.M. (2010). "I did what I was directed to do but he didn't touch me": The impact of being a victim of internet offending. *Journal of Sexual Aggression, 16*(2), 249–256.

Levine, J. (2002). *Harmful to minors: The perils of protecting children from sex*. Minneapolis: University of Minnesota Press.

Levine, P. (1997). *Waking the tiger: Healing trauma*. Berkeley, CA: North Atlantic Books.

Lewis, H.B. (Ed.). (1987). *The role of shame in symptom formation*. Hillsdale, NJ: Erlbaum.

Linehan, M.M. (1993). *Cognitive-behavioral treatment of Borderline Personality Disorder*. New York: Guilford Press.

Liotti, G. (1999). Disorganization of attachment as a model of understanding dissociative psychopathology. In J. Solomon & C. George (Eds.), *Attachment disorganization* (pp. 291–317). New York: Guilford Press.

Liotti, G. (2009). Attachment and dissociation. In P. Dell & J. O'Neil (Eds.), *Dissociation and the dissociative disorders: DSM V and beyond* (pp. 53–65). New York: Routledge.

Lipton, B.H. (2005). *The biology of belief: Unleashing the power of consciousness, matter and miracles*. Carlsbad, CA: Hay House.

Loewenstein, R. J. (2006). A hands-on clinical guide to the stabilization phase of Dissociative Identity Disorder treatment. *Psychiatric Clinics of North America, 29*(1), 305–333.

Ludäscher, P., Valerius, G., Stiglmayr, C., Mauchnik, J., Lanius, R.A., Bohus, M., & Schmahl, C. (2010). Pain sensitivity and neural processing during dissociative states in patients with borderline personality disorder with and without comorbid posttraumatic stress disorder: A pilot study. *Journal of Psychiatry & Neurosciences, 35*(3), 177–184.

Luther, J. S., McNamara, J. O., Carwile, S., Miller, P., & Hope, V. (1982). Pseudoepileptic seizures: Methods and video analysis to aid diagnosis. *Annals of Neurology, 12*, 458–462.

Macfie, J., Cicchetti, D., & Toth, S.L. (2001). The development of dissociation in maltreated preschool-aged children. *Development and Psychopathology, 13*, 233–254.

Main, M., & Solomon, J. (1990). Procedures for identifying infants as disorganized/disoriented during the Ainsworth strange situation. In M. Greenberg, D. Cichetti, & E.M. Cummings (Eds.), *Attachment in the preschool years* (pp. 121–160). Chicago: University of Chicago Press.

Malenbaum, R., & Russell, A.T. (1987). Multiple personality disorder in an eleven-year-old boy and his mother. *Journal of the American Academy of Child & Adolescent Psychiatry, 26*, 436–439.

Marks, R. P. (2011). Jason (7 years old)—Expressing past neglect and abuse: Two-week intensive therapy for an adopted child with dissociation. In S. Wieland (Ed.), *Dissociation in traumatized children and adolescents: Theory and clinical interventions* (pp. 97–140). New York: Routledge.

McDonald, R., Jouriles, E. N., Ramisetty-Mikler, S., Caetano, R., & Green, C. (2006). Estimating the number of American children living in partner-violent families. *Journal of Family Psychology, 20*, 137–142.

McHugh, P. R. (2008). *Try to remember: Psychiatry's clash over meaning, memory, and mind.* Washington, DC: Dana Press.

McLewin, L.A., & Muller, R. T. (2006). Childhood trauma, imaginary companions and the development of pathological dissociation. *Aggression & Violent Behavior, 11*, 531–545.

Mehta, M.A., Golembo, N. I., Nosarti, C., Colvert, E., Mota, A., Williams, S.C., … Sonuga-Barke, E. J. (2009). Amygdala, hippocampal and corpus callosum size following severe early institutional deprivation: The English and Romanian Adoptees study pilot. *Journal of Child Psychology and Psychiatry, and Allied Disciplines, 50*, 943–951.

Meier, J. (2009). *Parental Alienation Syndrome and parental alienation: Research reviews.* Harrisburg, PA: VAWnet, a project of the National Resource Center on Domestic Violence. Retrieved from http://www.vawnet.org

Miller, A. L., Rathus, J. H., & Linehan, M.M. (2007). *Dialectical Behavior Therapy with suicidal adolescents.* New York: Guilford Press.

Monsen, J.T., & Monsen, K. (1999). Affects and affect consciousness: A psychotherapy model integrating Silvan Tomkin's affect and -script theory within the framework of self-psychology. In A. Goldberg (Ed.), *Pluralism in self psychology: Progress in self psychology* (Vol. 15, pp. 287–306). Hillsdale, NJ: The Analytic Press.

Moskowitz, A., Read, J., Farrely, S., Rudegeair, T., & Williams, O. (2009). Are psychotic symptoms traumatic in origin and dissociative in kind? In P. Dell & J. O'Neil (Eds.), *Dissociation and the dissociative disorders: DSM V and beyond* (pp. 521–533). New York: Routledge.

Myrick, A.C., Brand, B.L., McNary, S.W., Loewenstein, R.J., Classen, C.C., Lanius, R.A., … Putnam, F.W. (in press). An exploration of young adults' progress in treatment for dissociative disorder. *Journal of Trauma and Dissociation.*

Nathan, D. (2011). *Sybil exposed: The extraordinary story behind the famous multiple personality case.* New York: Free Press.

Nathanson, D. (1992). *Shame and pride: Affect, sex, and the birth of the self.* New York: Norton.

Neustein, A., & Lesher, M. (2005). *From madness to mutiny: Why mothers are running from the family courts—and what can be done about it.* Boston, MA: Northeastern University Press.

Nijenhuis, E. R. S. (2004). *Somatoform dissociation: Phenomena, measurement, and theoretical issues.* New York: Norton.

Nijenhuis, E. R. S., Vanderlinden, J., & Spinhoven, P. (1998). Animal defensive reaction as a model for trauma-induced dissociative processes. *Journal of Traumatic Stress, 11,* 243–260.

Nilsson, D., & Svedin, C. G. (2006). Dissociation among Swedish adolescents and the connection to trauma: An evaluation of the Swedish version of Adolescent Dissociative Experience Scale. *Journal of Nervous and Mental Disease, 194,* 684–689.

Noll, J. G. (2005). Forgiveness in people experiencing trauma. In E. L. Worthington, Jr., (Ed.), *Handbook of forgiveness* (pp. 363–376). New York: Brunner-Routledge.

Norretranders, T. (1998). *The user illusion: Cutting consciousness down to size.* New York: Viking.

Ogawa, J. R., Sroufe, L. A., Weinfield, N. S., Carlson, E. A., & Egeland, B. (1997). Development and the fragmented self: Longitudinal study of dissociative symptomatology in a nonclinical sample. *Developmental Psychopathology, 9,* 855–979.

Ogden, P., & Minton, K. (2000). Sensorimotor psychotherapy: One method for processing traumatic memory. *Traumatology, 6*(3). Retrieved from http://www.fsu.edu/~trauma/v6i3/v6i3a3.html

Ogden, P., Pain, C., Minton, K., & Fisher, J. (2005). Including the body in mainstream psychotherapy for traumatized individuals. *Psychologist Psychoanalyst, 25*(4), 19–24. Retrieved from http://www.sensorimotorpsychotherapy.org/article%20APA.html

Olafson, E., & Lederman, J. C. S. (2006). The state of the debate about children's disclosure patterns in child sexual abuse cases. *Juvenile and Family Court Journal, 57,* 27–40.

Parry, P. I., & Levin, E. C. (2012). Pediatric Bipolar Disorder in an era of "mindless psychiatry." *Journal of Trauma & Dissociation, 13*(1), 51–68.

Pearlman, L. A., & Courtois, C. A. (2005). Clinical applications of the attachment framework: Relational treatment of complex trauma. *Journal of Traumatic Stress, 18*(5), 449–459.

Pearlman, L. A., & Saakvitne, K. W. (1995). *Trauma and the therapist: Countertransference and vicarious traumatization in psychotherapy with incest survivors.* New York: Norton.

Perry, B. D. (2002). *Adaptive responses to childhood trauma.* Retrieved from http://74.52.31.127/~oldnew/fasa/FASA%20PDF/For%20Professionals/Neurodevelopment%20&%20Trauma.pdf

Perry, B. D. (2006). The Neurosequential Model of Therapeutics: Applying principles of neuroscience to clinical work with traumatized and maltreated children. In N. B. Webb (Ed.), *Working with traumatized youth in child welfare* (pp. 27–52). New York: Guilford Press.

Perry, B. D. (2009). Examining child maltreatment through a neurodevelopmental lens: Clinical application of the Neurosequential Model of Therapeutics. *Journal of Loss and Trauma, 14,* 240–255.

Perry, B. D., Pollard, R., Blakely, T., Baker, W., & Vigilante, D. (1995). Childhood trauma, the neurobiology of adaptation and use-dependent development of the brain: How states become traits. *Infant Mental Health Journal, 16,* 271–291.

Peterson, G. (1998). Diagnostic taxonomy: Past to future. In J.L. Silberg (Ed.), *The dissociative child: Diagnosis, treatment and management* (2nd ed, pp. 3–26). Lutherville, MD: Sidran Press.

Phillips, M., & Frederick, C. (1995). *Healing the divided self: Clinical and Ericksonian hypnotherapy for post-traumatic and dissociative conditions.* New York: Norton.

Pica, M. (1999). The evolution of alter personality states in Dissociative Identity Disorder. *Psychotherapy, 30,* 404–415.

Pine, D.S., Mogg, K., Bradley, B.P., Montgomery, L., Monk, C.S., McClure, E., ... Kaufman J. (2005). Attention bias to threat in maltreated children: Implications for vulnerability to stress-related psychopathology. *American Journal of Psychiatry, 162,* 291–296.

Pollak, S.D., & Sinha, P. (2002). Effects of early experience on children's recognition of facial displays of emotion. *Developmental Psychology, 38,* 784–791.

Porges, S.W. (2003). The Polyvagal Theory: Phylogenetic contributions to social behavior. *Physiology and Behavior, 79,* 503–513.

Putnam, F.W. (1991). Dissociative disorders in children and adolescents: A developmental perspective. *Psychiatric Clinics of North America, 14,* 519–532.

Putnam, F.W. (1997). *Dissociation in children and adolescents: A developmental approach.* New York: Guilford Press.

Putnam, F.W. (2003). Ten-year research update review: Child sexual abuse. *Journal of the American Academy of Child & Adolescent Psychiatry, 42,* 269–278.

Putnam, F.W., Helmers, K., & Trickett, P.K. (1993). Development, reliability, and validity of a child dissociation scale. *Child Abuse and Neglect, 17,* 731–741.

Putnam, F.W., Hornstein, N., & Peterson, G. (1996). Clinical phenomenology of child and adolescent dissociative disorders: Gender and age effects. *Child and Adolescent Psychiatric Clinics of North America, 5,* 303–442.

Ratner, S.C. (1967). Comparative aspects of hypnosis. In J.E. Gordon (Ed.), *Handbook of clinical and experimental hypnosis* (pp. 550–587). New York: Macmillan.

Rhue, J.W., Lynn, S.J., & Sandberg, D. (1995). Dissociation, fantasy, and imagination in childhood: A comparison of physically abused, sexually abused and non-abused children. *Contemporary Hypnosis, 12,* 131–136.

Riley, R.L., & Mead, J. (1988). The development of symptoms of multiple personality in a child of three. *Dissociation, 1,* 41–46.

Rind, B., Tromovitch, P., & Bauserman, R. (1998). A meta-analytic examination of assumed properties of child sexual abuse using college samples. *Psychological Bulletin, 124,* 22–53.

Rivera, M. (1996). *More alike than different: Treating severely dissociative trauma survivors.* Toronto: University of Toronto Press.

Rothchild, B. (2000). *The body remembers: The psychophysiology of trauma and trauma treatment.* New York: Norton.

Ruths, S., Silberg, J.L., Dell, P.F., & Jenkins, C. (2002, November). *Adolescent DID: An elucidation of symptomatology and validation of the MID.* Paper presented at the 19th meeting of the International Society for the Study of Dissociation, Baltimore, MD.

Sar, V. (2011). Developmental trauma, complex PTSD, and the current proposal of DSM-5. *European Journal of Psychotraumatology, 2,* 5662.

Saxe, G.N., Ellis, B.H., & Kaplow, J.B. (2006). *Collaborative treatment of traumatized child and teens: The trauma systems therapy approach.* New York: Guilford Press.

Schiffer, F., Teicher, M.H., & Papanicolaou, A.C. (1995). Evoked potential evidence for right brain activity during the recall of traumatic memories. *The Journal of Neuropsychiatry and Clinical Neurosciences, 7,* 169–175.

Schore, A. (2009). Attachment trauma and the developing right brain. In P. Dell & J. O'Neil (Eds.), *Dissociation and the dissociative disorders: DSM V and beyond* (pp. 107–144). New York: Routledge.

Seligman, M. E. P., Steen, T. A., Park, N., & Peterson, C. (2005). Positive psychology progress: Empirical validation of interventions. *American Psychologist, 60*, 410–421.

Seuss, T. G. (1982). *Hunches and bunches*. New York: Random House.

Shin, J. U., Jeong, S. H., & Chung, U.S. (2009). The Korean version of the Adolescent Dissociative Experience Scale: Psychometric properties and the connection to trauma among Korean adolescents. *Psychiatry Investigation, 6*(3), 163–172.

Shirar, L. (1996). *Dissociative children: Bridging the inner and outer worlds*. New York: Norton.

Siegel, D. J. (1999). *The developing mind: Toward a neurobiology of interpersonal experience*. New York: Guilford Press.

Siegel, D. J. (2010). *The mindful therapist: A clinician's guide to mindsight and neural integration*. New York: Norton.

Silberg, J. L. (Ed.). (1998a). *The dissociative child: Diagnosis, treatment and management* (2nd ed.). Lutherville, MD: Sidran Press.

Silberg, J. L. (1998b). Interviewing strategies for assessing dissociative disorders in children and adolescents. In J. L. Silberg (Ed.), *The dissociative child: Diagnosis, treatment and management* (2nd ed., pp. 47–68). Lutherville, MD: Sidran Press.

Silberg, J. L. (1998c). Dissociative symptomatology in children and adolescents as displayed of psychological testing. *Journal of Personality Assessment, 71*, 421–439.

Silberg, J. (1998d). Psychological testing with dissociative children and adolescents. In J. L. Silberg (Ed.), *The dissociative child: Diagnosis, treatment and management* (2nd ed., pp. 85–102). Lutherville, MD: Sidran Press.

Silberg, S. L. (1999). Parenting the dissociative child. *Many Voices, 11*(1), 6–7.

Silberg, J. L. (2001a). Treating maladaptive dissociation in a young teenage girl. In H. Orvaschel, J. Faust, & M. Hersen (Eds.), *Handbook of conceptualization and treatment of child psychopathology* (pp. 449–474). Oxford, UK: Elsevier Science.

Silberg, J. L. (2001b). A president's perspective: The human face of the diagnostic controversy. *Journal of Trauma and Dissociation, 2*(1), 1–5.

Silberg, J. L. (2001c). An optimistic look at childhood dissociation. *ISSD NEWS, 19*(2), 1.

Silberg, J. L. (2004). Treatment of dissociation in sexually abused children: A family/attachment perspective. *Psychotherapy: Theory, Research, Practice & Training, 41*, 487–496.

Silberg, J. L. (2011). Angela (14 to 16 years old)—Finding words for pain: Treatment of a dissociative teen presenting with medical trauma. In S. Wieland (Ed.), *Dissociation in children and adolescents: Clinical case studies* (pp. 263–284). New York: Routledge Press.

Silberg, J. L., & Dallam, S. J. (2009). Out of the Jewish closet: Facing the hidden secrets of child sex abuse and the damage done to victims. In A. Neustein (Ed.), *Tempest in the temple: Jewish communities and child sex scandals* (pp. 77–104). Waltham, MA: Brandeis University Press.

Silberg, J. L., & Ferentz, L. (2002, November). *Dissociation and self-injury in teens*. Presentation at the 18th International Meeting, The International Society for Traumatic Stress Studies, Baltimore, MD.

Silberg, J. L., & Waters, F. W. (1998). Factors associated with positive therapeutic outcome. In J. L. Silberg (Ed.), *The dissociative child: Diagnosis, treatment and management* (2nd ed., pp. 105–112). Lutherville, MD: Sidran Press.

Silverman, A.B., Reinherz, H.Z., & Giaconia, R.M. (1996). The long-term sequelae of child and adolescent abuse: A longitudinal community study. *Child Abuse & Neglect, 20*(8), 709–723.

Silverstien, S. (1974). *Where the sidewalk ends*. New York: HarperCollins.

Singer, D.G., & Singer, J.L. (1990). *The house of make-believe: Children's play and the developing imagination*. Cambridge, MA: Harvard University Press.

Sobol, B., & Schneider, K. (1998). Art as an adjunctive therapy in the treatment of children who dissociate. In J.L. Silberg (Ed.), *The dissociative child: Diagnosis, treatment and management* (2nd ed., pp. 219–230). Lutherville, MD: Sidran Press.

Soukup, J., Papežová, H., Kuběna, A.A., & Mikolajová, V. (2010). Dissociation in non-clinical and clinical sample of Czech adolescents: Reliability and validity of the Czech version of the Adolescent Dissociative Experiences Scale. *European Psychiatry, 25*, 390–395.

Spiegel, D., Loewenstein, R.J., Lewis-Fernández, R., Sar, V., Simeon, D., Vermetten, E., ... Dell, P.F. (2011). Dissociative disorders in DSM-5. *Depression & Anxiety, 28*, 824–852.

Spinazzola, J., Ford, J.D., Zucker, M., van der Kolk, B.A., Silva, S., Smith, S.F., & Blaustein, M. (2005). Survey evaluates complex trauma exposure, outcome, and intervention among children and adolescents. *Psychiatric Annals, 35*(5), 433–439.

Sroufe, L.A. (2012, January 28). Ritalin gone wrong. *New York Times*. Retrieved from http://www.nytimes.com/2012/01/29/opinion/sunday/childrens-add-drugs-dont-work-long-term.html?_r=2

Steinberg, M. (1994). *Structured clinical interview for DSM-IV dissociative disorders* (SCID-D). Washington, DC: American Psychiatric Press.

Stien, P., & Kendall, J. (2004). *Psychological trauma and the developing brain: Neurologically based interventions for troubled children*. Binghamton, NY: Haworth Press.

Stolbach, B.C. (1997). The Children's Dissociative Experiences Scale and Posttraumatic Symptom Inventory: Rationale, development, and validation of a self-report measure. *Dissertation Abstracts International, 58*(3), 1548B.

Stolbach, B.C. (2005). Psychotherapy of a dissociative 8-year-old boy burned at age 3. *Psychiatric Annals, 35*, 685–694.

Stout, M. (2001). *The myth of sanity: Divided consciousness and the promise of awareness*. New York: Penguin Books.

Taylor, M. (1999). *Imaginary companions and the children who create them*. New York: Oxford University Press.

Taylor, M., Carlson, S.M., Maring, B.L., Gerow, L., & Charley, C.M. (2004). The characteristics and correlates of fantasy in school-age children: Imaginary companions, impersonation, and social understanding. *Developmental Psychology, 40*, 1173–1187.

Tedeschi, R.G., & Calhoun, L.G. (2004). Posttraumatic growth: Conceptual foundations and empirical evidence. *Psychological Inquiry, 15*(1), 1–18.

Teicher, M. (2010, October). *Does child abuse permanently alter the brain?* Plenary at 27th International Conference of the International Society for the Study of Trauma and Dissociation, Atlanta, GA.

Teicher, M.H., Andersen, S.L., Dumont, N.L., Ito, Y., Glod, C.A., Vaituzis, C., & Giedd, J.N. (2000, November). Childhood neglect attenuates development of the corpus callosum. *Society for Neuroscience Abstracts, 26*, 549.

Teicher, M.H., Andersen, C.M., & Polcari, A. (2012). Childhood maltreatment is associated with reduced volume in the hippocampal subfields CA3, dentate gyrus, and subiculum. *Proceedings of the National Academy of Sciences*. Retrieved from www.pnas.org/cgi/doi/10.1073/pnas.1115396109

Teicher, M. H., Andersen, S. L., Polcari, A., Anderson, C. M., Navalta, C. P., & Kim, D. M. (2003). The neurobiological consequences of early stress and childhood maltreatment. *Neuroscience and Biobehavioral Reviews, 27*, 33–44.

Teicher, M. H., Ito, Y., Glod, C. A., Andersen, S. L., Dumont, N., & Ackerman, E. (1997). Preliminary evidence for abnormal cortical development in physically and sexually abused children using EEG coherence and MRI. *Annals of the New York Academy of Sciences, 821*, 160–175.

Teicher, M., Samson, J. A., Polcari, A., & McGreenery, C. E. (2006). Sticks and stones and hurtful words: Relative effects of various form of childhood maltreatment. *American Journal of Psychiatry, 163*, 993–1000.

Teicher, M., Samson, J. A., Sheu, Y. S., Polcari, A., & McGreenery, C. E. (2010). Hurtful words: Association of exposure to peer verbal abuse with elevated psychiatric symptom scores and corpus callosum abnormalities. *American Journal of Psychiatry, 167*, 1464–1471.

Terr, L. (1988). What happens to early memories of trauma? A study of 20 children under age 5 at the time of documented traumatic events. *Journal of the American Academy of Child & Adolescent Psychiatry, 27*(1), 96–104.

Terr, L. (1994). *Unchained memories: True stories of traumatic memories, lost and found.* New York: Basic Books.

Thoennes, N., & Tjaden, P. G. (1990). The extent, nature, and validity of sexual abuse allegations in custody and visitation disputes. *Child Sexual Abuse & Neglect, 14*(2), 151–163.

Tomkins, S. S. (1962). *Affect imagery consciousness: Vol. 1. The positive affects.* New York: Springer.

Tomkins, S. S. (1963). *Affect imagery consciousness: Vol. 2. The negative affects.* New York: Springer.

Tomoda, A., Suzuki, H., Rabi, K., Sheu, Y. S., Polcari, A., & Teicher, M. H. (2009). Reduced prefrontal cortical gray matter volume in young adults exposed to harsh corporal punishment. *Neuroimage, 47*(Suppl. 2), T66–T71.

Trickett, P. K., Noll, J. G., & Putnam, F. W. (2011). The impact of sexual abuse on female development: Lessons from a multi-generational, longitudinal study. *Development and Psychopathology, 23*, 453–476.

Trujillo, K., Lewis, D. O., Yeager, C. A., & Gidlow, B. (1996). Imaginary companions of school boys and boys with Dissociative Identity Disorder/ Multiple Personality Disorder: A normal to pathological continuum. *Child and Adolescent Psychiatric Clinics of North America, 5*, 375–391.

Turkus, J. A., & Kahler, J. A. (2006). Therapeutic interventions in the treatment of Dissociative Disorders. *Psychiatric Clinics of North America, 29*(1), 245–262.

U.S. Department of Health and Human Services, Administration for Children and Families, Administration on Children, Youth and Families, Children's Bureau. (2011). *Child Maltreatment 2010.* Retrieved from http://www.acf.hhs.gov/programs/cb/stats_research/index.htm#can

van der Hart, O., Nijenhuis, E. R. S., & Steele, K. (2006). *The haunted self: Structural dissociation and the treatment of chronic traumatization.* New York: Norton.

van der Kolk, B. A. (2005). Developmental trauma disorder: Toward a rational diagnosis for children with complex trauma histories. *Psychiatric Annals, 35*(5), 401–408.

van der Kolk, B., Pynoos, R., Cicchetti, D., Cloitre, M., D'Andrea, W., Ford, J., … Teicher, M. (2009, February). *Proposal to include a Developmental Trauma Disorder diagnosis for children and adolescents in DSM-V.* Unpublished manuscript. Retrieved from http://www.traumacenter.org/announcements/DTD_papers_Oct_09.pdf

van der Kolk, B.A., Roth, S., Pelcovitz, D., Sunday, S., & Spinazzola, J. (2005). Disorders of extreme stress: The empirical foundation of a complex adaptation to trauma. *Journal of Traumatic Stress, 18,* 389–399.

Waters, F.S. (1998). Parents as partners in the treatment of dissociative children. In J.L. Silberg (Ed.), *The dissociative child: Diagnosis, treatment and management* (2nd ed., pp. 273–296). Lutherville, MD: Sidran Press.

Waters, F.S. (2005a). Atypical DID adolescent case. *ISSTD News, 23*(3), 1–2, 4–5.

Waters, F.S. (2005b). Recognizing dissociation in preschool children. *ISSTD News, 23,* 4.

Waters, F.S. (2011). Ryan (8 to 10 years old)—Connecting with the body: Treatment of somatoform dissociation (encopresis and multiple physical complaints) in a young boy. In S. Wieland (Ed.), *Dissociation in traumatized children and adolescents: Theory and clinical interventions* (pp. 141–186). New York: Routledge.

Waters, F.S., & Silberg, J.L. (1998a). Promoting integration in dissociative children. In J.L. Silberg (Ed.), *The dissociative child: Diagnosis, treatment and management* (2nd ed., pp. 167–190). Lutherville, MD: Sidran Press.

Waters, F.S., & Silberg, J.L. (1998b). Therapeutic phases in the treatment of dissociative children. In J.L. Silberg (Ed.), *The dissociative child: Diagnosis, treatment and management* (2nd ed., pp. 135–156). Lutherville, MD: Sidran Press.

Watkins, J.G., & Watkins, H.H. (1993). Ego-state therapy in the treatment of dissociative disorders. In R.P. Kluft & C.G. Fine (Eds.), *Clinical perspectives on multiple personality disorder* (pp. 277–299). Washington, DC: American Psychiatric Press.

Weiss, M., Sutton, P.J., & Utecht, A.J. (1985). Multiple personality in a 10 year old girl. *Journal of the American Academy of Child & Adolescent Psychiatry, 24,* 495–501.

Wester, II, W.C. (1991). Induction and deepening techniques with children. In W.C. Wester II & D.J. O'Grady (Eds.), *Clinical hypnosis with children* (pp. 34–40). New York: Brunner/Mazel.

Whitaker, R. (2010). *Anatomy of an epidemic: Magic bullets, psychiatric drugs, and the astonishing rise of mental illness in America.* New York: Crown.

Widom, C.S. (1989). Child abuse, neglect, and violent criminal behavior. *Criminology, 27*(2), 251–271.

Wieland, S. (1998). *Techniques and issues in abuse-focused therapy.* Thousand Oaks, CA: Sage.

Wieland, S. (Ed.). (2011a). *Dissociation in traumatized children and adolescents: Theory and clinical interventions.* New York: Routledge.

Wieland, S. (2011b). Joey (11 to 12 years old)—Moving out of dissociative protection: Treatment of a boy with Dissociative Disorder Not Otherwise Specified following early family trauma. In S. Wieland (Ed.), *Dissociation in traumatized children and adolescents: Theory and clinical interventions* (pp. 197–262). New York: Routledge.

Williams, D. (1992). *Nobody nowhere: The remarkable autobiography of an autistic girl.* London: Jessica Kingsley.

Williams, D. (1994). *Somebody somewhere: Breaking free from the world of autism.* New York: Random House.

Williams, D. (1999). *Like color to the blind: Soul searching and soul finding.* London: Jessica Kingsley.

Williams, D.T., & Velazquez, L. (1996). The use of hypnosis in children with dissociative disorders. *Child and Adolescent Psychiatric Clinics of North America, 5,* 495–508.

Winnicott, D. (1953). Transitional objects and transitional phenomena. *International Journal of Psychoanalysis, 34*, 89–97.

Wolff, P. H. (1987). *The development of behavioral states and the expression of emotions in early infancy*. Chicago: University of Chicago Press.

Yates, T. M. (2004). The developmental psychopathology of self-injurious behavior: Compensatory regulation in posttraumatic adaptation. *Clinical Psychology Review, 24*, 35–74.

Yehuda, N. (2011). Leroy (7 years old)—"It's almost like he is two children": Working with a dissociative child in a school setting. In S. Wieland (Ed.), *Dissociation in traumatized children and adolescents: Theory and clinical interventions* (pp. 285–343). New York: Routledge.

Zelechoski, A., Warner, E., Emerson, D., & van der Kolk, B. (2011, November). *Innovative approaches to the treatment of Developmental Trauma Disorder in children and adolescents*. Paper presented at pre-meeting institute, 27th international conference, International Society for the Study of Trauma and Dissociation, Baltimore, MD.

Zoroglu, S., Sar, V., Tuzun, U., Tutkun, H., & Savas, H. A. (2002). Reliability and validity of the Turkish version of the adolescent dissociative experiences scale. *Psychiatry & Clinical Neurosciences, 56*, 551–556.

Zoroglu, S., Yargic, L. M., Tutkun, H., Ozturk, M., & Sar, V. (1996). Dissociative Identity Disorder in childhood: Five cases. *Dissociation, 11*, 253–260.

Appendix A

A Guide to Dissociation-Focused Interventions: EDUCATE

E: Educate about dissociation and traumatic processes

1. Behaviors and symptoms have a meaning or purpose.
2. Trauma causes disconnections in the mind.
3. A healthy mind has the most connections.
4. The whole self must work together.
5. Voices or imaginary friends are signals or feelings that "talk."
6. No part of the self can be dismissed.

D: Dissociation motivation: Address and analyze the factors that keep the client tied to dissociative strategies

1. Build hope.
2. Confront need for dissociation: pros and cons.
3. Encourage realistic consequences and central responsibility.

U: Understand what is hidden: Unravel the secret pockets of automatically activated affect, identity, or behavioral repertoires

1. Encourage drawing, symbolic play, or describing hidden states with welcoming approach.
2. Encourage child to "listen in."
3. Describe child's unremembered actions with gentle confrontation.

C: Claim as own these hidden aspects of the self

1. Reframe negative dissociated content.
2. Encourage gratefulness—the "thank-you note" technique.
3. Make bargains with hidden parts of the self.
4. Facilitate memory with environmental contingencies.
5. Destigmatize forgotten behaviors.
6. Highlight feelings with role-plays.

7.   Imagine together to fill in blanks in autobiographical (not trauma) memory.
8.   Collect data, and document context cues.

A: Arousal modulation/affect regulation/attachment: Learning to regulate arousal and the ebb and flow of feelings in the context of loving relationships

1.   Hyperarousal

     a.   Reinforce safety.
     b.   Connect on a symbolic level.
     c.   Breathing and calming imagery.
     d.   Sensorimotor activities.

2.   Numbing and Hypoarousal

     a.   Connect to body.
     b.   Arousing the child from dissociative shutdown.
     c.   Identifying the triggering moment and precursors.
     d.   Unraveling the hidden traps and dilemmas that keep patients reliant on these avoidant strategies.
     e.   Changing the environment to release the child from those traps.
     f.   Practicing a "redo" of the moment.
     g.   Rehearsing "staying connected" strategies.
     h.   Honoring motivations to stay dissociative.
     i.   Rewarding awareness and connection.

3.   Affect Regulation

     a.   Affect education: Feelings are the body's signals—anger is a self-defense emotion, feelings do not have to be contagious.
     b.   Highlight awareness at transition moments.
     c.   Identify triggers.
     d.   Establish a feeling vocabulary.
     e.   Imagery to practice affect tolerance and behavior choice.
     f.   Provide alternative behavioral choices.
     g.   Reinforce increasing self-control and mastery.
     h.   Build attachment across states.
     i.   Reinforce and evaluate safety.
     j.   Help family tolerate child's expression of intense feelings.
     k.   Build reciprocity in relationships

T: Triggers and trauma: Identifying precursors to automatic trauma-based responding and processing associated traumatic memories

1. Encourage discussion of trauma content.
2. Process sensorimotor memory.
3. Process traumatic meaning of the event and develop alternate view.
4. Process affect associated with the event with loving caregiver or therapist.
5. Encourage mastery experiences both in life and symbolically.
6. Find purpose of flashback, and replace with mastery scenario.
7. Escape cycle of traumatic attachment.

E: Ending stage of treatment

1. Reinforcement of differences between "now" and "then."
2. Escape cycle of traumatic demoralization.
3. Explore existential questions.
4. Use symbols and metaphors to reinforce integration.
5. Use experiences to help others.

Appendix B

Interview Guide for Dissociative Symptoms in Children

A: Perplexing Shifts in Consciousness

1. (If observing a momentary lapse): What are you doing when you are spaced out like that?
2. What were you thinking just before that happened? Have you noticed what your thoughts or feelings are right before you space out?
3. Do you ever find yourself blanking out, not paying attention at all? What are you doing at those times? What are you thinking, hearing, seeing, feeling?
4. Do you have an imaginary place you like to go to in your mind? Do you have imaginary friends you like to talk to?
5. Do you ever have times when you feel like you are reliving something from the past? What does that feel like?
6. Where are you when you are not paying attention?
7. Have you been told you do strange things in your sleep?
8. Do you have trouble waking in the morning? Tell me about that.
9. Do you sometimes feel like you change after going into a deep sleep?
10. Do you ever feel like you are not really there, like you are watching yourself from a distance?
11. Do you ever feel like you are looking through a fog?

B: Vivid Hallucinatory Experiences

1. Many times children who have lost someone special to them, still hear them talking to them in their mind. Does this happen to you? What does he/she say?
2. Some children feel like their brain is fighting with itself. Does yours? Do you ever hear the fight?
3. Sometimes mean words that children heard over and over and over again seem to be stuck in the children's minds. Does this happen to you?
4. Sometimes children do things they wish they had not done. Has that happened to you?
5. Sometimes they feel like they didn't want to but someone or something made them feel like they had to. Do you have anything like that?

6.   Some children have toys that they have had for a long time that are particularly special to them. Do you have a special toy? Can you talk to it? Can you hear it talk to you?

7.   Some children have invisible friends that others can't see. Do you have friends like this now? Did you have them when you were younger? Do you feel sometimes like the friends are still there? Can you see them?

C: Marked Fluctuations in Knowledge, Moods, or Patterns of Behavior and Relating

1.   Do you feel sometimes like you can do something one day, and have great trouble doing it the next day?

2.   Does it surprise you when your moods change? Give examples.

3.   Do your tastes change from day to day?

4.   Do your feelings about family members seem to go through changes? What are some examples of this?

D: Perplexing Memory Lapses for One's Own Behavior or Recently Experienced Events

1.   Do you forget things you should remember—what you did with friends, places you went, birthday parties?

2.   Do you sometimes forget what you did when you are angry? Let's try together to remember one of these. [Therapist should make sure to emphasize how logical the anger was to destigmatize the shame associated with the events.]

3.   Assess whether you can get the child to remember something about past behavior he or she has forgotten, using incentives and gentle encouragement.

4.   Do your friends say you have done things that you cannot remember doing?

5.   Do you ever forget good things that happened to you?

E: Abnormal Somatic Experiences

1.   Do you notice that you do not experience pain the way other children do?

2.   Do you find yourself injuring your body in some way repeatedly? How does this feel after you do this?

3.   Do you have a pain or disability for which no medical reason can be found?

4.   Do you have unusual weakness in your body, or unusual strength at times?

5.   Do you have bathroom accidents?

Appendix C

Imaginary Friends Questionnaire 2.0

Joyanna L. Silberg, PhD

1. My imaginary friend(s) is more than just a pretend friend.

    T   F

2. My imaginary friend(s) gives good advice.

    T   F

3. I have more than one imaginary friend and they disagree.

    T   F

4. My imaginary friend bugs me and I wish it would go away.

    T   F

5. My imaginary friend(s) takes over and makes me do things I don't want to do.

    T   F

6. My imaginary friend(s) tells me to keep secrets.

    T   F

7. My imaginary friend(s) tries to boss me.

    T   F

8. My imaginary friend(s) has knowledge about my life that I don't have.

    T   F

9. My imaginary friend(s) has skills or abilities that I don't have.

    T   F

10. My imaginary friend(s) does not like others to know about him/her.

    T   F

11. My imaginary friend plays with me when I am lonely.

    T   F

12. I wish everyone could see my imaginary friend(s) like I do.

T   F

13. My imaginary friend helps me when I am afraid.

T   F

14. My imaginary friend comes to me when I am angry.

T   F

15. My imaginary friend comes to me when I am happy.

T   F

SCORING THE IMAGINARY FRIENDS QUESTIONNAIRE

The Imaginary Friends Questionnaire can be used to help make the differentiation between normal imaginary friend phenomena and pathological dissociative phenomena. Research suggests that item numbers 1, 3, 4, 5, 7, 10 and 14 are more characteristic of hospitalized children with severe behavioral and emotional problems and who have been diagnosed with dissociative symptoms and disorders.

Appendix G

Clinician Checklist for Autobiographical Amnesia

Have you ruled out neurological or drug-related causes of the amnesia?
Has the environment made it worthwhile for memory to be achieved?
Have you emphasized the importance of autobiographical memory for safe functioning?
Have you identified any dissociated parts of the self who might hold this memory?
Have you validated feelings associated with the forgotten episode?
Have you used role play to explore what it might be like to have those feelings?
Have you tried to imagine together what a person might do if they had those feelings?
Have you helped to build context clues about the missing events?
Have you helped the client disconnect any painful traumatic memories from the autobiographical events through containment imagery?

Appendix H

Therapist Checklist for Managing Urinary and Bowel Incontinence

Have you explained that these symptoms are common and destigmatized them for the child and parent?
Have you identified ways that the behavior is being reinforced in the environment and reversed this pattern (e.g., negative attention from parents or avoidance of unpleasant consequences?)
Have you helped the parent understand that these behaviors are mostly involuntary even if they have a small voluntary component?
Have you helped to identify any traumatic thoughts associated with the onset of the behavior?
Have you identified any hidden states, imaginary friends, or voices associated with the behavior and enlisted these as allies?
Have you helped the child focus on sensations associated with urinating or defecating?
Have you rewarded even very small steps toward having more sensory awareness and control?
Have you identified any traumatic occurrences happening now in the environment and reduced the child's exposure to these?

Appendix J

Clinician Checklist for Managing Aggressive Children and Teens

Does the client know that anger is a necessary survival feeling, and not bad?
Has the client been helped to feel gratefulness for her anger and rage, even if it is now getting her in trouble?
Does the client understand the realistic consequences of his current rage-filled behavior?
Have you identified any internal states that harbor the rage?
Are contingencies in place to make change worthwhile for the whole child, including the perceptions and goals of the dissociated self?
Have you identified a source of the rage?
Have you identified beliefs about lack of safety that may be underlying the rage? (e.g., the perpetrator will return, I will be returned to an orphanage)
Have you provided and practiced an alternative action plan when triggered (e.g., a calm-down space)?
Have you helped the child attach fully to the caregiver, including the dissociated, angry part of the self?
Have you identified the triggers for the behavior that may relate to past trauma and validated the feelings associated with these triggers?
Have you given opportunities for direct communication of justifiable anger in family sessions and given the child some feeling of power by facilitating family changes?
Have you practiced imagery techniques related to choice points and change, or safe places for the dissociated part of self?

Appendix K

Clinician Checklist for Family Work

Have you explained the nature and purpose of affects, the effects of trauma, and the nature of dissociation?
Have you helped the parents understand the struggles of the child as survival tactics and explained they should not take the child's extreme behaviors personally?
Have you worked to identify triggers in the family to traumatic reactions and intense affective states and tried to mitigate these?
Have you desensitized automatic reactions to facial expressions, or phrases?
Have you instructed the family on keeping appropriate boundaries?
Have you given the child some power in the relationship with the parent, to reverse the child's sense of helplessness and ineffectuality in relationships?
Have you helped the child communicate distressing feelings without overreaction or defensiveness on the part of the parents and helped the parents show empathy?
Have you explained the importance of peers and helped the family encourage normal peer activities?
Have you identified any family dynamics that serve to reinforce dissociation and tried to reverse these?
Have you helped the family believe in the child and a positive future?
Have you helped the parents extend love to the whole child, including any angry or alienated dissociative states, imaginary friends, or voices?
Have you modeled respectful responses to dissociative states that promote the appropriate expression of feelings without regression or acting out?

Index